SHANIKA GRAHAM-WHITE

Orchids + Sweet Tea

PLANT-FORWARD
Recipes *with*
Jamaican Flavor
& Southern
Charm

VICTORY BELT PUBLISHING

LAS VEGAS

Cover design by Justin-Aaron Velasco

Interior design by Justin-Aaron Velasco, Yordan Terziev, and Boryana Yordanova

Illustrations by Yordan Terziev and Boryana Yordanova

Back cover photo and photos on pages 2, 6, 7, 14, 18, 20, 34, 154, 242, 319 by Matt Ellis

Printed in Canada

TC 0121

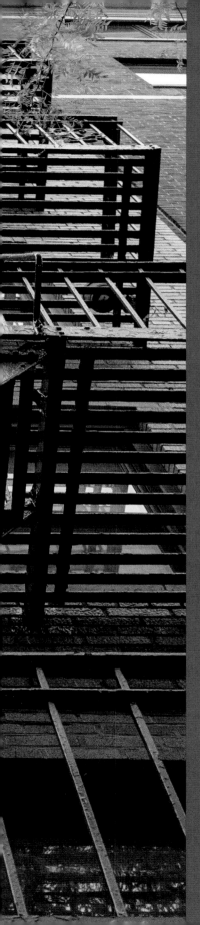

Table of
CONTENTS

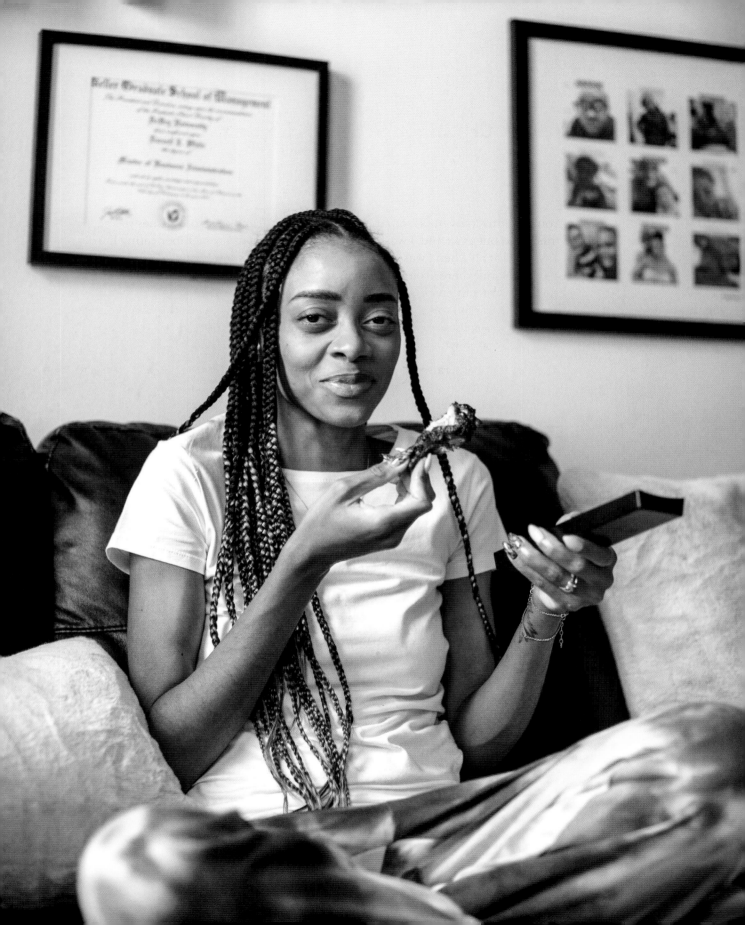

INTRODUCTION

THE GIRL WITH A CHICKEN WING IN HER HAND

You wouldn't know this from the array of beautiful and delicious dishes you see in this book, but as a child, I was an extremely picky eater. I remember eating hardly any foods at all when I was growing up. Looking back now, I believe I suffered from anxiety. Somewhere around the ages of five to eight, I was so anxious when it came to eating away from home that sometimes I would be sick to my stomach just thinking about being asked to eat something my body and mind didn't want to allow. It wasn't until I reached adulthood and later became a mother myself that I was able to wrap my head around what was happening to me back then.

The fact that I was raised by a young single mother in an era when anxiety wasn't really talked about—and wasn't even a "thing"—certainly didn't help. My life circumstances weren't conducive to understanding anxiety, how to deal with it, or how not to let it dictate my eating habits. At one point, I would go days and weeks without eating solid foods, preferring to get my nutrients from creamy ice pops or meal replacement shakes.

When I did eat solid foods, my choices weren't the healthiest. Junk foods were the only things I would eat. Think chips, candy, cookies, cakes, donuts, ice cream, along with easy Southern dishes that my maternal step-grandmother would make or purchase, such as French toast, banana pudding, hot sausages, and fried pork chops— all of which were the complete opposite of the traditional Jamaican dishes enjoyed by most of my Jamaican family members.

More than any of those things, I loved chicken, which was one of the few things that I found tasty. I also took comfort in its versatility, which allowed me to enjoy it fried, baked, barbecued, jerked, and so on. I ate chicken nuggets from McDonald's, fried chicken from Popeyes, chicken wings, and more chicken! In fact, my childhood nickname was "Chicken Wing." That says a lot about my undying love for chicken. I was known as the girl with a chicken wing in her hand (and maybe a cookie in the other).

While my love for food has evolved over the years, my love for chicken has remained constant. It was and still is my kryptonite.

Since I started on my own love journey with food, I have come to a better understanding of what healthy eating looks like for me. This reflects my current choice not to restrict myself entirely to one diet, but rather to create a good enough structure to keep healthy plant-based ingredients at the forefront while incorporating meat, dairy, and other animal foods as the "background."

My Food
DISCOVERY

As I grew older and finally began to let go of my angst, my love for food grew. From mainly eating junk—tons of it—throughout childhood, I was able to expand my palate to enjoy a wider variety of foods.

I also started connecting more with my Jamaican roots after meeting my dad, who was born and raised in Jamaica, for the first time when I was nine years old. With my father being very much tied to traditional Jamaican cuisine, my eating habits started to shift. I had a lot more home-cooked meals and fewer fast-food moments. It was during this time that I became familiar with staple Jamaican fare, such as stew chicken, rice and peas, oxtail, stew peas, curry shrimp, and jerk chicken.

Once I reached my teenage years, I began experimenting in the kitchen, making the things that I wanted to eat instead of the traditional Jamaican dishes that were often prepared in my home. After a series of attempts and failures, I finally mastered simple things like pancakes, biscuits, and chicken wings. I began to realize just how much I enjoyed cooking and seeing what I could come up with in the kitchen. However, since I didn't have much exposure to anything outside of my Southern and Jamaican roots, my cooking and eating repertoire was still pretty limited.

Then our family moved from central Florida (Orlando, to be exact) to New York when I was thirteen, and everything changed for me. Unlike central Florida, New York was a place where it was easy to get around independently, which meant that I was able to explore different foods after school with friends. By the time I reached my junior year of high school and met my now-husband, my life revolved around food. Though my husband came from the same Jamaican background, he was raised in Brooklyn, and he'd been exposed to more global cuisines and cultures than I was growing up. We had fun exploring the different boroughs of New York and sampling cheesecake, Philly cheesesteak sandwiches, sugar pretzels, hero sandwiches, brick-oven pizzas,

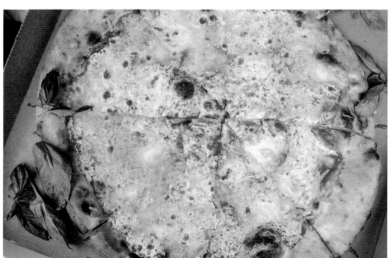

pasta in vodka sauce, and a wide array of foods the city has to offer. Food became our "thing" and our love language.

In those moments, I realized just how much bigger the world was when it came to food—and life. That notion has stayed with me, and I've evolved into someone who seeks the finest food experiences possible, even if that means I have to create them myself at home. Food has become art for me.

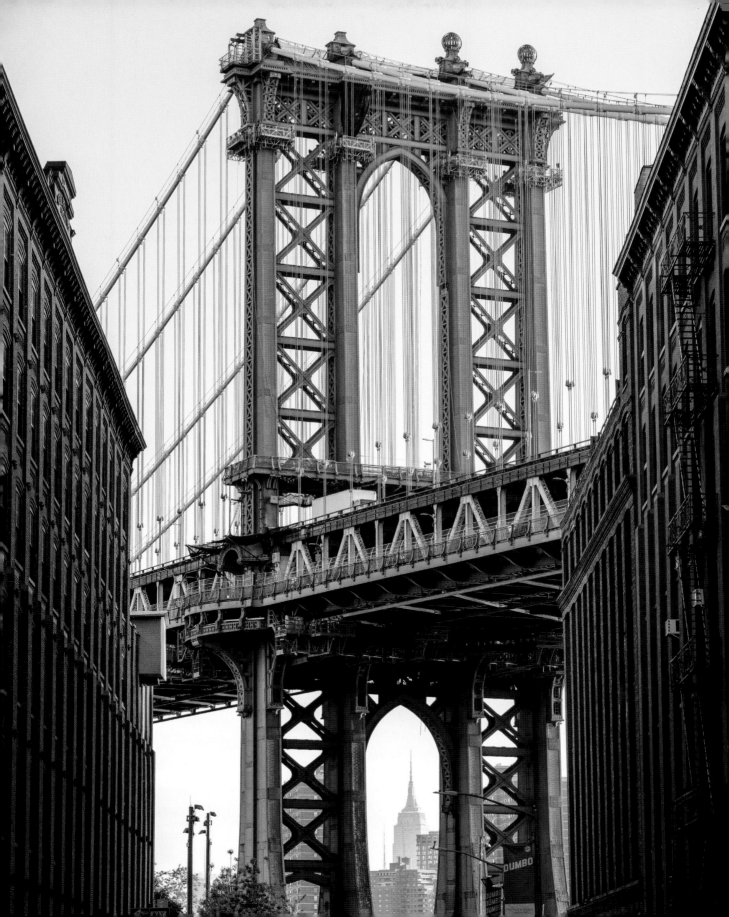

My Food PHILOSOPHY

Since starting my family (which consists of my husband, our five-year-old son, and our puppy), I've become more conscious about living a healthy lifestyle. Four years ago, I began experimenting even more with cooking and stumbled upon a real passion for creating food, and thus *Orchids + Sweet Tea* was born. Shortly after starting *Orchids + Sweet Tea*, while still on my postpartum journey, I realized that my body was having a hard time bouncing back to its pre-pregnancy self and that my hormones were really out of whack. Some of the signs of my hormonal imbalance were ovarian cyst pain, extreme lower abdominal/pelvic pain, painful menstruation, constipation, and nausea, which were draining to suffer through for most of each month for almost two years. I also struggled with hair loss and calcium deficiency, which showed up in my teeth, bones, and brittle nails. Countless doctor visits resulted in no solution besides hormonal medications, such as birth control.

One thing I couldn't shake was that I could no longer digest dairy and gluten effectively; they seemed to be the biggest culprits in making my symptoms worse. It was then that I decided to change my diet and lifestyle to a healthier one.

Because dairy was a problem for me, a vegan diet seemed like the perfect solution, but it felt too restrictive, and I found myself supplementing with not-so-great ingredients like processed sugars and carbs. Vegetarianism was less restrictive, but I found myself consuming higher levels of dairy along with processed sugars, carbs, and breads, which weren't ideal for my goal of eating healthier. After much trial and error, I realized that there was no one diet that completely fit my condition or lifestyle, and I decided to tailor my eating habits to my personal needs. I created a mix of dairy-free, gluten-free, and vegan meals for my family while still having the ability to consume meat, dairy, and gluten in moderation, ensuring that those ingredients were organic. Fast-forward to the newly trendy plant-forward diet, which falls in line with my decision not to restrict the foods I eat, but rather to focus on consuming more plants and other healthy ingredients.

Today, I take great pride in having discovered so many amazing ingredients that have helped my condition in such significant ways. A great deal of discipline and intentionality go into what I consume and expose my body to daily. Thankfully, most of my symptoms have either subsided considerably or disappeared. Yes, it has been a journey, but it's one that I am learning to embrace and fight through—one plate at a time!

Orchids + SWEET TEA

Growing up, one of the main ways that my family came together was through food, music, and laughter, and this upbringing inspired me to create a space that both uplifts and feeds those who choose to visit my little corner of the web.

Before *Orchids + Sweet Tea* became a full-fledged food and lifestyle blog, it was just an online platform where I would write about my life and thoughts and posted my dinners for my closest family and friends. Soon enough, my simple iPhone snapshots became a social media sensation, which led me to turn my blog into a complete food-centered platform where I educate others on healthier food choices.

I don't come from a line of trained cooks or bakery owners, and everything I've created was through my experience of being self-taught. As a novice cook and baker, I was limited in my knowledge of ingredients. All-purpose flour, for example, was once my go-to type of flour, and the range of my food creations was limited to what I could do with it. Well, I still love using all-purpose flour (I prefer organic now), but I've expanded my options to include gluten-free alternatives such as almond, coconut, quinoa, buckwheat, and oat flour, to name a few. Likewise, my range of sweetener options now includes healthier ingredients like pure maple syrup, agave nectar, and date syrup. I'm sure you'll see from the recipes in this book that I have come a long way from when I started *Orchids + Sweet Tea* and my childhood eating habits.

Although I started *Orchids + Sweet Tea* because of my personal need to alter my diet, it continues to evolve based on my discovery of new ingredients, innovative twists on old favorites, my community's love for specific recipes and trends, as well as my son's own picky-eating phase, which sometimes mirrors my struggle as a child—pushing me to get creative in making healthier foods taste and look great.

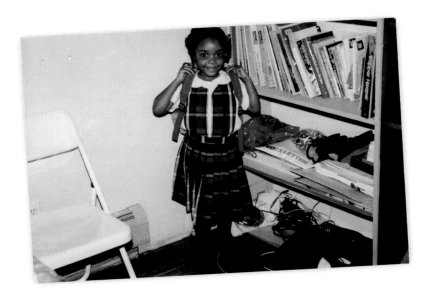

About THIS BOOK

Understanding my food journey and seeing just how long the road has been for me to become my best self both inside and out, I wanted to share what I've learned with you.

I want to share easy and flavorful dishes that my family loves and show you how you can personalize them to fit your preferences. I also want to show you the dishes from my Southern and Jamaican background that have made me the happiest in this plant-based way of life.

Through this book, I want to come alongside you in the kitchen to guide and encourage you so that you walk out feeling more confident on your journey to health. All along my journey, I've learned that even though things aren't always easy, they are possible. And I want you to leave knowing that it is possible to create delicious, exciting meals without having any fancy skills or a boatload of ingenious ideas.

First and foremost, I want this cookbook to be useful to everyone—plant-based eaters and meat-eaters alike. I want you to feel that you don't have to be an advanced cook or baker to make my recipes. The cookbook is a collection of my favorite plant-forward dishes, featuring combinations of bold flavors that I've experimented with, refined through trial and error, and added to my repertoire along my journey. I've also included recipes influenced by my Southern and Jamaican heritage. These are dishes that my grandma, grandpa, aunts, and uncles lovingly prepared as I was growing up.

And that is to say you'll find here a lot of my childhood favorites—updated, refreshed, and made in a way that reflects who I am today. I remember having weekend brunches with my grandmother and watching her put together delicious French toast or pancakes, and then our favorite banana pudding for our movie night later that evening. As a nod to those moments and my grandmother's knack for Southern classics, I've included an easy yet flavorful Dairy-Free Strawberry Pecan French Toast Casserole (page 124) in her honor. While my grandmother's rendition was simple and straightforward, I make mine with a more buttery type of bread, such as challah or brioche, for a more decadent bite, and I load it with strawberries and pecans, my two favorite ingredients by far.

There are a few savory staples like Southern collard greens (page 176) and some Cajun-inspired dishes. I've also included a lot of Southern-inspired pancakes and waffles, since eating these comfort foods at my local Waffle House or all-you-can-eat restaurants was such an important part of my childhood.

However, the South is only part of who I am; there's also the Jamaican part. Once I started living in the same house with my dad, I was exposed to staple Jamaican fare like ackee and saltfish, cooked kidney, steamed fish with veggies, and curry shrimp. Being a picky eater, I didn't embrace all of those dishes, but I quickly fell in love with Jamaican spicy beef patties, soups, flavored drinks, dumplings, and many others.

Therefore, to honor my Jamaican heritage, I've included a lot of hearty Jamaican-inspired recipes as well—full of spices and fresh, bold flavors. You'll get to try amazing recipes like a vegan version of a Jamaican classic, Irish (Sea) Moss (page 312), a traditional drink used to keep the body nourished, healthy, and strong. Also, I keep things interesting with my Jerk BBQ Pineapple Black Bean Burgers (page 220), which are made from black beans and carrots; a beautiful jade-colored Jamaican "Pepperpot" Soup (page 180); Ginger Cupcakes with Chai Cream Cheese Frosting (page 260) that play on the sweet and spicy flavors; and so much more goodness.

Overall, these plant-forward recipes are my way of helping others discover their love of food while keeping true to their own personal journey, with the ultimate goal of a healthier lifestyle—all with a bit of Brooklyn flair, bursts of Jamaican flavors, and a whole lot of Southern charm.

Therefore, you can expect everything from easy essentials (vegan buttermilk, seasoning mixes, pie crusts, etc.) that can fit within various recipes without question, to delicious Morning Eats for your early mornings, to family-friendly main dishes, and everything in between. Oh, and I have some amazing homemade drinks in here, too. Some of my personal favorites include

- **Cucumber Ginger Lemon Detox Juice (page 284)**

- **Jamaican Hibiscus Drink (aka sorrel) (page 288)**

- **Slim's Grapefruit Rosemary Mocktail (page 294)—a special nod to my late grandpa**

- **Spicy Kiwi Lime Mocktail (page 296)**

- **Honey Lemon Ginger Tea (page 306)**

Cheers to that! Plus, I'm sharing a special section, "Food Love Affairs," which pairs together my favorite recipe types for a delicious food love experience (be sure to swipe your way toward the end of the book).

All in all, every recipe does a great job at highlighting plant-based ingredients while gently incorporating others like dairy and meat (unless it's your "cheat day," which means that you can eat a fully jam-packed meal so that you aren't completely boxed into one strict diet). It's a book of my "faves of all faves" when it comes to cooking and baking as well as homemade drinks. They are flavorful (never lacking that, actually), colorful, easy, and full of true character.

However, before you grab your best wooden spoon or pull your nonstick skillet out of the cabinet and have some fun cooking and baking, let's get into what it means to live a plant-forward way of life.

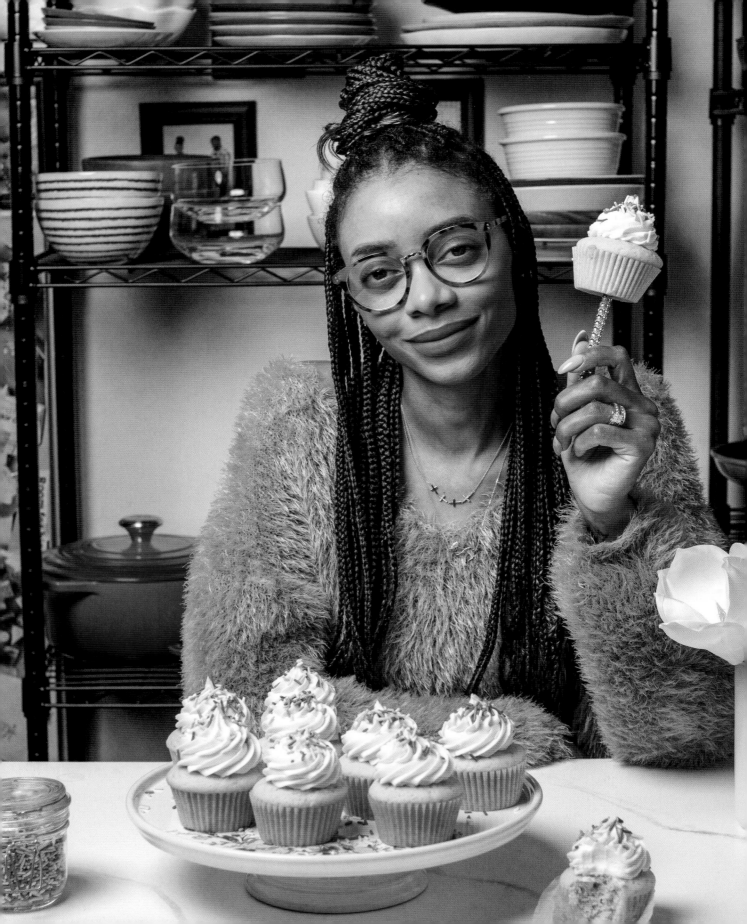

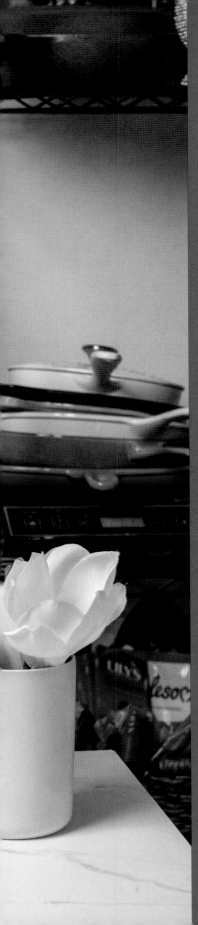

Chapter 1:

WELCOME TO THE PLANT-FORWARD WAY OF LIFE

Whether you're new to a plant-forward diet or you're familiar with it but need a refresher—or, like me, you simply try to eat healthy without necessarily subscribing to any specific diet—I'd like to establish what it means.

Plant-forward just means that plant foods are the stars of your daily meals. They're not all you eat, however. In addition to unprocessed or minimally processed foods such as vegetables, fruits, whole grains, legumes, nuts, seeds, healthy fats from plants, herbs, and spices, you can consume moderate amounts of organic meat and dairy products that are produced responsibly and on a small scale. For example, stuffed shells has been one of my favorite dishes in recent years. While traditional stuffed shells include loads of cheese and often ground meat as well, my Fire-Roasted Tomato Deconstructed Stuffed Shells recipe (page 212) greatly reduces the use of animal products by including only a base of ricotta cheese (heavy on the lemon flavor) that is smeared on the bottom of the plate, while the pasta, sauce, and fresh herbs are plated at the forefront.

Make sense? Good. So, in a nutshell, you're simply taking the longstanding traditions of vegetarianism and veganism and creating a new way of eating that also emphasizes unprocessed or minimally processed foods.

Why PLANT-FORWARD?

The biggest question you might be asking as you read the introduction to this cookbook is "Why should I eat plant-forward?" Well, to keep things simple, I'll say that plant-forward eating reduces the risk of many serious health conditions, such as heart disease, stroke, obesity, high blood pressure, high cholesterol, and many cancers, that are often tied to high levels of meat consumption. The best part about a plant-forward approach is that while you aren't necessarily restricted from eating meat, the structure of the diet keeps your consumption low because plant foods are highlighted.

In addition, a plant-forward diet is said to have a positive impact on energy levels, weight management, digestion, and the health of the gut microbiome. Besides the many health benefits, a plant-forward diet tends to be less expensive because you do not need to invest in meats and prepackaged convenience foods.

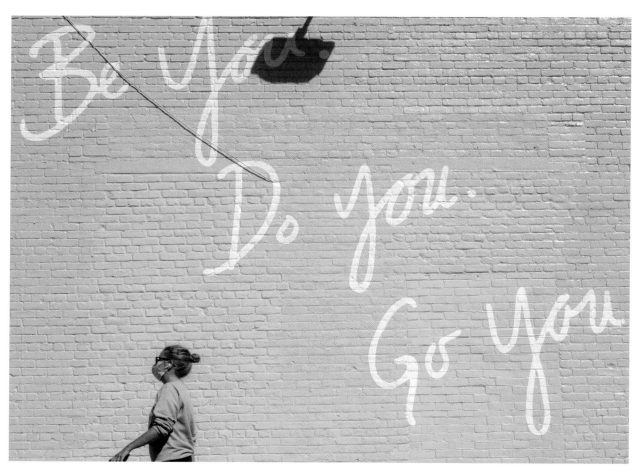

Transitioning to A PLANT-FORWARD WAY OF EATING

Now that you've got a clear picture of what a plant-forward diet entails, let's talk about how to easily transition if you aren't already eating this way. I'll break it down into six easy steps.

1. Gradually add more plant-based and unprocessed ingredients to your diet.

When it comes to transitioning, I've learned that a slow pace is best. (Well, not too slow, since it's super important to do just that—transition. I'll be elaborating more in point #2.) Going cold turkey can backfire, as it frequently leads to relapsing into old eating habits. Trust me—I learned this lesson the hard way, having gone through several diets which all failed because I didn't allow myself time to transition at my own pace. Pressure, pressure, pressure! I highly recommend slowly adding more plant-based and unprocessed ingredients to your current diet to get your taste buds used to the new, healthier stuff before fully delving in.

2. Find ways to swap animal products for plant-based ones.

Research has shown that when you jump right into a new way of eating, there will be a "bidding war" of sorts between your brain and your diet. When you feel deprived, your mind encourages you to binge—no doubt as a defense mechanism against what the body perceives as starvation. Therefore, while it's super important to make your brain comfortable with the change in your eating habits by not giving up all of your favorite foods right away, I think it's even more important to understand how to swap certain ingredients with plant-based ones so that you don't feel like you're giving up your favorites without a reward.

Today, there are so many food blogs and cookbooks like this one that offer a variety of ingredient options for healthier eating. Although a plant-forward approach doesn't omit animal products entirely, it does require that we eat more plant foods; therefore, finding new ingredients that fit this plan helps us keep our meals interesting. For example, in this book, I've re-created traditional favorites as plant-forward options with a flavorful twist, such as Creamy Cajun Pumpkin Mac & "Cheese" (page 172), Spicy Sesame Plant-Based Meatballs with Cauliflower Rice (page 222), Vegan Jerk BBQ Meatball Po' Boys (page 230), Vegan Oat Cupcakes with Strawberry Buttercream (page 258), and Vegan Spiced Hot Chocolate (page 278).

3: Research your ingredient options.

Again, it's all about the transition. And knowing your ingredient options is very important in the process of transitioning to a healthier plant-forward diet. The key is to work them into your diet little by little. Surprisingly, there are so many ingredients that make it almost impossible to feel deprived even in the absence of meat and/or processed foods, from dairy-free milks and coconut whipped cream to quinoa, beans, jackfruit, and mushrooms. It's even easier with a plant-forward diet since we are simply choosing healthier animal-based ingredients while emphasizing plant foods as opposed to eliminating anything entirely.

4: Find recipes that cater to your taste buds, and expose yourself to more variety.

Forcing yourself to eat what you don't truly enjoy can only last for so long. You're more likely to stay on track when you're aware of what great alternatives and ingredients are out there and know how to use them to create meals you truly love. For this reason, I've made sure this cookbook is jam-packed with all kinds of delicious food and drink options so you'll never feel deprived on a plant-forward diet.

5: Adopt the "out with the old, in with the new" attitude.

Once you've eased into this way of eating, it's time to decide to just do it! One of the best ways to get rid of temptation is to not have anything around that will tempt you. I understand that it can be a lot of stuff to toss. However, once you're fully acclimated to the new diet, you'll be content with the new way of preparing food, and you won't need those unhealthy food options any longer!

6: Give yourself grace.

Lastly, here's the heart of the matter: give yourself the grace to mess up and have the courage to begin again! It's as simple as that. One of the hardest things about being on a strict diet is that there isn't much wiggle room; you can't mess up—even slightly—without completely breaking the rules of that particular diet. On a plant-forward diet, since you aren't eliminating any specific ingredient, there's a lot of room for flexibility. You might "mess up a bit" by eating more meat or other ingredients than you should, but it's OK—you get right back on the right track! So don't be super hard on yourself about following everything to a "T." Food should be fun, engaging, and fulfilling, not rigid and guilt-inducing. So let's have some fun in the kitchen!

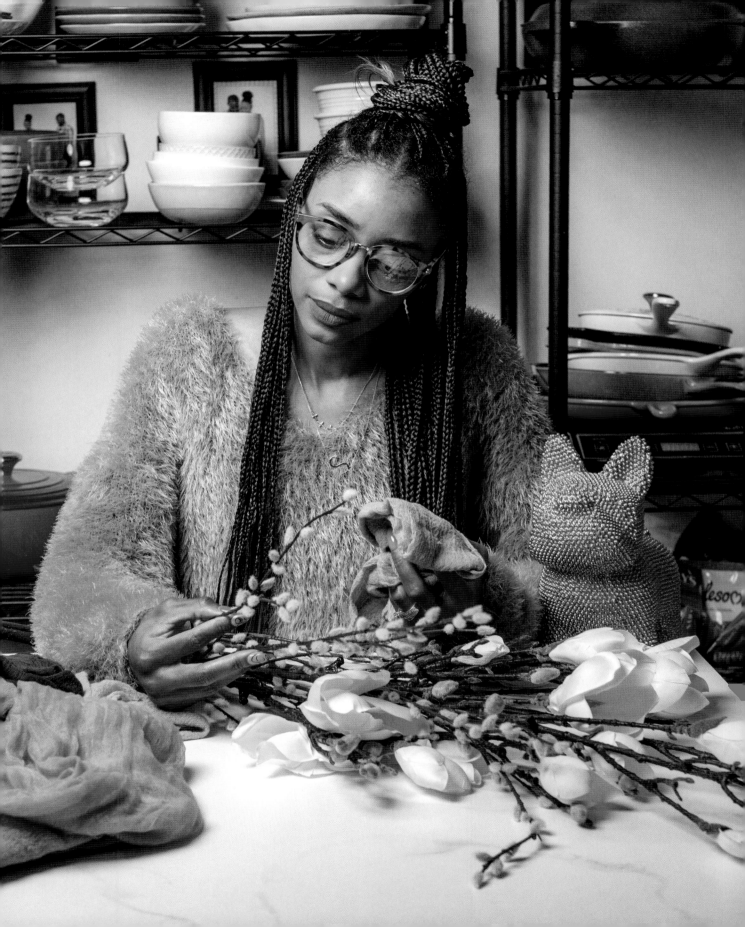

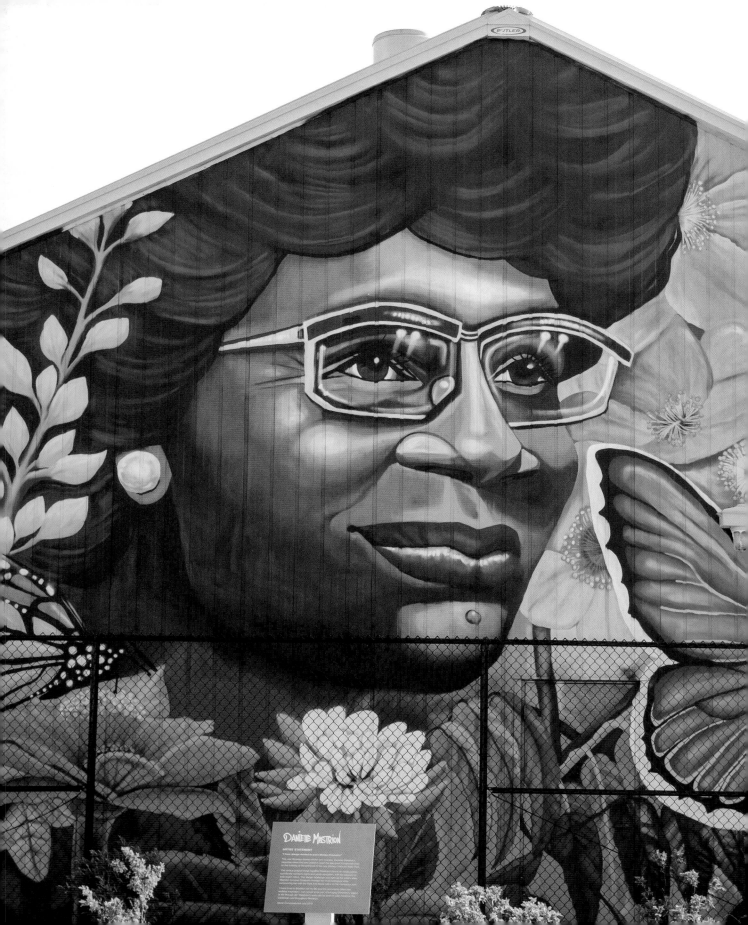

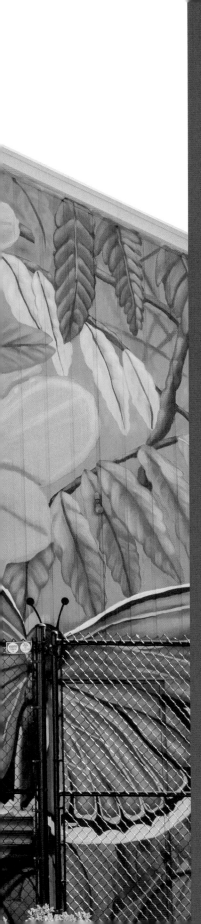

Chapter 2:
THE PLANT-FORWARD KITCHEN

I wrote this chapter to help you better understand some of the great options for cooking plant-forward meals. While the following review of ingredients does not reflect all of the ingredients used in the recipes in this book, it does supply you with a number of options for your plant-forward kitchen.

Awesome
MEAT SUBSTITUTES

Whether you just want to take a short break from eating like a carnivore, or you've decided to take the plunge into an entirely meatless diet and you just want some ideas to keep things exciting and fun, you can get some or all of the protein your body needs from these fantastic meat substitutes.

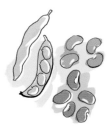

Beans

The best meat substitutes on a plant-forward diet are beans! Anything from black beans to lima beans to pinto beans to red kidney beans to chickpeas to soybeans—they're all good for you. Most of these little beauties offer lots of protein, fiber, potassium, and other nutrients that will keep you fueled and strong. Besides, beans have a nice "meaty" texture and flavor (they make a great burger!), so that those taste buds are left satisfied after every bite.

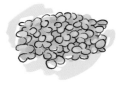

Lentils

Like beans, lentils are a significant source of protein and fiber. They make amazing burgers and side dishes, too. I don't include any recipes using lentils in this book, but you can find a ton of lentil-based dishes on my blog, *Orchids + Sweet Tea.*

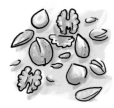

Nuts and Seeds

Nuts and seeds are often tossed in salads, sprinkled on desserts, added to pastas—you name it! But did you know that they are a great meat substitute? Yes, they are! And they're just as filling as meat.

Organic Tofu and Tempeh

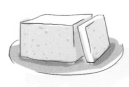

Tofu is made from soy milk, whereas tempeh is made from fermented soybeans. However, they're similar in many ways. They're both versatile, and they both can be cooked in a variety of ways (pan-fried, sautéed, etc.); they're high in protein and make great meat substitutes. Personally, I am not a huge fan of tofu and don't use this ingredient specifically; however, it is a great option if you enjoy it.

Avocados

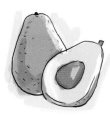

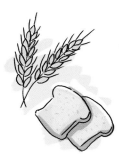

Once considered the "best-kept secret" for many, avocados have become an "it" ingredient. Think avocado toast, avocado salad, avocado burger buns (yes, that's a thing!), avocado and eggs, avocado fries, avocado ice cream—and the list goes on. However, just because avocado is a trendy ingredient doesn't mean that it can't be taken seriously. This fruit is packed with proteins and heart-healthy monounsaturated fatty acids! All the better reason to eat a few of these in place of meat.

Whole Grains

While some people aren't able to consume whole grains and need to follow a gluten-free diet because of celiac disease or other health reasons, those of us who are able to eat grains should! Not only do grains provide an amazing amount of protein—especially when paired with other foods, such as eggs, almonds, chicken breast, and broccoli—but they also provide a lot of fiber, help with digestion, help lower cholesterol and blood pressure, maintain blood sugar levels, protect teeth and gums, and can help control weight, and they may reduce asthma risks. So many benefits wrapped in such small packages!

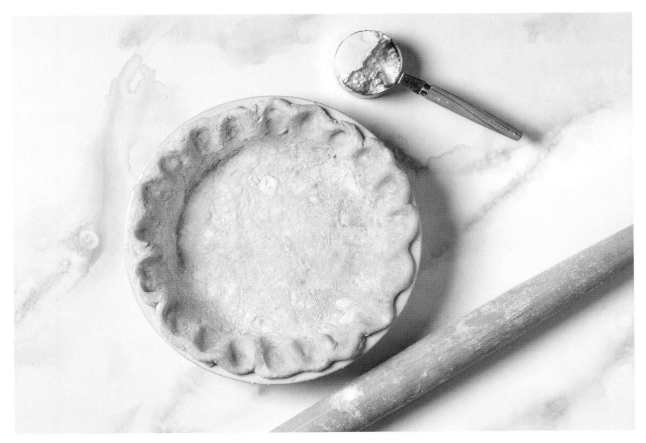

Dairy & EGG SUBSTITUTES

Regardless of your reason for wanting to substitute for dairy, there are many options to ensure that you are able to enjoy your favorite foods without compromising your intention to eat healthy. Due to my Southern background, I grew up on all things dairy, and in the beginning, I found it incredibly hard to eliminate dairy to help with some of my health issues, such as recurring ovarian cysts, endometriosis-like symptoms, and irritable bowel syndrome (IBS) symptoms, all of which seem to be linked to hormonal imbalances, stress, and sensitivity to certain ingredients. As scientific research has shown, the foods we consume play a major role with not only our digestive systems, but also the major systems that regulate sleep, stress levels, the reproductive system, and so on. Many of our systems are linked, which further explains why eating, physical activity, stress management, and much more all work together to determine our physical and mental health. However, as I discovered more and more new ingredients, I realized just how easy it was to replace my favorite dairy products with some pretty great substitutes, which are now my staples.

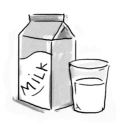

Milk

I've never been a huge fan of whole milk (except for chocolate milk); therefore, I don't miss having it in my diet now. However, I've had to find substitutes for heavy cream, whipped cream, and so on. Rest assured, I've discovered some amazing ingredients that work in the same way as their dairy-based counterparts in recipes but don't wreak havoc on my body or digestive system. When it comes to milk, I love using almond and coconut milks as well as oat and cashew milks (you'll find recipes for making homemade versions of the latter two on my blog). In addition to my go-to milk alternatives, the following are handy options: soy milk, rice milk, flaxseed milk, and hemp milk.

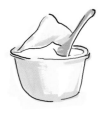

Yogurt

We all know just how essential yogurt is for our digestive system, especially when it comes to women and our hormonal shifts. Consuming probiotics in our diet is imperative for keeping the "good" bacteria in our microbiome balanced, so it's important to have a great substitute for dairy yogurt that offers the same benefits. My go-to dairy-free yogurt is coconut yogurt; I love its lightness and creaminess. In addition to these, there are almond milk, soy milk, and hemp milk yogurt products as well.

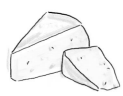

Cheese

One of the hardest dairy products for me to reduce by far was cheese. Honestly, cheese makes everything taste better, or at least that was what I felt growing up. Not being able to fully indulge in one of my favorite foods was tough, but I truly love the fact that I can sometimes use cheese while substituting plant-based ingredients in many other instances to keep my consumption of cheese in check. Over the years, I've discovered some amazing cheese alternatives. I mostly make them at home, and it has changed my life! While many store-bought nondairy shreds look and work like cheese, I've become a big fan of making cheese sauce out of cashews (see my recipe on page 48) and incorporating nutritional yeast, which adds a nice "cheesy" flavor, into my recipes.

Butter

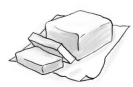

Butter plays such an important role in cooking and baking. In baking, butter adds not just flavor but also fat, which interacts with other ingredients, affecting the texture, appearance, and so on. However, these days there are amazing plant-based butter alternatives, including plant-based butter and dairy-free buttery sticks made by Earth Balance that work well in cooking and baking. I recommend testing different brands to see which tastes the best to you and keeping an eye out for hidden dairy derivatives like whey, which can be easily overlooked.

Cream

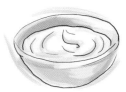

My go-to substitute for heavy cream is canned full-fat and unsweetened coconut milk; it is such a lifesaver! You can use it at room temperature right out of the can as a substitute for cream in a simple cream-based recipe. However, when you need something creamier and sturdier—when making whipped cream, for example—you can refrigerate a can of coconut milk overnight and scoop out the thick and solid part that has risen to the top to use. Dairy-free yogurts, cheeses, and milks can serve as substitutes for cream in some recipes as well.

Ice Cream

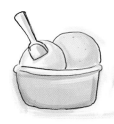

Most of us love a good scoop of ice cream, and this dairy type is very special to me! Growing up, I had weekly ice cream adventures with my grandfather when we both enjoyed vanilla ice cream with sprinkles, which is still my absolute favorite today. And while I hardly ever have a scoop of regular ice cream these days, I regularly enjoy dairy-free ice cream; my go-to brands are So Delicious Dairy-Free and Oatly. There are so many options made with different plant-based milk alternatives, and they are just as creamy, decadent, and delicious as their dairy counterparts.

Eggs

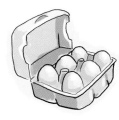

Flax "eggs," made with flaxseed meal and water, are an indispensable egg substitute. You can find a recipe for making them on page 38. Other good egg substitutes are chia seeds soaked in warm water (see page 39 for a recipe), aquafaba (the liquid from a can of chickpeas), egg substitute powder, and tapioca starch or arrowroot mixed with 3 tablespoons of warm water. Applesauce and mashed banana double as sweeteners and are favorites of mine to use in cookies when I'm looking for a binder plus a sweetener in one. It adds a nice chewiness and softness, too. The best kind to use is organic with no sugar added. Of course, you can always make your own at home as well—homemade is always best!

Healthy SWEETENERS

When it comes to desserts, I hate the idea of giving them up completely. Throughout my healthy food journey, I've learned how to make certain foods healthier without entirely compromising their flavor and texture! Sugar has been a part of the human diet for centuries; it's nothing new. However, in recent years, sugar has become the highlight of scientific studies due to rising obesity rates, especially in the U.S. Not only that, but specific types of sugar, including white sugar and added sugar (high-fructose corn syrup), are believed to increase the risk of heart disease and metabolic syndrome.

While a plant-forward diet doesn't eliminate any type of ingredient, it greatly minimizes the use of processed ones. With that being said, I'm sharing a nice short list of awesome sweetener substitutes that can be incorporated in almost anything you want to make.

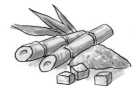

Raw Cane Sugar & Brown Sugar

While raw cane sugar and brown sugar aren't exactly sugar substitutes, you can use them in a plant-forward diet as healthier alternatives to white sugar. I often use the vegan-approved organic versions, which don't contain the harmful additives that conventional sugars do.

Agave & Pure Maple Syrup

Agave is said to have a lower glycemic index, which makes it perfect for people with diabetes. On the other hand, pure maple syrup packs tons of antioxidants. I often use them interchangeably, although I prefer maple syrup due to its clean and complex flavor profile, which includes hints of caramel, vanilla, and prune.

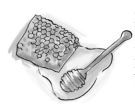

Raw Honey

Raw honey is another great sweetener that has tons of antioxidants. In addition, it has prebiotic properties, which help keep your gut healthy and improve the microbial balance in your gut.

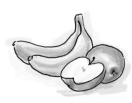

Fruits

Fruits make great sugar substitutes due to their natural sugars. Different fruits offer different levels of sweetness—and sometimes they come with tartness, as in the case of cranberries—so use your judgment when determining in which recipes and in what amounts to use them. Two of the most versatile fruits when it comes to sweetening recipes (and often binding them as well) are apples and bananas. Both banana puree, prepared from fully ripe bananas, and applesauce (essentially apple puree) work perfectly. In my vegan cookies, I love using applesauce as a binder and sweetener to get the cookies soft and chewy. I recommend organic applesauce with no sugar added. You can make your own applesauce at home as well.

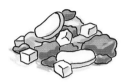

Raisins & Dates

You read that right—raisins and dates make awesome sweeteners! They offer health benefits as well. Both raisins and dates are great sources of antioxidants and fiber. Dates are also believed to boost brain and bone health, promote natural labor in pregnant women, and help with blood sugar control.

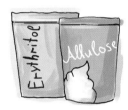

Erythritol & Allulose

Erythritol and allulose are considered to be excellent alternatives to sugar, especially for those who suffer from diabetes, because they are known for not raising blood sugar levels. Both can be used in baking or for sweetening drinks and foods. Because these sweeteners aren't as sweet as regular sugar, when using them to replace sugar in a recipe, you may need to use 1⅓ cups for every 1 cup of regular sugar. My go-to brand for both types is Whole Earth Sweetener.

While I don't specifically call for these sugar alternatives in any of the recipes in this book, you can easily incorporate either of them in my Citrus Whole-Wheat Breakfast Loaf (page 132), Vegan Pecan Chia Banana Bread (page 134), Gluten-Free Double Chocolate Muffins (page 138), Easy Fudgy Vegan Avocado Brownies (page 244), Ginger Cupcakes with Chai Cream Cheese Frosting (page 260), and so many other recipes.

My Favorite
SOUTHERN INGREDIENTS

When it comes to eating healthy, I'm such a big believer in staying true to your roots, which is why I wanted to highlight my favorite Southern ingredients in this chapter. I use most of these ingredients on a daily basis. Some of them are included in the recipes in this book, while others can be found in recipes on my blog. Either way, this list showcases the best plant-forward and healthy swaps for cooking Southern dishes.

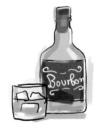

Bourbon

Bourbon is a huge staple in the South. While I rarely use alcohol when creating dishes, I do enjoy incorporating bourbon into Southern-inspired dishes because it adds such a beautiful hint of vanilla, oak, and caramel flavor to both savory and sweet dishes.

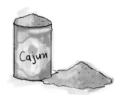

Cajun Seasoning

This is one of my favorite seasonings to add to savory dishes, such as pasta, seafood, and rice dishes. Although I sometimes purchase the store-bought blend, I enjoy making my own from scratch (see page 43) and storing it in an airtight container for several months, using it as desired. Because I use herbs and spices often, stocking the necessary components to create this seasoning isn't hard to do at all.

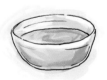

Chicken or Vegetable Broth

I love to use both chicken and vegetable broth for many of my cream-based soups and other dishes. I prefer the low-sodium versions because they allow me to control the amount of salt in any dish that I create.

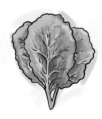

Collard Greens

I use a variety of greens, such as kale, spinach, arugula, and many different types of lettuce. However, whenever I decide to make a Southern-inspired recipe, collard greens are my go-to! Besides the traditional collard greens dish often served in the South, I enjoy sautéing collard greens and adding them to other dishes for a nice balance of flavor and nutrients.

Hot Honey

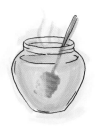

This ingredient is one of my new loves. I find myself using it on a daily basis, especially as a condiment. Although you can purchase hot honey from my go-to brand, Mike's Hot Honey, I do mention in the Hot Honey Skillet Cornbread recipe (page 174) the option of creating your own vegan version using agave as a substitute. I thoroughly enjoy the light kick of heat and sweetness that this ingredient adds to many Southern dishes.

Pecans & Walnuts

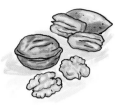

I talk about nuts in the list of plant-forward ingredients later in this chapter, but when it comes to Southern dishes, my favorite nuts to use are pecans and walnuts. I often toast my nuts to create a more intense flavor profile.

Vegetable Oil (for Baking)

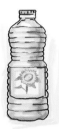

As you may know, baking is a huge part of Southern tradition. I'm talking everything from cakes to pies to donuts to cupcakes and everything in between. One of the essential ingredients for baking is an oil of some sort. And while I often substitute a healthier alternative, such as coconut oil or melted vegan butter, when I'm keeping things more traditional, I love to use vegetable oil. It works great for keeping baked goods moist.

Whole-Wheat Flour

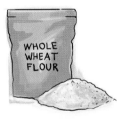

Whenever I get the chance, I try to substitute whole-wheat flour for all-purpose flour, especially in Southern-inspired recipes. As we know, whole-wheat flour is a healthier option, and although I don't use it on a daily basis, I do enjoy it in personal favorites such as my Vegan Blueberry Whole-Wheat Pancakes (page 104) and my Citrus Whole-Wheat Breakfast Loaf (page 132).

Yogurt

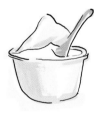

While many of my recipes (especially the ones in this book) call for dairy-free alternatives to milk, cheese, yogurt, and so on, when I do use dairy, I love using full-fat Greek yogurt. Again, so that I can control the flavor in my dishes, I stick with an unsweetened plain version unless otherwise stated specifically in the recipe.

My Favorite
JAMAICAN INGREDIENTS

In Jamaican culture, there aren't as many health-conscious ingredients as we find in the United States. Rather, many typical Jamaican ingredients (such as vegetables and fruits) are minimally processed and come directly from farms or backyard gardens. That being said, when it comes to Jamaican-inspired dishes, a lot of common ingredients fit perfectly into my healthier way of eating, especially when eating plant-forward.

Bananas

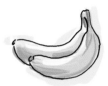

Banana is a staple ingredient in many Jamaican dishes. Normally, ripe yellow bananas are used to make breads, fritters, cakes, and even breakfast dishes like porridge or pancakes. However, green bananas and plantains are often used as well. Both ripe and green bananas and plantains can be boiled, fried, or incorporated into a recipe in some other way. My favorite Jamaican-inspired recipe that includes bananas is my Jamaican-Inspired Banana Oatmeal Porridge (page 96).

Coconut

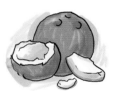

Coconut has a great island-y flavor that adds a subtle nuttiness and sweetness to any dish. Growing up, whenever I visited Jamaica, coconut was a common ingredient used in baked goods such as cakes, puddings, and a dessert staple called "coconut drops," which was made from shredded coconut and brown sugar. Therefore, when cooking Jamaican-inspired dishes, I love to include coconut in some way or to highlight it as a main ingredient when I can.

Cornmeal

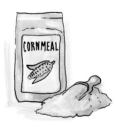

Cornmeal is something that I ate growing up, especially on Sunday mornings when we enjoyed a big breakfast. Specifically, my mom would make traditional Jamaican porridge, which honestly wasn't my favorite at the time; however, I've since grown to love it and now make a healthier version—my Creamy Cornmeal Porridge (page 94), which has a vegan option as well.

Ginger

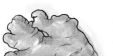

In Jamaican culture, ginger is a heavily used ingredient in many dishes and drinks, from traditional teas to soups to savory and sweet dishes. It has awesome health benefits and medicinal properties, improving heart disease risk factors and treating digestive issues. My Ginger Cupcakes with Chai Cream Cheese Frosting recipe (page 260) is a great nod to bold ginger flavor.

Hibiscus

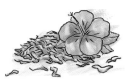

I use this floral ingredient whenever I make my version of the traditional Jamaican drink sorrel (see page 288). Usually, this drink is made on occasions such as Christmas, Thanksgiving, or a special family gathering; however, I enjoy making it every so often on a regular day.

Jerk Seasoning

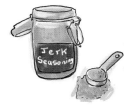

Jerk anything is a staple in Jamaican cuisine, and while jerk chicken is one of the most consumed dishes, I love adding jerk seasoning (see page 42) to plant-forward dishes that include chickpeas, roasted vegetables, veggie burgers, and so on.

Rum

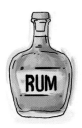

I don't usually drink alcohol or use it in my cooking; however, I couldn't create a Jamaican dish without incorporating rum in some way. Rum is one of the many staple ingredients, especially in drinks and dessert recipes.

Sea Moss

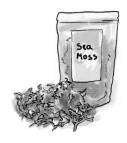

Dried and gel sea moss are go-to ingredients for Jamaican-inspired recipes like my Vegan Jamaican Sea Moss Drink (page 312). Sea moss has great health benefits and immune-boosting properties. The awesome thing about using sea moss is that you can add it to smoothies, juice drinks, oatmeal, soups, and sauces.

Scotch Bonnet (aka Habanero) Pepper

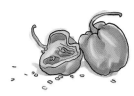

Scotch bonnet pepper is the main type of hot pepper used in Jamaican cooking. Because these peppers are often grown in personal gardens, they are readily accessible to many households, which makes them the perfect convenient ingredient. While the heat factor can get pretty intense (especially when the seeds are added), Scotch bonnet pepper adds a nice kick of heat to many Jamaican dishes, including my Jamaican Rice & Peas recipe (page 170) and Plant-Based Jamaican "Pepperpot" Soup (page 180).

My Favorite
PLANT-FORWARD INGREDIENTS

If there's one thing I've learned along my journey as a plant-forward recipe developer, it's that a well-stocked pantry and fridge will save you so much time and headache. The following ingredients are my favorites, and I use them frequently in my recipes.

Fruits

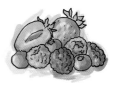

I have a long list of favorite fruits! The more common ones include strawberries, blueberries, blackberries, raspberries, cherries, citrus fruits, mangoes, pineapples, apples, peaches, bananas, cranberries, plums, and grapes. I also love lesser-known fruits like durian (yes!), papaya, and pomegranate.

Veggies

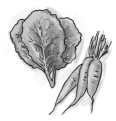

Vegetables come with many nutrients and are very good for you. Some of my favorites include spinach, carrots, arugula, celery, tomatoes, bell peppers, olives, cauliflower, broccoli or broccolini, kale, corn, Brussels sprouts, Swiss chard, asparagus, red cabbage, butternut squash, zucchini, collard greens, different types of lettuce, sweet potatoes, russet potatoes, avocados, and cucumbers.

Fresh Herbs & Aromatics

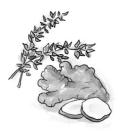

Fresh aromatics and seasoning produce are versatile; they add a punch of flavor to just about any dish. Garlic, onion, and ginger are some of the most frequently used aromatics you should have on hand. Also included in this category are flavor-enhancing ingredients like fresh chili peppers (I love jalapeños!). You'll find I sometimes use fresh herbs—most often as a garnish or when a recipe would not be the same without them (what would a Green Goddess dressing be without fresh green herbs?). But most often, for their convenience and ready availability, I use dried herbs.

Dried Herbs & Spices

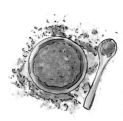

Dried herbs and spices are small ingredients with big flavors that I use in all of my recipes; a little goes a long way. Some dried herbs that you should have on hand are bay leaves, basil, oregano leaves, parsley, rosemary (although I often use fresh leaves), and thyme leaves. Handy spices include allspice, black pepper, cayenne pepper, chili powder, curry powder, garlic power, ginger powder, ground cardamom, ground cinnamon, ground cloves, ground cumin, ground nutmeg, onion powder, paprika (smoked or sweet), red pepper flakes, and turmeric powder.

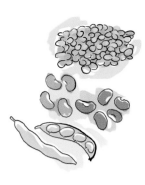

Beans & Legumes

Beans and legumes are some of the best meat substitutes on those days when you don't feel like eating meat. Besides, they are an excellent source of essential vitamins and minerals, including thiamine, folic acid, riboflavin, vitamin B6, copper, phosphorus, manganese, magnesium, potassium, and iron. They come in handy when I want to create meatless yet exciting and flavorful dishes. Great options include kidney beans, black beans, white beans, navy beans, pinto beans, mature soybeans, young soybeans (edamame), chickpeas (my fave!), peas, lentils, and many more.

Nuts, Seeds, and Nut & Seed Butters

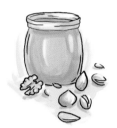

For most of my adulthood, I wasn't a fan of nuts at all. Now I enjoy pecans, walnuts, almonds, and cashews. In addition to these, there are various other nuts, such as acorns, hazelnuts, pistachios, chestnuts, macadamia, peanuts (technically a legume, but used as a nut), and more.

With seeds, there are several excellent options to choose from. I love using ground flax seeds (aka flaxseed meal) and chia seeds in place of eggs in baking (they're also listed in the substitute ingredient list on page 23). Other amazing seeds to try include hemp seeds, poppy seeds, pumpkin seeds, sesame seeds, sunflower seeds, wild rice (considered a grain, but actually the seed of an aquatic grass), and quinoa.

Peanut butter is one of my favorite ingredients of all time. However, if you don't like peanut butter or can't have it, you can easily replace it with any of the many nut or seed butters available on the market, such as almond butter, cashew butter, pecan butter, sunflower seed butter, and sesame butter (tahini).

Healthy Fats & Oils

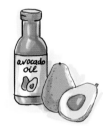

Healthy fats are a vital part of a plant-forward diet. They are good for your heart, cholesterol levels, and overall health. Most people assume that you can't get adequate healthy fats from plant-based foods, but this isn't true at all. Healthy plant-based fats and oils to keep on hand include avocados, avocado oil, chia seeds, coconut oil, olive oil, flax oil, grapeseed oil, peanut oil, and sunflower oil. As noted on page 27, I also like to use vegetable oil (which is typically soybean oil) for traditional Southern baking.

Flours

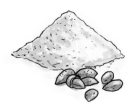

When it comes to flours, I choose organic ones (especially from my go-to brand, Bob's Red Mill). In some recipes, I use artisan bread and cake flours as well as gluten-free 1-to-1 baking flour, almond flour, cassava flour, coconut flour, and oat flour.

Leaveners

I always have leavening agents like baking soda, aluminum-free baking powder, active dry yeast, and cream of tartar in my pantry, as they are super important in baking. To make sure they are fresh, I recommend replacing them every six months.

Sweeteners

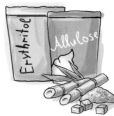

While the point of a plant-forward diet is to keep processed foods and ingredients to a minimum, sugars are an essential ingredient in baking that you can't just leave out entirely. However, we now have several healthy sugar alternatives to choose from (discussed earlier in this chapter). I also recommend organic raw cane sugar, organic brown sugar, organic powdered (confectioner's) sugar, coconut sugar, allulose, and erythritol.

Thickeners

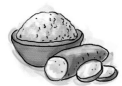

My go-to thickener is arrowroot starch. I frequently use this gluten-free starch to thicken sauces and other dishes. If you don't have arrowroot starch, you can use tapioca flour, all-purpose flour, cornstarch, or potato starch.

OTHER INGREDIENTS THAT I USE FREQUENTLY

- Artisan and rustic breads

- Breadcrumbs

- Brown rice

- Butter breads like brioche and challah

- Canned coconut milk (my favorite dairy-free option for cream-based recipes)

- Cheeses (organic): Gouda, mild cheddar, mozzarella, Parmesan, ricotta, etc.

- Chocolate bars and chips (both dairy-free and regular)

- Coconut flakes

- Coconut whipped cream

- Cream cheese (organic)

- Curry paste

- Dairy-free ice cream

- Dairy-free yogurt and Greek yogurt

- Date syrup

- Eggs (organic)

- Ghee

- Granola

- Low-sodium broths: vegetable, beef, and chicken

- Low-sodium soy sauce

- Meat and seafood: organic chicken, organic short ribs, turkey bacon, wild salmon, and shrimp

- Molasses

- Natural jams and preserves

- Oatmeal

- Oils: avocado, olive oil, grapeseed, and coconut

- Pastas and noodles: spaghetti, rigatoni, pappardelle, fettuccine, penne, macaroni, orzo, and ramen

- Polenta, grits, and cornmeal

- Pumpkin puree (organic)

- Pure maple syrup

- Pure vanilla extract

- Raw cacao powder

- Raw honey

- Ripe plantains

- Taco shells and tortillas

- Tomato paste

- Unsalted butter (organic)

- Vegan butter

- Vegan cream cheese

- Vinegars: apple cider, balsamic, red wine, white wine

- Whipped cream

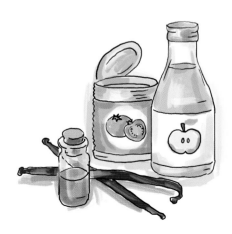

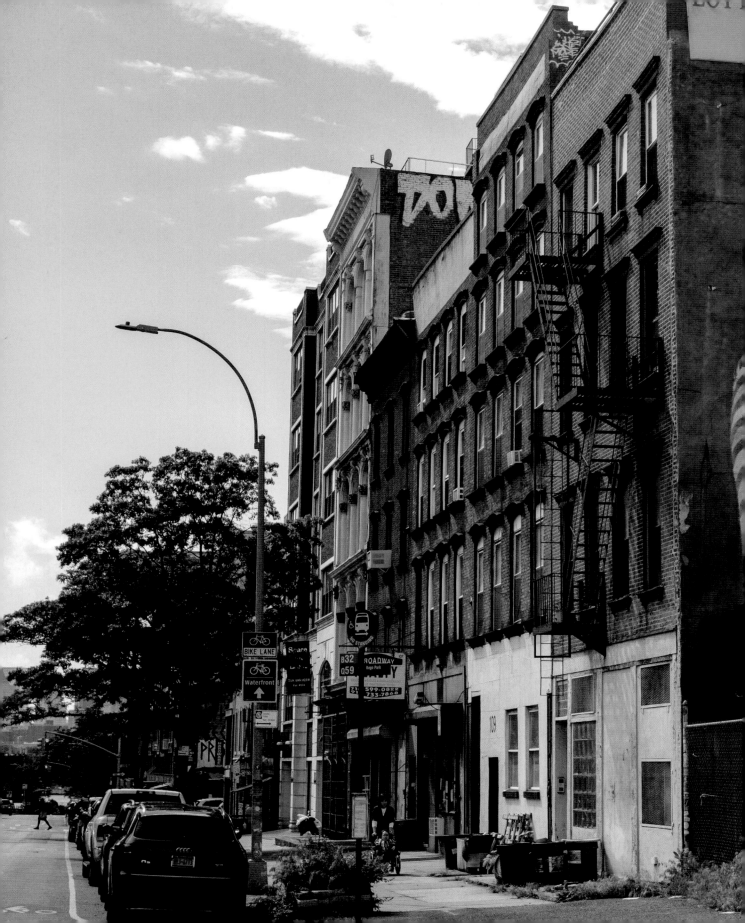

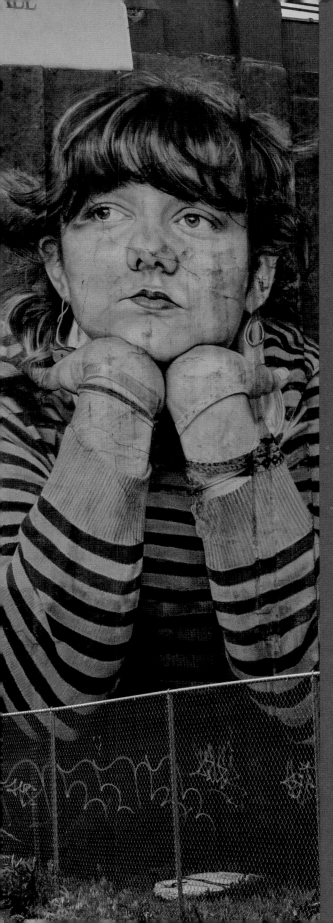

Vegan Buttermilk

This simple recipe is my go-to for all vegan baking and is by far the easiest substitute for regular buttermilk. The recipe can easily be scaled up or down as needed; just be sure to use the ratio of 1 tablespoon vinegar or lemon juice to 1 cup milk. For example, if a recipe calls for 1½ cups of buttermilk, you would use 1½ tablespoons of vinegar or lemon juice to 1½ cups milk; if only ½ cup of buttermilk is required, you would use 1½ teaspoons of vinegar or lemon juice to ½ cup milk. Rest assured, this buttermilk acts just the same as regular buttermilk, adding a nice acidic/sour touch to cakes, muffins, cupcakes, pancakes, waffles, and more. All it takes is 6 minutes of your time, and you can use any of your favorite dairy-free milks.

1 cup unsweetened, unflavored almond milk or other dairy-free milk of choice

1 tablespoon apple cider vinegar or lemon juice (see Tip)

1. In a 2-cup liquid measuring cup or small glass or ceramic bowl, whisk together the milk and vinegar or lemon juice; let the mixture sit for 5 minutes or so, until curdled.

2. Use right away in any recipe that calls for buttermilk. Vegan buttermilk does not store well.

Tip: Apple cider vinegar and lemon juice have different flavors, which subtly affect the flavor of the buttermilk. Depending on the recipe, this slight difference may be apparent. You can experiment with using each one to complement the flavor of the dish you're making. In general, I prefer apple cider vinegar for sweet preparations and lemon juice for savory.

If you don't have apple cider vinegar or lemon juice, you can use distilled white vinegar; it will work just as well, but the flavor of the buttermilk won't be as rich.

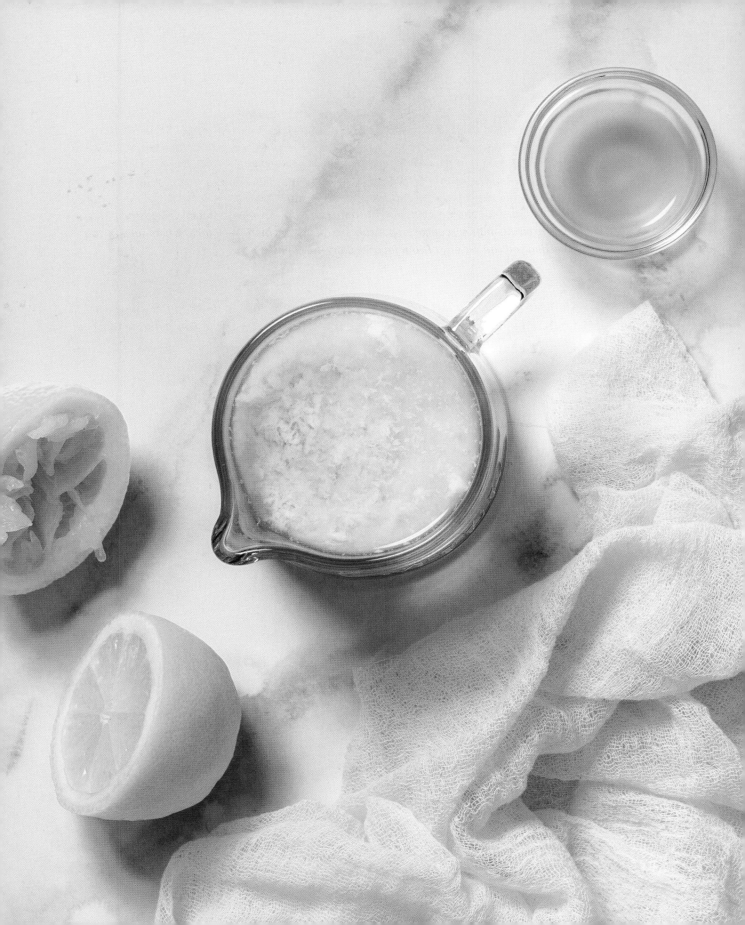

Flaxseed Egg

MAKES
1 flaxseed egg

PREP TIME
1 minute, plus 10 minutes to activate

Learning the art of vegan baking after much trial and error, I've come to use flaxseed eggs as a binder that also helps keep baked goods moist. While there are plenty of other binders, such as mashed bananas, applesauce, and egg substitute powder, a flaxseed egg is one of the best substitutes when you don't want any added sweetness. My favorite trick is to use warm water instead of cold, which helps the flaxseed meal activate and thicken a bit quicker. When a recipe calls for more than 1 flaxseed egg, simply multiply the ingredients as needed, using a 1:3 ratio. For example, if a recipe calls for 3 flaxseed eggs, you would use 3 tablespoons of flaxseed meal plus 9 tablespoons of warm water to create 3 flaxseed eggs. It's that easy!

1 tablespoon flaxseed meal

3 tablespoons warm water

Put the flaxseed meal and water in a small bowl and stir until combined. Let the mixture sit until thickened and pastelike, 5 to 10 minutes.

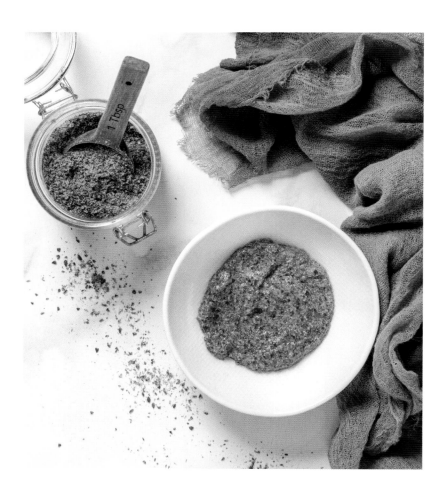

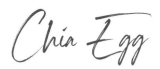

Chia Egg

MAKES
1 chia egg

PREP TIME
1 minute, plus
5 minutes to gel

Another of my favorite binders for baking and cooking is a chia egg. Much like a flaxseed egg, this vegan egg substitute is an easy and convenient way to create a really quick binder. I fell in love with chia seeds once I realized how much of a great superfood this ingredient is and how versatile it is as a binder for baked goods and a thickening agent for foods and drinks. A single tablespoon does wonders nutritionally, and due to chia seeds' tendency to swell and thicken when combined with liquid, they make a great thickening/binding agent as well. As with the flaxseed egg recipe, if you need more than one chia egg, simply multiply the ingredients using a 1:2.5 ratio. For example, if you need 2 chia eggs, use 2 tablespoons of chia seeds and 5 tablespoons of water.

1 tablespoon chia seeds

2½ tablespoons warm water

Put the chia seeds and water in a small bowl and stir until combined. Let the mixture sit until it has a thick gelled consistency, about 5 minutes.

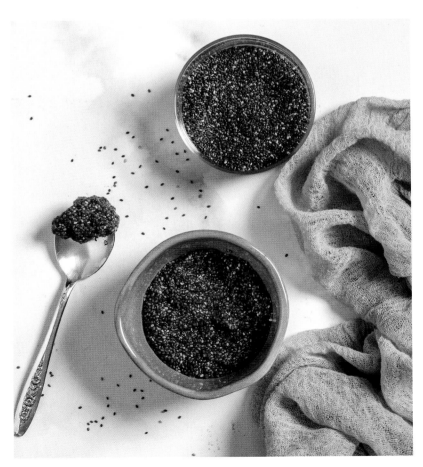

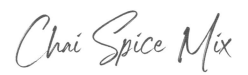

Chai Spice Mix

MAKES
¾ cup

PREP TIME
5 minutes

This DIY chai spice mix is my absolute favorite. The best thing about this blend is that you can store it in a small spice container or jar for continual use, making things much easier when a recipe calls for chai spice mix. Confession: I became obsessed with all things chai after having my son and transitioning to a dairy-free option during my Starbucks run. A venti chai latte has been my go-to morning pick-me-up ever since. If you're a lover of warm spices, then this mix is perfect for you. Add it to your favorite homemade lattes, smoothies, breakfast foods, or baked goods and enjoy!

2 tablespoons ground cinnamon

2 tablespoons ginger powder

2 teaspoons ground allspice

2 teaspoons ground cardamom

2 teaspoons ground cloves

2 teaspoons ground nutmeg

½ teaspoon finely ground black pepper

Put all the ingredients in a small bowl and stir until combined. Store in an airtight spice jar or small container for up to 6 months.

Tip: I like to make my chai spice mix with ground spices because it gives me the flexibility to use it not just to make tea but also as a garnish on lattes, creamy oats, and more. If you're using a store-bought blend made with whole spices, be sure to grind it in a small food processor before using it in the recipes in this book.

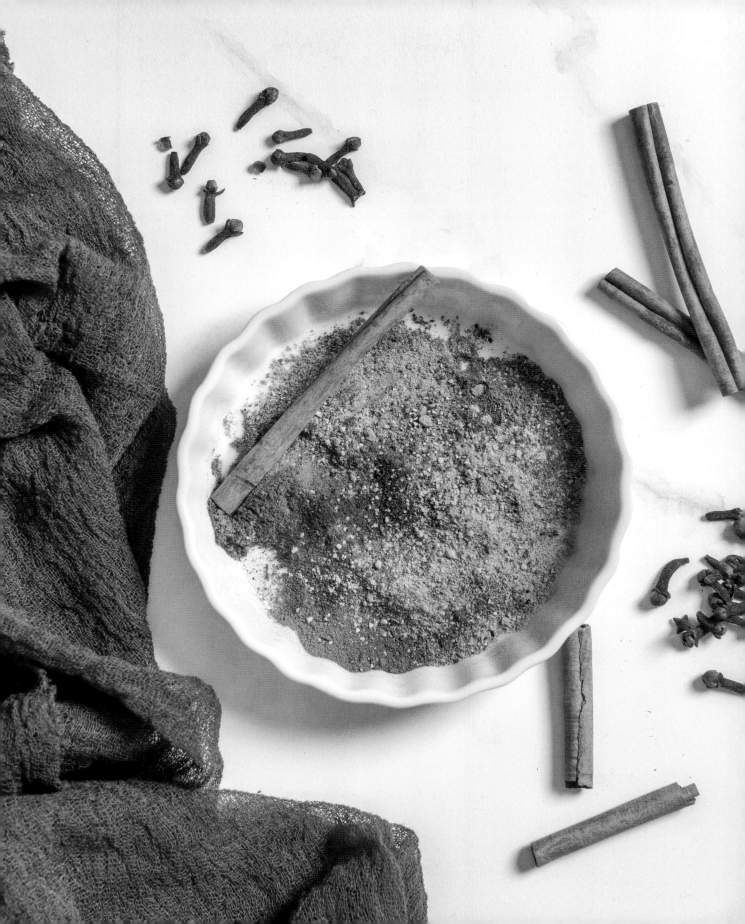

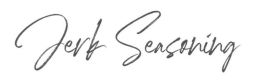

Jerk Seasoning

MAKES
10 tablespoons

PREP TIME
5 minutes

I'm so excited to share this DIY mix with you. Jerk seasoning is such a staple in Jamaican cuisine, and while a wet rub is commonly used, this dry option adds just as much flavor, spicy kick, and overall sweetness that makes chicken, fish, red meats, veggies, and more taste irresistible! All it takes is a quick mixing together of the ingredients to create this handy staple. Of course, you can always adjust the ingredients based on your taste preferences—whether you like things spicier or on the sweeter side.

1 tablespoon garlic powder

1 tablespoon onion powder

1 tablespoon cane sugar or lightly packed brown sugar

1 tablespoon dried parsley

2 teaspoons cayenne pepper

2 teaspoons paprika (smoked or regular)

2 teaspoons finely ground sea salt

2 teaspoons ground black pepper

2 teaspoons dried thyme leaves

1 teaspoon ground allspice

1 teaspoon red pepper flakes

½ teaspoon ground cinnamon

½ teaspoon ground cloves

½ teaspoon ground cumin or cumin seeds

½ teaspoon ground nutmeg

Put all the ingredients in a small bowl and stir until combined. Store in an airtight spice jar or small container for up to 6 months.

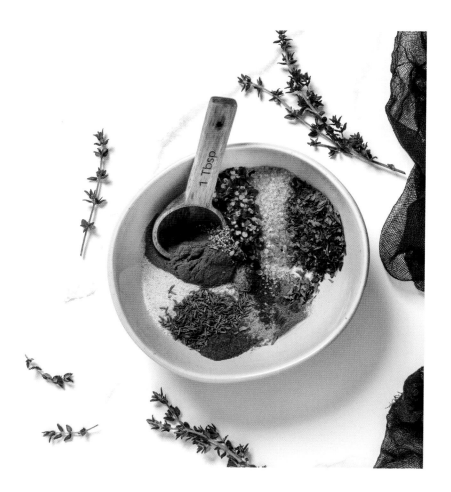

Cajun Seasoning

MAKES
10 tablespoons

PREP TIME
5 minutes

This Cajun seasoning mix comes together in just 5 minutes and adds a great spicy flavor to any food you choose to use it on. This savory and complex blend of spices and herbs elevates just about any of your favorite dishes—pasta, burgers, soups, sides, meats, seafood, you name it!

2 tablespoons garlic powder

2 tablespoons Italian seasoning

2 tablespoons smoked paprika

1 tablespoon cayenne pepper

1 tablespoon ground dried thyme

1 tablespoon onion powder

1 teaspoon finely ground sea salt

1 teaspoon ground black pepper

Put all the ingredients in a small bowl and stir until combined. Store in an airtight spice jar or small container for up to 6 months.

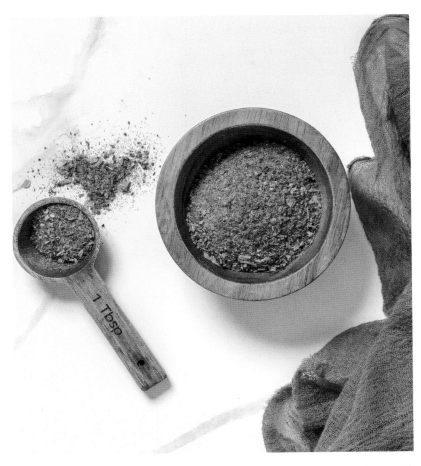

Easy Pizza Dough

MAKES
1 large pizza crust

PREP TIME
10 minutes, plus 1 hour to rise

I grew up eating a lot of pizza in Florida. My favorite place to enjoy a good slice was Pizza Hut. Now that I'm living in NYC, I don't find many Pizza Huts; however, there are lots of authentic mom-and-pop pizza shops that make the best pizzas I've ever tasted. There's nothing like a good homemade pizza, and I really enjoy the fact that you can customize your pie to suit your taste buds. If you love homemade pizza, then this easy dough recipe will become a staple. Plus, this recipe can easily be transformed into a flavored crust (think herbs, spices, purees, etc.), or you can make a gluten-free version by substituting your favorite gluten-free 1-to-1 baking flour for the all-purpose flour.

1 cup lukewarm water

1 tablespoon raw honey

1 tablespoon extra-virgin olive oil, plus more for the bowl

2¼ teaspoons instant yeast

1 teaspoon garlic powder

1 teaspoon dried parsley

2¾ cups all-purpose flour, plus more if needed

½ teaspoon finely ground sea salt

1. In a stand mixer fitted with the whisk attachment, whisk together the warm water, honey, olive oil, yeast, garlic powder, and parsley.

2. Change the attachment to the dough hook and, with the speed on low, slowly add the flour and salt until fully incorporated and a soft, smooth dough has formed, 3 to 4 minutes. If the dough is too sticky, add ½ cup of additional flour at a time until the dough can be stretched with your fingers without completely sticking.

3. Increase the mixer speed to high and knead the dough for about 10 minutes, until it becomes elastic and shiny looking. Form the dough into a ball. Lightly grease a large bowl with olive oil and put the dough ball in the bowl, rolling it around to coat it in the oil. Cover with plastic wrap or a towel and let rise until doubled in size, about 1 hour.

4. Use immediately or place in a plastic container with a lid or wrap in plastic wrap and store in the refrigerator for up to 3 days.

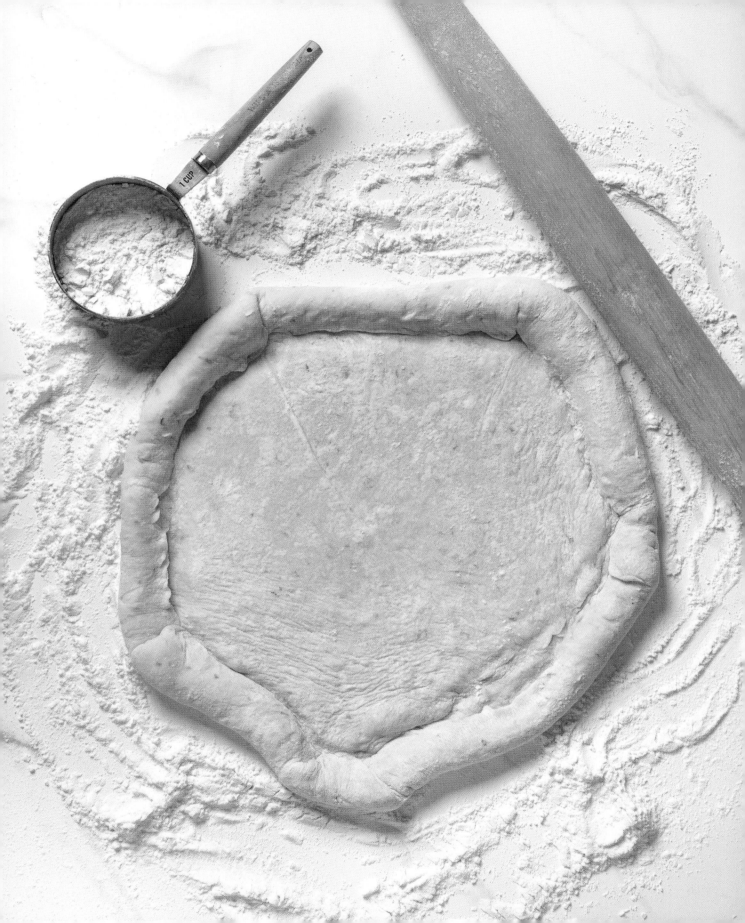

Everyday Pie Crust

MAKES
one 9-inch pie
crust

PREP TIME
10 minutes, plus
1 hour to rest

Throughout my recipe development career, pies were one of the few desserts that I felt extremely intimidated to make; cakes were another. It took a ton of trial and error before I finally mastered a simple pie crust, which is why I wanted to include this recipe in the book. I've learned that pie crusts aren't insanely hard, and this recipe is perfect for anything related to pies (whether just a bottom crust or both top and bottom), hand pies, and even galettes. This everyday recipe meets the needs of most pastry indulgences, whether sweet or savory—if using it for a savory dish, simply omit the cinnamon. The best part is that you can easily make it vegan by replacing the unsalted butter with vegan butter (or vegan buttery sticks). Plus, I love that you can add herbs, spices, and other ingredients such as cheese for a savory twist!

½ cup cold unsweetened almond milk or cold water, plus more if needed

1 teaspoon apple cider vinegar

1½ cups all-purpose flour

½ teaspoon finely ground sea salt

Pinch of ground cinnamon (optional; see Tip)

½ cup (1 stick) cold unsalted butter

1. Pour the almond milk and vinegar into a liquid measuring cup and whisk until combined. Set aside.

2. In a large bowl, whisk together the flour, salt, and cinnamon, if using, until combined.

3. Cut the butter into ½-inch pieces and add it to the dry ingredients. Using a pastry blender, blend the butter into the dry ingredients until the mixture appears crumbly and the butter is broken down into pea-size pieces.

4. While slowly pouring in the milk and vinegar mixture with one hand, use the other hand to work the ingredients together until the dry ingredients become moistened and the mixture transforms into a dough that holds together and has a smooth consistency, 3 to 4 minutes. If the dough feels a little too dry or doesn't come together easily, add 1 tablespoon of cold milk or water at a time until it's moistened enough to hold together.

5. Form the dough into a ball, then gently flatten it into a disk. Wrap the dough in plastic wrap and refrigerate for at least 1 hour or up to overnight before using. *Note:* If making a double quantity of this dough for a recipe that requires a top and bottom crust, simply divide the dough in half and form into two equal-size disks.

Tip: I love including a touch of cinnamon in pie crust for most sweet pies, especially ones that feature cinnamon in the filling, like apple or pumpkin pie; but feel free to omit it if the flavor doesn't suit the type of pie you're making. And of course, you should omit it if you're using this crust for a savory preparation, like the Mini Garlic Herb Tomato Galettes on page 168.

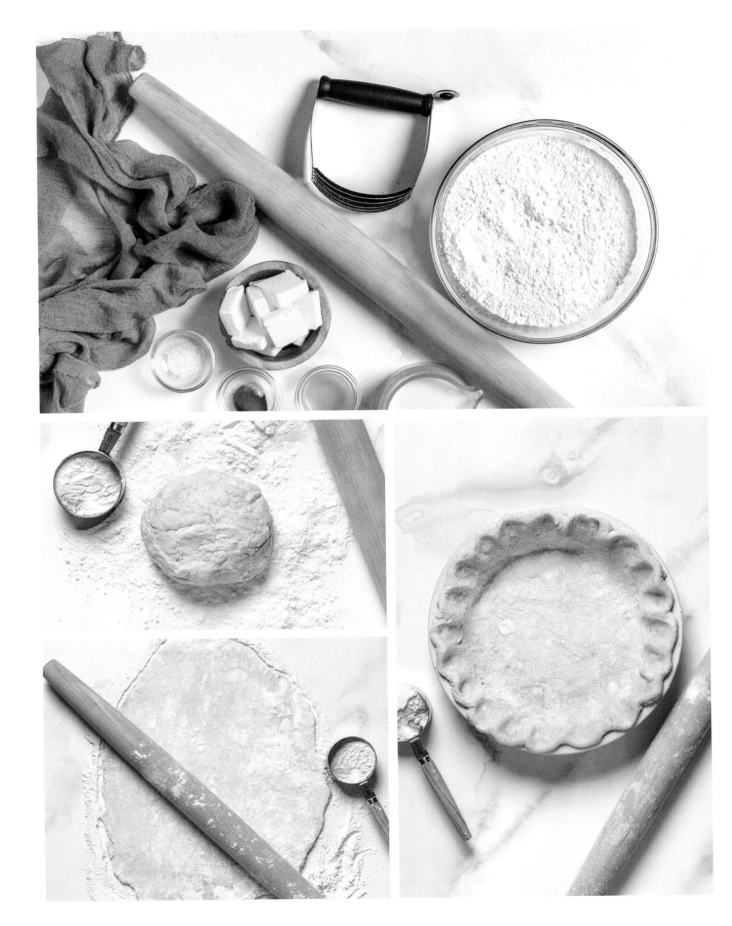

Vegan Cream Cheese Sauce

MAKES
2 cups

PREP TIME
5 minutes, plus
30 minutes or
overnight to
soak cashews

This luxuriously thick sauce is my go-to for creamy-style recipes. A touch of lemon juice gives it a bit of tang—think cream cheese—yet it is simple enough to be used as a replacement for a basic white sauce in recipes like macaroni and cheese. I love to make a double batch when I know that I'll be whipping up creamy dishes a few days in a row. This vegan recipe's base is soaked cashews that are blended with a bit of seasoning, oil, and the aforementioned lemon juice and . . . voilà. You're done!

2 cups raw cashews, soaked, drained, and rinsed (see note)

1 cup low-sodium vegetable stock or water

1 tablespoon extra-virgin olive oil

1 tablespoon freshly squeezed lemon juice

1 teaspoon finely ground sea salt

1. Put all the ingredients in a high-powered blender. Blend on medium-high speed for about 1 minute, until smooth and thick. The texture should be somewhere between whipped cream cheese and crème fraîche—just fluid enough to very slowly fall off a spoon; if it's chunky or too stiff, add a bit more water (1 tablespoon at a time) until the sauce is very smooth.

2. Use immediately or store in a tightly sealed jar in the refrigerator for up to 4 days, or freeze in a freezer-safe container for up to 3 months.

HOW TO SOAK CASHEWS:
Place the raw cashews in a medium-size bowl or 4-cup liquid measuring cup along with enough fresh cold water to fully cover the cashews. Cover with plastic wrap and let sit at room temperature overnight or until the cashews are swollen. When ready to use, drain and rinse the cashews, then drain again. The overnight method is best, creating softer soaked cashews; however, if you're short on time, you can use a shortcut method. For a quick soak, place the cashews in a medium-size heatproof bowl or 4-cup liquid measuring cup and cover with boiling water. Let sit for at least 30 minutes, or until the cashews are swollen. When ready to use, drain, rinse, and drain again.

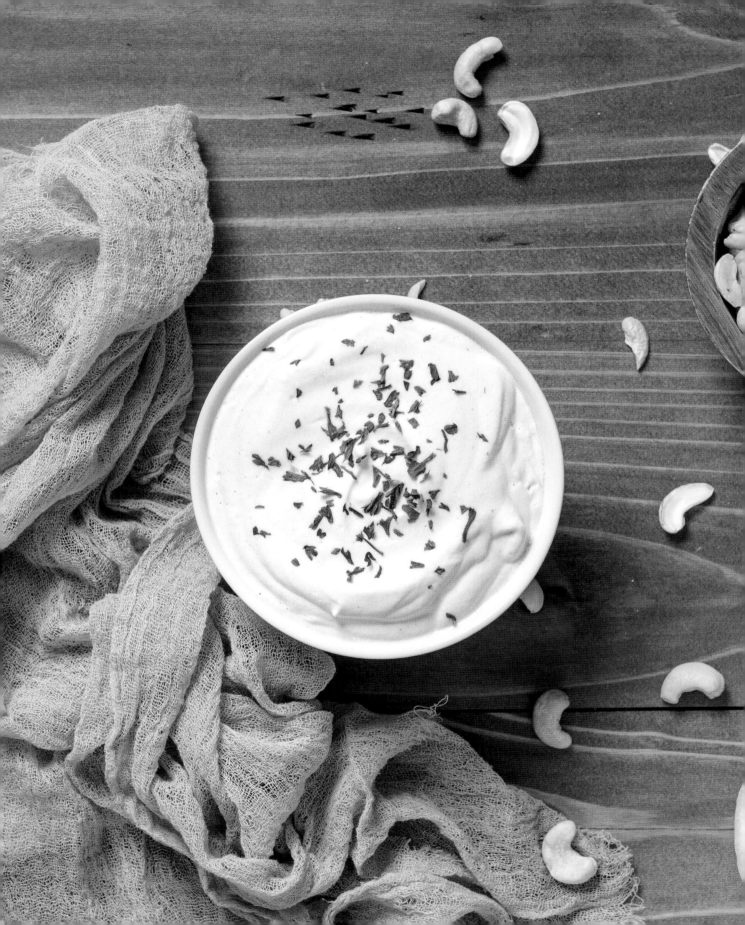

Smoky BBQ SAUCE

MAKES
1 cup

PREP TIME
5 minutes

COOK TIME
15 minutes

BBQ sauce is one of my favorite condiments, and even more so when it's homemade like this one. This sauce is the perfect balance of sweet, tangy, and smoky flavors, which creates the best flavor for burgers, sandwiches, sides, and more.

1 cup unsweetened ketchup

½ cup lightly packed brown sugar

¼ cup apple cider vinegar

2 tablespoons raw honey

1 teaspoon chili powder

1 teaspoon garlic powder

1 teaspoon onion powder

1 teaspoon smoked paprika

1 teaspoon finely ground sea salt

½ teaspoon ground black pepper

1. Put all the ingredients in a medium-size saucepan and whisk everything together. Bring to a boil over medium-high heat. Once at a boil, reduce the heat to low and let simmer for 10 minutes or so, stirring occasionally, until slightly thickened.

2. Remove the pan from the heat and set aside to cool before using. Store any remaining sauce in a sealed glass container or jar in the refrigerator for up to 2 weeks.

VARIATION: Vegan Smoky BBQ Sauce.
Substitute pure maple syrup or agave syrup for the honey, and be sure to use organic brown sugar.

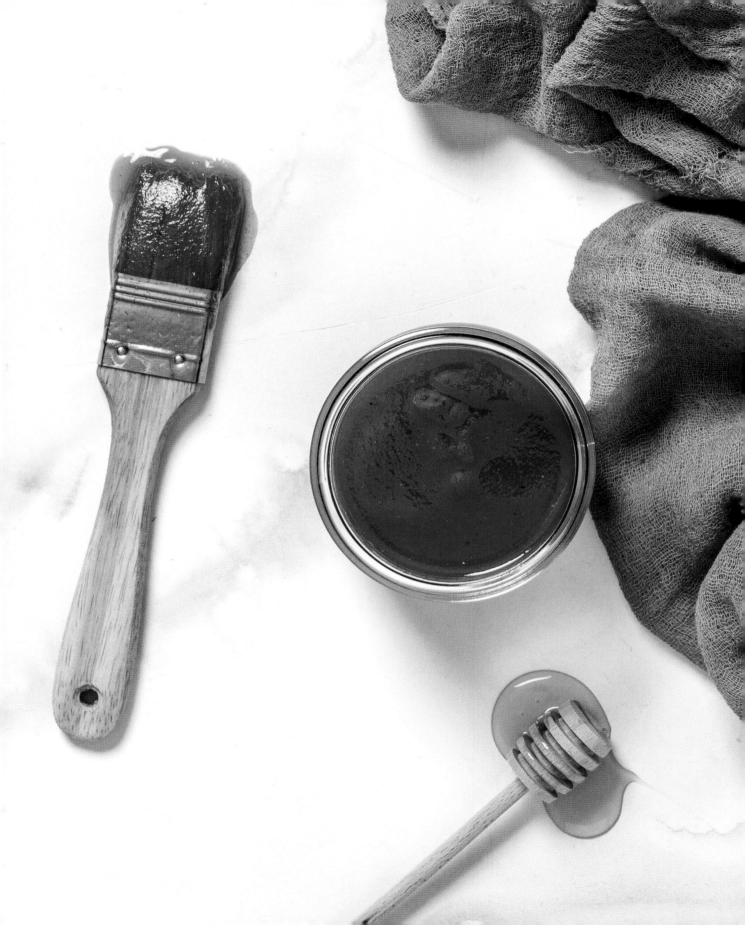

Jerk
BBQ SAUCE

MAKES
1 cup

PREP TIME
1 minute

Unlike traditional BBQ sauce, this recipe comes with a nice dose of spiciness that complements the sweetness already present. While you are able to find reputable Jamaican brands of jerk barbecue sauce (such as Grace or Walkerswood) at specialty grocers and online, making this sauce from scratch is easy, and, once the two components are made, it takes but a minute. Simply mix together BBQ sauce and jerk seasoning and voilà! If you use store-bought BBQ sauce and jerk seasoning, it's of course even faster.

1 cup BBQ sauce, homemade (page 50) or store-bought

3 to 4 tablespoons jerk seasoning, homemade (page 42) or store-bought

1. Put the BBQ sauce and 3 tablespoons of jerk seasoning in a medium-size bowl and whisk together until combined and the sauce darkens a bit. Taste the sauce and add up to an additional tablespoon of jerk seasoning if you'd like it spicier.

2. Store any leftover sauce in a sealed glass container or jar in the refrigerator for up to 2 weeks.

VARIATION: Vegan Jerk BBQ Sauce.
To make this sauce vegan, be sure to use a vegan BBQ sauce. If using the homemade BBQ sauce on page 50, follow the instructions there for making a vegan version.

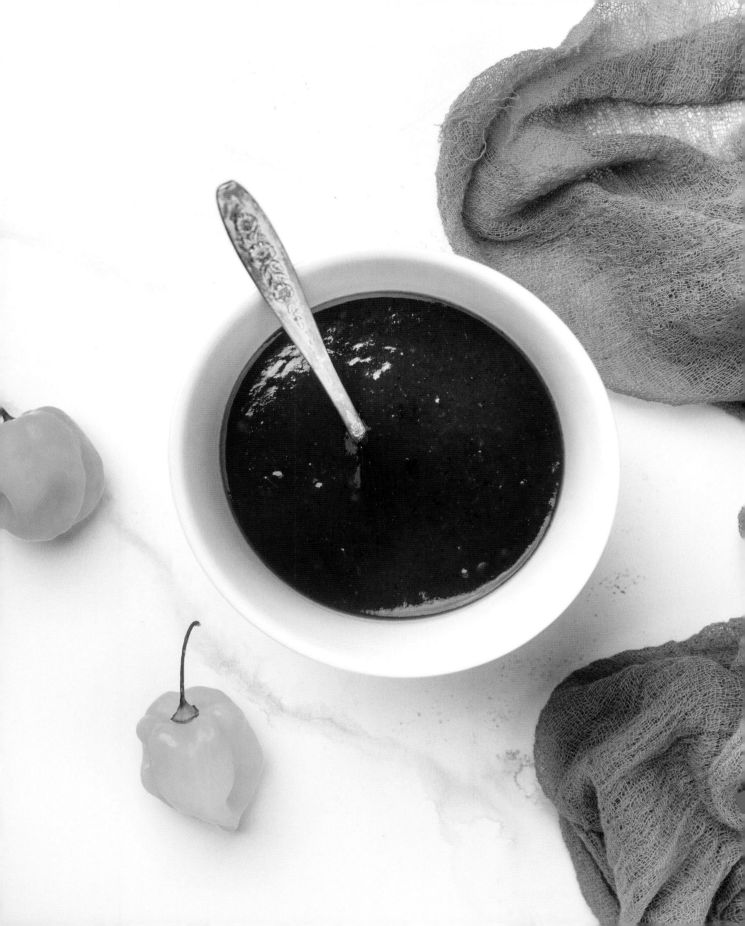

Simple Sweet Potato
PUREE/MASH

MAKES
about 3 cups

PREP TIME
10 minutes

COOK TIME
1 hour

Sweet potato puree or mash is one of my favorite ingredients to use as a binder and natural sweetener. I include it in all sorts of sweet and savory dishes ranging from pancakes and waffles to pasta, tacos, and brownies. I even include it in the occasional smoothie or drink! For that reason, I love having this puree (or mash) on hand stored tightly sealed in my refrigerator so that it's an easy "pull-out-and-add" ingredient. Growing up, I remember seeing the grown-ups cook sweet potatoes in boiling salted water before mashing them up and adding them to whatever dish they were making. However, it wasn't until I began to cook more and more that I realized while this method isn't wrong, you get better results from roasting the sweet potatoes rather than boiling them. Roasting reduces their moisture content, concentrating their flavor and creating a thick and creamy puree or mash.

2 large sweet potatoes (about 1 pound)

1 tablespoon extra-virgin olive oil

¼ cup water, plus more if needed, for the puree

1. Preheat the oven to 400°F. Line a sheet pan with parchment paper or foil.

2. Rinse and pat dry the sweet potatoes, then poke holes in them using a fork. Coat the potatoes with the olive oil and place on the prepared pan. Bake the potatoes for 45 minutes to 1 hour, until tender and juices begin to bubble outside of the skin. Remove the potatoes from the oven and let them cool until cool enough to handle, 20 to 30 minutes.

3. **To make sweet potato puree:** Cut the potatoes down the middle, then open them up and scoop the insides into a high-powered blender. Pour in the water and blend the sweet potato flesh until completely smooth and pureed, 2 to 3 minutes. If the potatoes are too thick to puree to a perfectly smooth consistency, add another tablespoon of water. Proceed to Step 4.

To make sweet potato mash: Cut the potatoes down the middle, then open them up and scoop the insides into a bowl. Using a hand-held potato masher or a fork, mash the sweet potatoes until smooth.

4. Use immediately. Store any leftovers in an airtight container in the refrigerator for up to 3 days or freeze for up to 3 months, thawing the puree or mash overnight in the refrigerator before use.

Tip: For some recipes, you want a sweet potato puree that has a completely smooth texture; this requires getting a blender out and adding a bit of water when pureeing the cooked sweet potato flesh. For other recipes, mashing the sweet potato by hand is all that's needed. When a recipe requires sweet potato puree, that is noted in the recipe.

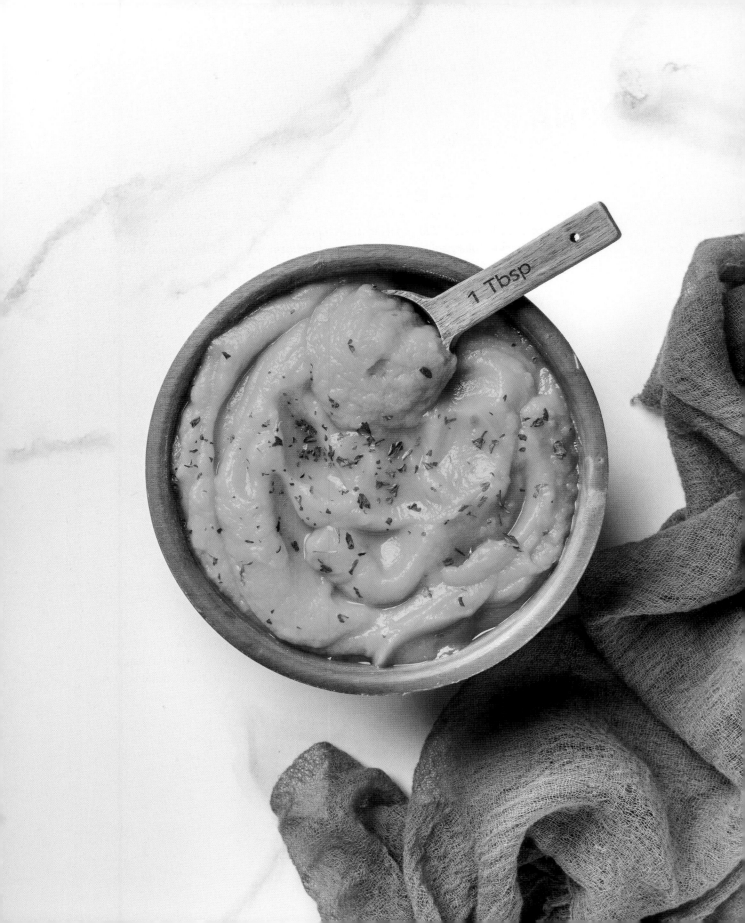

Easy 20-Minute
QUINOA

MAKES
3 cups

PREP TIME
5 minutes

COOK TIME
15 minutes

When it comes to cooking quinoa, it's super important to understand how to create both heartiness and flavor to avoid the blandness that most of us run from when we hear the word quinoa. I've found the trick is to cook quinoa in stock—usually veggie or chicken if not needing it to be vegan—and to season it well; doing so creates a nice flavorful side dish or component that really brightens the flavor profile of whatever dish you pair it with. Add this quinoa to tacos, burgers, meatballs, salads, quinoa bowls, and more.

1 cup red or tri-color quinoa

3 cups low-sodium chicken or vegetable stock or water

½ teaspoon finely ground sea salt

1. Rinse the quinoa under running water in a fine-mesh strainer, then put the quinoa in a medium-size saucepan. Pour in the stock and bring to a boil over medium-high heat, whisking continuously as it begins to boil.

2. Once boiling, season with the salt and reduce the heat to low. Cover and let simmer for 10 to 15 minutes, whisking every 3 to 4 minutes, until the quinoa is cooked. It is done when the water is fully absorbed and the quinoa has increased in size and is fluffy. Fluff with a fork and serve immediately. Store any leftovers in an airtight container in the refrigerator for up to 1 week or freeze for up to 6 months.

Tip: This recipe can be made in a half-batch quantity if you prefer.

As directed in Step 1, be sure to whisk continuously while the quinoa and cooking liquid are coming to a boil; doing so ensures that the liquid won't boil over.

Many recipes call for using 1 part quinoa to 2 parts cooking liquid; however, to create a soft and fluffy quinoa, I've had the best success using 3 parts liquid. If you find that there is too much water remaining at the bottom of the pot or the quinoa is too mushy, try reducing the quantity of stock or water to 2 cups. Due to variabilities in cookware and stovetops, you may need to experiment with the ratio of quinoa to liquid to arrive at perfectly cooked quinoa.

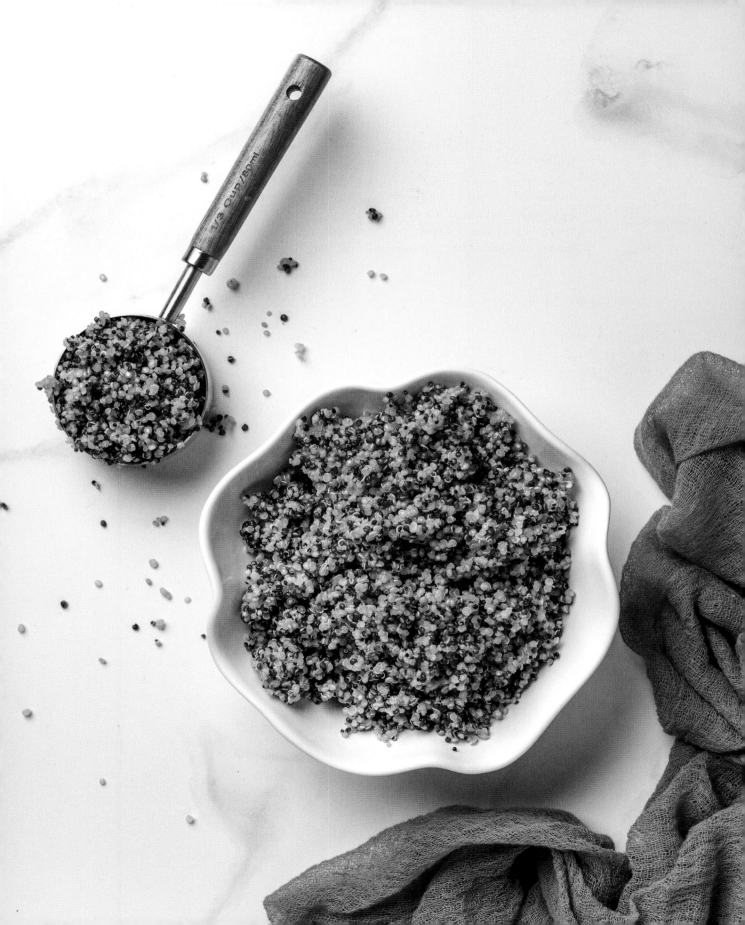

Shredded Jerk Chicken

MAKES
1 cup

PREP TIME
5 minutes, plus
5 minutes to
marinate

COOK TIME
30 minutes

Having shredded chicken made ahead is a convenient way to add a touch of animal protein to salads and wraps, but also to pizzas and even a savory scone or two (see my recipe on page 144). Seasoning the chicken with my jerk spice mix takes it from ordinary to extra special. The iconic Jamaican dish jerk chicken is traditionally prepared on the bone. Here, boneless chicken is smothered in jerk seasoning and baked to perfection in just 30 minutes. This recipe can easily be scaled up to suit your needs.

1 (6-ounce) boneless, skinless chicken breast

3 to 4 tablespoons jerk seasoning, homemade (page 42) or store-bought

1. Preheat the oven to 400°F.

2. Put the chicken breast in a medium-size bowl and sprinkle both sides with the jerk seasoning. *Note:* If you like moderate heat, use 3 tablespoons of jerk seasoning; add up to 1 additional tablespoon if you enjoy things spicy. Turn the chicken a few times to make sure it's well coated in the seasoning. Let the chicken sit for 5 minutes to marinate, then place it on a sheet pan.

3. Place the chicken in the oven and bake for 30 minutes, or until cooked through (when the juices run clear when cut into), turning it over midway through cooking. Remove the chicken from the oven and shred it using two forks. Leftovers will keep in the fridge for up to 4 days.

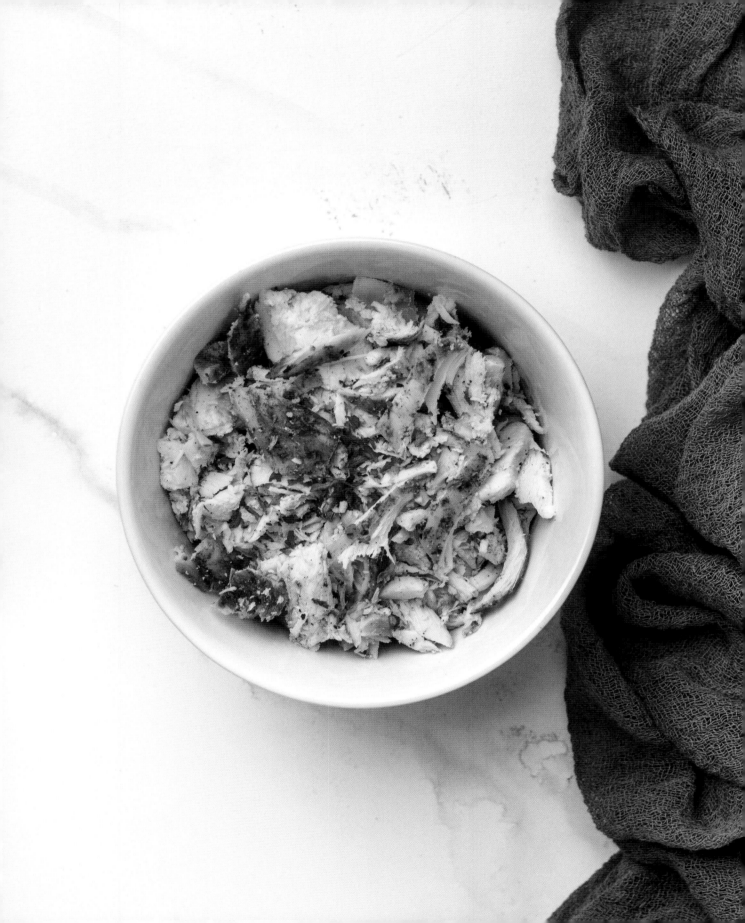

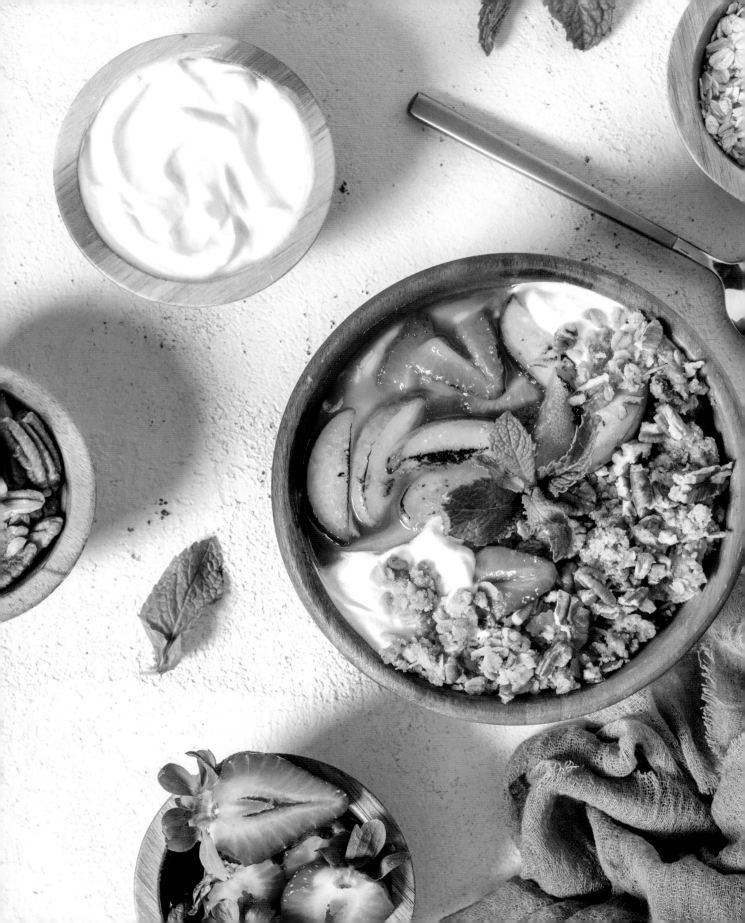

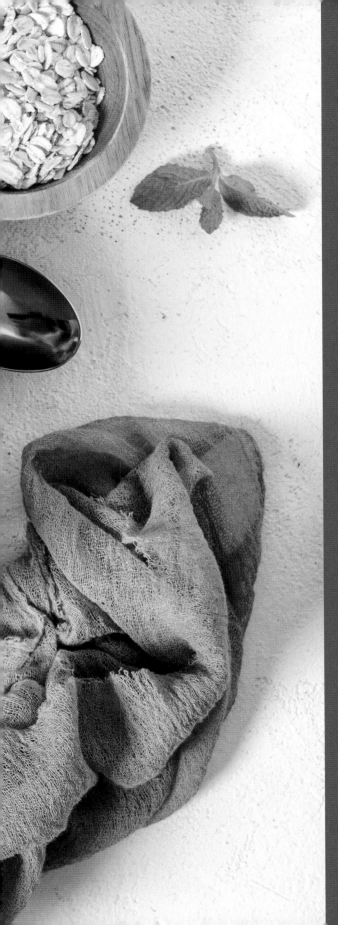

Chapter 4:

MORNING EATS

Overnight Oats Four Ways:
BANANA PEANUT BUTTER, ALMOND BLUEBERRY, PUMPKIN CHAI LATTE, AND CACAO

SERVES
2 (each)

PREP TIME
5 minutes, plus
8 hours to chill

When I first tasted overnight oats a few years ago, I remember thinking, "Why didn't I try this sooner?" Honestly, overnight oats have become my go-to easy-to-whip-together breakfast. This recipe is dear to my heart because it can be personalized in so many ways, allowing you to explore four different flavors—Banana Peanut Butter, Almond Blueberry, Pumpkin Chai Latte, and Cacao—from one base of foundational ingredients. Made in a single bowl with a few quick stirs, these creamy oats are the perfect healthy option (think vegan and gluten-free) for the entire family.

BANANA PEANUT BUTTER OATS

1 cup rolled oats (gluten-free)

1 cup unsweetened almond milk

1 ripe banana, mashed

¼ cup natural peanut butter, softened

2 tablespoons pure maple syrup (see Tip)

1 tablespoon flaxseed meal

2 teaspoons vanilla extract

1 teaspoon ground cinnamon

¼ teaspoon ground nutmeg

Pinch of finely ground sea salt

TOPPINGS (OPTIONAL):

Sliced ripe bananas

½ cup chopped pecans, toasted (see note, page 107)

2 tablespoons natural peanut butter, melted

ALMOND BLUEBERRY OATS

1 cup rolled oats (gluten-free)

1 cup unsweetened almond milk

¼ cup natural almond butter, softened

2 tablespoons pure maple syrup (see Tip)

1 tablespoon flaxseed meal

2 teaspoons almond extract

1 teaspoon ground cinnamon

¼ teaspoon ground nutmeg

Pinch of finely ground sea salt

1 cup fresh blueberries

TOPPINGS (OPTIONAL):

Sliced almonds

Fresh blueberries

PUMPKIN CHAI LATTE OATS

1 cup rolled oats (gluten-free)

1 cup brewed chai tea, using almond milk (see Tip)

¼ cup canned pumpkin puree

¼ cup natural peanut butter, softened

2 tablespoons pure maple syrup (see Tip, page 69)

1 tablespoon flaxseed meal

2 teaspoons vanilla extract

1 teaspoon chai spice mix, homemade (page 40) or store-bought

Pinch of finely ground sea salt

TOPPINGS (OPTIONAL):

Coconut whipped cream

Pinch of chai spice mix, homemade (page 40) or store-bought

(Recipe continues on page 69)

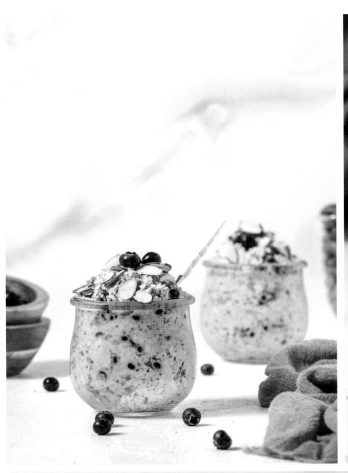
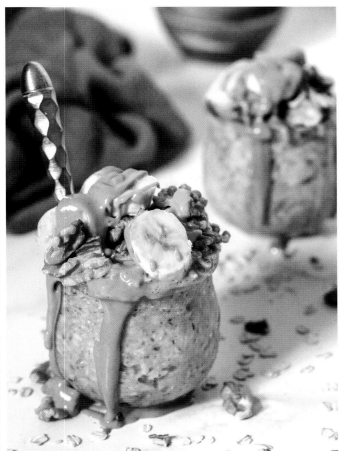
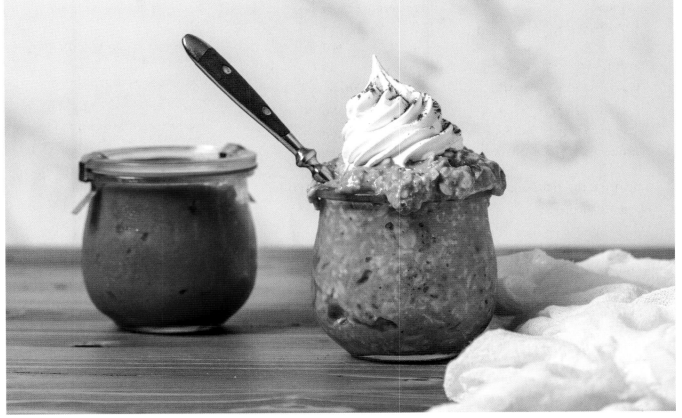

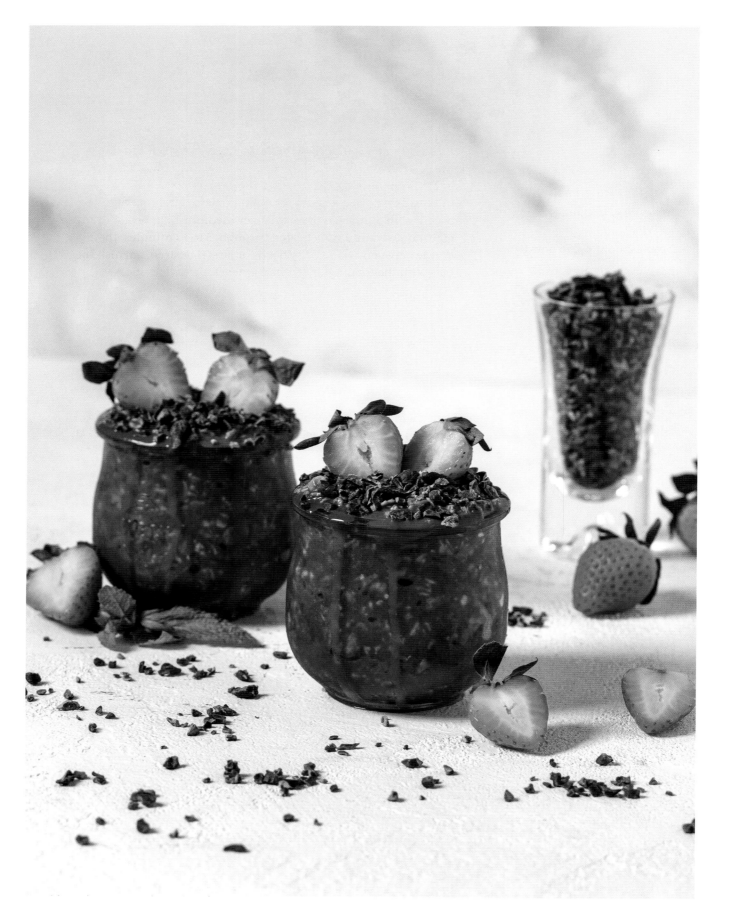

CACAO OATS

1 cup rolled oats (gluten-free)

1 cup unsweetened almond milk

¼ cup natural almond butter, softened

2 tablespoons cacao powder

2 tablespoons pure maple syrup (see Tip)

1 tablespoon flaxseed meal

2 teaspoons vanilla extract

½ teaspoon ground cinnamon

Pinch of finely ground sea salt

TOPPINGS (OPTIONAL):

Sliced strawberries

Chopped vegan chocolate, cacao nibs, or pinch of cacao powder

Put all the ingredients in a medium-size mixing bowl and stir until well combined. Tightly cover the bowl with plastic wrap and refrigerate overnight (or at least 8 hours). To serve cold, divide the oats between two bowls or jars; to serve hot, put the oats in a medium-size saucepan over medium-high heat and stir continuously until fully heated through, 5 to 10 minutes, then divide between two serving bowls or jars. If desired, garnish the oats with the toppings suggested for each flavor variation.

 Tip: Instead of maple syrup, you can use agave syrup or, for the Banana Peanut Butter flavor, add another ½ cup of mashed banana to the oat mixture.

HOW TO MAKE CHAI TEA:

Bring 1 cup of unsweetened almond milk to a rolling boil in a medium-size saucepan over medium-high heat. Remove the pan from the heat, add 2 black tea bags, and let steep for 5 to 6 minutes. Once fully steeped, remove the tea bags and whisk in 1 tablespoon of chai spice mix until well combined.

Cinnamon Quinoa Breakfast Bowl
WITH CARAMELIZED APPLES & POMEGRANATE ARILS

SERVES
2

PREP TIME
5 minutes

COOK TIME
10 minutes

When it comes to breakfast, I often get excited about over-the-top dishes like waffles, pancakes, and French toast. However, for the past year or two, I've made it a mission to try new hearty breakfast meals. Quinoa bowls were something I stumbled upon and fell completely in love with. I enjoy how comforting these bowls are and the versatility of being able to fully customize the ingredients to fit your immediate needs. This recipe is super easy to make: it uses my Easy 20-Minute Quinoa as a base, which is bulked up and sweetened with chia seeds, maple syrup, and cinnamon and topped with spiced caramelized apples and fresh pomegranate arils.

CINNAMON QUINOA:

2 cups cooked red or tri-color quinoa (see page 58)

1 cup unsweetened almond milk

2 tablespoons pure maple syrup

2 tablespoons chia seeds

1 tablespoon ground cinnamon

CARAMELIZED APPLES:

3 tablespoons vegan butter

¼ cup lightly packed brown sugar

1 teaspoon ground cinnamon

½ teaspoon ground nutmeg

⅛ teaspoon ground cloves

Pinch of ground allspice

Pinch of finely ground sea salt

2 medium Granny Smith apples, peeled and diced

FOR TOPPING:

Arils from ½ pomegranate

Fresh rosemary sprigs (optional)

MAKE THE QUINOA:

1. Put the cooked quinoa, milk, maple syrup, chia seeds, and cinnamon in a medium-size saucepan over medium-high heat, stirring until the ingredients are well combined and the mixture begins to boil, 2 to 3 minutes.

2. Once boiling, reduce the heat to medium-low and cook until the liquid reduces greatly and the quinoa is nice and fluffy and moist, 5 to 6 minutes. Meanwhile, caramelize the apples.

MAKE THE CARAMELIZED APPLES:

3. Melt the butter in a large skillet over medium-high heat, then add the brown sugar, spices, and salt and stir until well combined and it begins to bubble.

4. Add the diced apples and cook until golden brown, 3 to 4 minutes, stirring occasionally. At this point, the sauce should begin to thicken and become more caramel-like in consistency. Remove the pan from the heat and set aside.

5. To serve, divide the quinoa between two bowls and top each with the caramelized apples and pomegranate arils and, if desired, fresh rosemary sprigs.

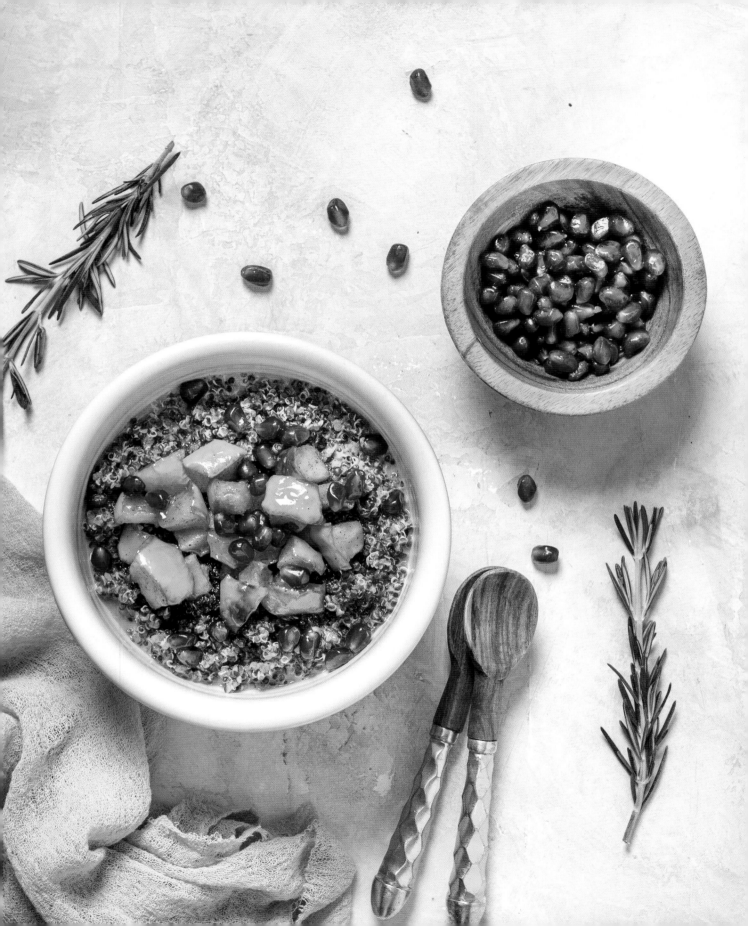

Mocha Chia Pudding
WITH COCONUT FLAKES

SERVES
2

PREP TIME
5 minutes, plus
15 minutes to
set

Much like overnight oats, chia pudding is a quick and easy fix for breakfast. This creamy pudding is whipped together in literally 5 minutes and then sits at room temperature for 15 minutes or so, until thickened. I never thought I would be a fan of chia pudding because of the gel-like texture; however, it has become my newest staple when I'm not eating overnight oats. If you're a lover of coffee and chocolate, this recipe is for you; it pays homage to a nice cup of joe in a delicious chocolate-laced spoonful.

1 cup unsweetened almond milk

½ cup chia seeds

¼ cup freshly brewed coffee

2 tablespoons agave syrup

2 tablespoons cacao powder

Pinch of ground cinnamon

TOPPINGS:

Unsweetened coconut flakes

Roughly chopped vegan chocolate

1. Put all the ingredients in a medium-size bowl and stir until well combined.

2. Tightly cover the bowl with plastic wrap and let it sit at room temperature for 15 minutes, until the mixture has thickened and becomes gel-like.

3. To serve, divide the chia pudding between two 4-ounce glasses (short and wide is best) or jars and top with coconut flakes and chopped chocolate.

VARIATION: Overnight Mocha Chia Pudding with Coconut Flakes.
Put all the ingredients for the pudding in a medium-size bowl, stir, and cover the bowl with plastic wrap. Refrigerate overnight. To serve, spoon the pudding into glasses and top with coconut flakes and chopped chocolate.

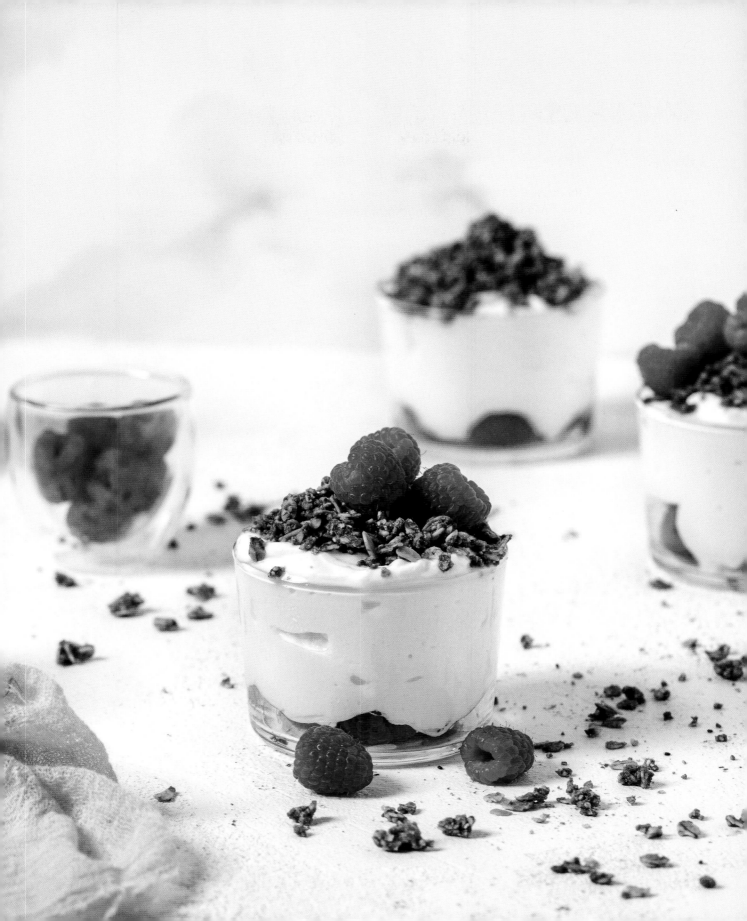

Peanut Butter Banana
OAT SMOOTHIE

SERVES
2

PREP TIME
5 minutes

I've always been a fan of peanut butter and banana, so putting them together in a smoothie seemed like the right thing to do. This is a delicious way to enjoy a quick and easy morning pick-me-up while gaining health benefits from the simple ingredients that marry so well, creating a powerful kick of flavor. (I've included turmeric for its powerful anti-inflammatory properties.) This vegan and gluten-free smoothie is the perfect meal substitute for the entire family.

2 large ripe bananas, sliced and frozen

1 cup unsweetened almond milk

⅓ cup rolled oats (gluten-free), plus more for topping if desired

3 tablespoons natural peanut butter

1 teaspoon flaxseed meal

1 teaspoon vanilla extract

½ teaspoon turmeric powder

1. Put all the ingredients in a high-powered blender and blend until smooth and creamy, 2 to 3 minutes.

2. To serve, pour the smoothie into two 16-ounce glasses and top with additional oats, if desired.

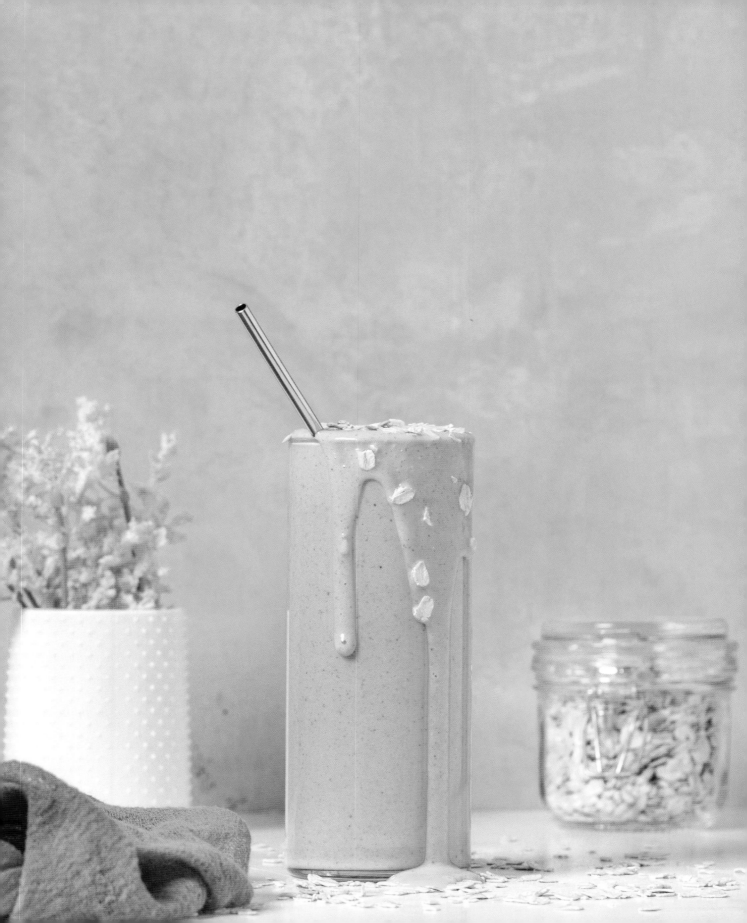

Sweet Potato OAT SMOOTHIE

SERVES
2

PREP TIME
5 minutes

I'm obsessed with sweet potatoes. I'm sure it has a lot to do with having been raised in the South. Sweet potato pie is my absolute favorite type of pie, and I actually love most things that include sweet potato; therefore, this smoothie is something special. This flavor-packed recipe is also nutrient-dense, which is sure to keep you filled for longer. To spice things up further, you can add additional spices such as chai spice mix (page 40), ginger powder, or ground cloves, or you can simplify things by using just ground cinnamon—it's up to you.

1 cup Simple Sweet Potato Mash (page 56)

1 ripe banana, sliced and frozen

1 cup unsweetened almond milk

2 tablespoons rolled oats (gluten-free)

1 tablespoon natural almond butter

1 tablespoon pure maple syrup

1 teaspoon vanilla extract

1 teaspoon ground cinnamon

1 teaspoon ground nutmeg

¼ teaspoon ground allspice

Pinch of finely ground sea salt

TOPPINGS (OPTIONAL):

Chopped pecans, toasted (see note, page 107)

Cacao nibs

1. Put all the ingredients in a high-powered blender and blend until smooth and creamy, 2 to 3 minutes.

2. To serve, pour the smoothie into two 16-ounce glasses and top with chopped pecans and cacao nibs, if desired.

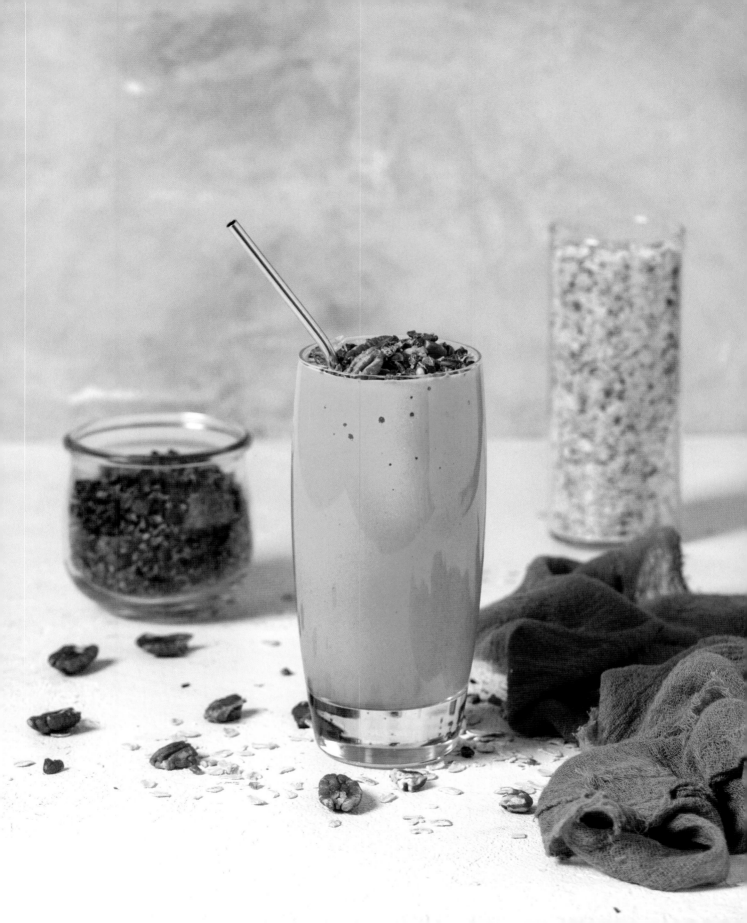

Sunrise Smoothie
(CARROT, STRAWBERRY & ORANGE)

SERVES
2

PREP TIME
5 minutes

I remember not being able to start my morning without whipping together a quick smoothie for my husband and me. It was the quickest and easiest thing to make while getting ready for work. And though our careers have changed a bit, I still make a morning smoothie at least once per week. This recipe adds such brightness to your morning, and the fresh citrusy flavors work so well together!

2 medium carrots, peeled and roughly chopped

1 medium navel orange, peeled

1 ripe banana, sliced and frozen

2 cups frozen strawberries

1½ cups unsweetened almond milk

¼ cup agave syrup

¼ cup plain Greek yogurt (full-fat)

1 tablespoon flaxseed meal

1 teaspoon vanilla extract

1. Put all the ingredients in a high-powered blender and blend until smooth and creamy, 2 to 3 minutes.

2. To serve, pour the smoothie into two 16-ounce glasses and enjoy!

Tip: To make this smoothie vegan, replace the Greek yogurt with unsweetened coconut yogurt.

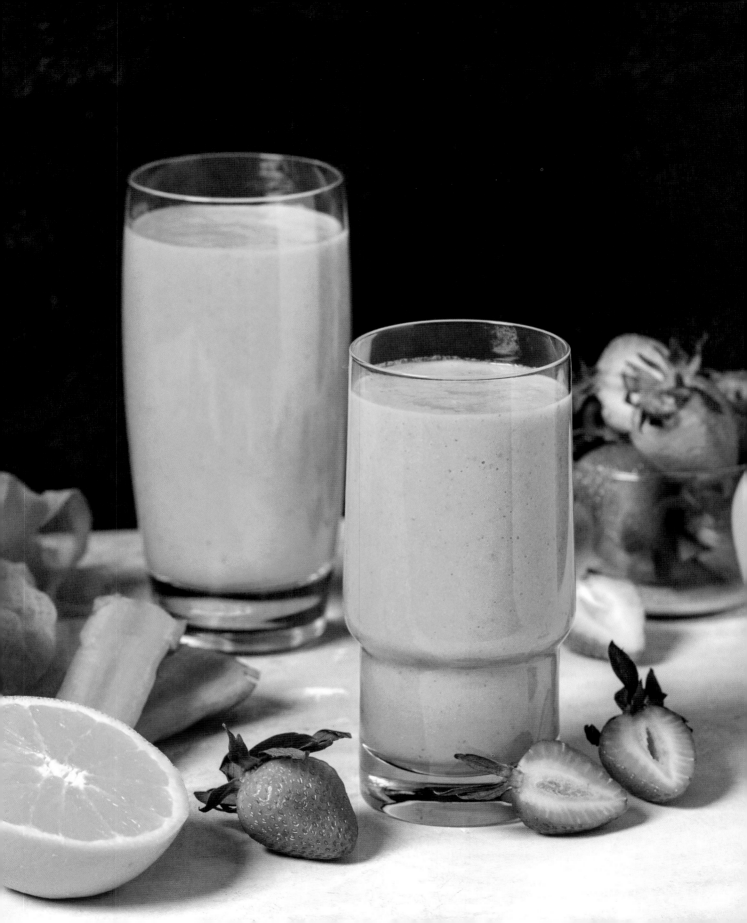

Cashew Date MORNING SHAKE

SERVES
2

PREP TIME
5 minutes, plus
10 minutes
to soak dates
(not including
time to soak
cashews)

This vegan shake is simply the best. It's made from cashews, oats, dates, bananas, plant-based milk, and warm spices and comes completely naturally sweetened, courtesy of the dates. Plus, it's a smooth and creamy drinking experience and makes the perfect post-workout shake or meal replacer to kick-start your day. If you're into smoothies or protein shakes, then this recipe will be right up your alley.

8 Medjool dates, pitted

1 cup boiling water

1¼ cups unsweetened almond milk

1 cup raw cashews, soaked, drained, and rinsed (see note, page 48)

1 ripe banana, peeled

¼ cup rolled oats (gluten-free)

1 teaspoon vanilla extract

½ teaspoon ground cinnamon, plus more for topping if desired

¼ teaspoon ground nutmeg

Pinch of finely ground sea salt

TOPPINGS (OPTIONAL):
Coconut whipped cream

Roughly chopped vegan chocolate

1. Put the dates in a medium-size heatproof bowl or 2-cup liquid measuring cup and cover with the boiling water. Let sit until swollen and softened, about 10 minutes, then drain and rinse.

2. Put the soaked dates and the rest of the ingredients in a high-powered blender and blend until smooth and creamy, 2 to 3 minutes.

3. To serve, pour the shake into two 16-ounce glasses and top with coconut whipped cream, a pinch of cinnamon, and chopped chocolate, if desired.

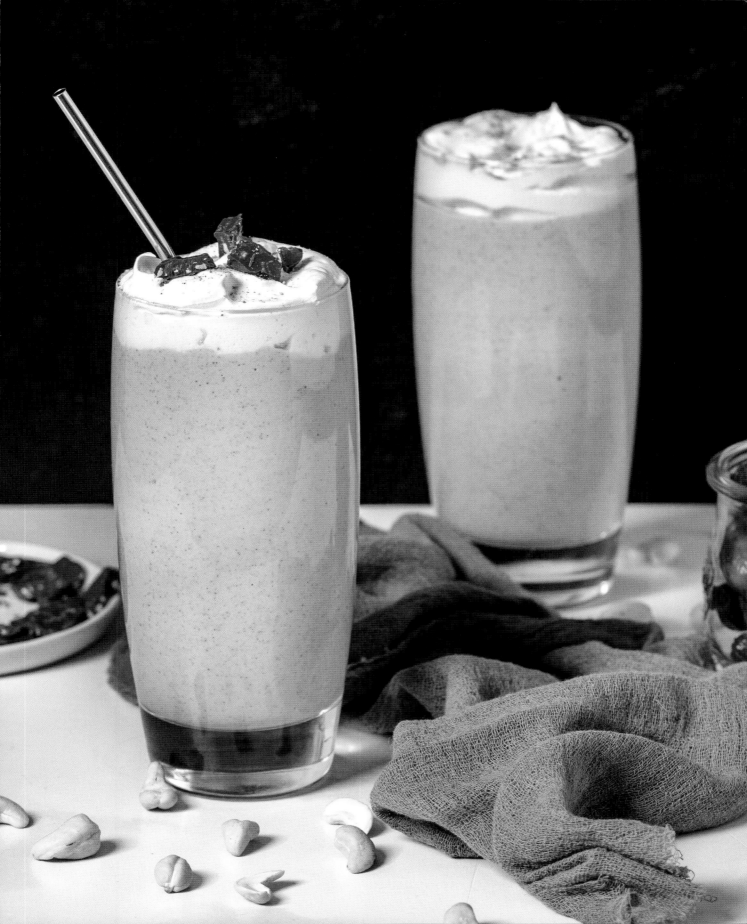

Dairy-Free Strawberry-Peach Crisp YOGURT BOWL

SERVES
2 or 4

PREP TIME
15 minutes

COOK TIME
45 minutes

There's something about a warm crisp of any flavor, but when peaches are in season, they're always what I turn to. While this recipe showcases a "deconstructed" crisp, it is totally fine to make it a more traditional crisp by baking everything together in the same dish. I usually enjoy my crisp with a scoop (or two) of my favorite dairy-free ice cream; however, you'll be eating this crisp over creamy coconut yogurt. This recipe is the perfect excuse to eat a crisp for breakfast. I love combining peaches and strawberries because they complement each other's sweet and tart flavors. This yogurt bowl is a new way of enjoying yogurt, and I make it at least once per week, changing up the fruit through the seasons.

STRAWBERRY-PEACH COMPOTE:

½ cup canned coconut cream or full-fat coconut milk

3 tablespoons pure maple syrup

2 cups sliced strawberries (fresh or frozen)

2 medium peaches, peeled and sliced

1 teaspoon ground cinnamon

½ teaspoon ground nutmeg

¼ teaspoon ginger powder

CRISP TOPPING:

1½ cups rolled oats (gluten-free)

¼ cup all-purpose flour

¼ cup lightly packed brown sugar

3 tablespoons vegan butter, room temperature, plus more for the pan

YOGURT:

2 cups unsweetened vanilla-flavored coconut yogurt

2 tablespoons agave syrup

1 tablespoon freshly squeezed lemon juice

TOPPINGS (OPTIONAL):

Chopped pecans, toasted (see note, page 107)

Fresh mint leaves

MAKE THE STRAWBERRY-PEACH COMPOTE AND CRISP TOPPING:

1. Have one oven rack in the middle position and another rack in the bottom position. Preheat the oven to 350°F. Lightly grease a 10-inch ovenproof skillet with butter, then line a sheet pan with parchment paper.

2. Combine the ingredients for the compote in a large bowl and stir using a rubber spatula until the fruit is well coated.

3. Put the ingredients for the crisp in a medium-size bowl and stir with a fork until the mixture looks crumbly.

4. Spoon the fruit mixture into the prepared skillet, then spread it out evenly. Spread the crisp topping in the prepared sheet pan.

5. Bake both the fruit and oats mixture for 40 to 45 minutes, or until the fruit has become bubbly and the oats mixture is golden brown. Once done, remove both from the oven and let them cool slightly, 5 to 10 minutes.

MAKE THE YOGURT BOWL:

6. In a medium-size bowl, stir together the yogurt, agave, and lemon juice until creamy and smooth.

7. To serve, divide the yogurt between two or four bowls, then top with the strawberry-peach crisp and, if desired, toasted pecans and mint leaves.

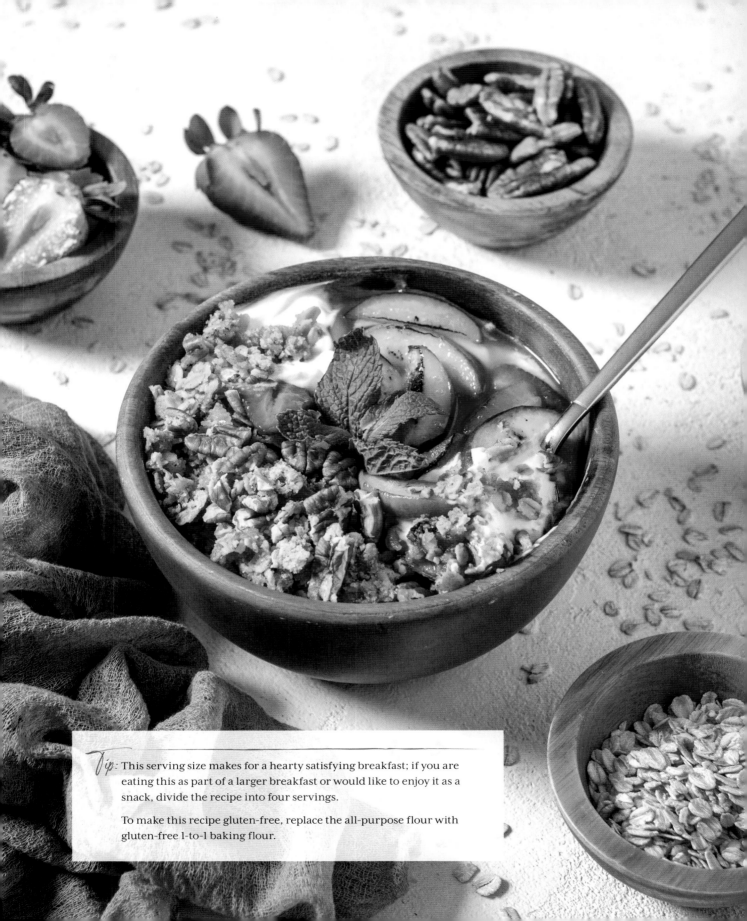

Tip: This serving size makes for a hearty satisfying breakfast; if you are eating this as part of a larger breakfast or would like to enjoy it as a snack, divide the recipe into four servings.

To make this recipe gluten-free, replace the all-purpose flour with gluten-free 1-to-1 baking flour.

Meatless
BREAKFAST TACOS

SERVES
3

PREP TIME
15 minutes

COOK TIME
15 minutes

Whether you're in search of a new breakfast recipe to fit the theme of Meatless Mondays, Taco Tuesdays, or any other day, these tacos will do the trick! I enjoy making meatless tacos for my family because regardless of diet, the "meatiness" of these tacos leaves everyone satisfied, without missing meat at all. Plus, this recipe is so easy to make and can easily be personalized by substituting red beans, kidney beans, chickpeas, lentils, or other great options for the black beans. And while I always opt to scramble my egg, you can top your taco with a fried egg if you prefer. Topped with your favorite taco garnishes and served with lime wedges, these tacos are a hearty and flavorful meat-free morning meal!

BLACK BEANS:

1 tablespoon extra-virgin olive oil

1 (15-ounce) can black beans, drained and rinsed

1 teaspoon garlic powder

1 teaspoon ground cumin

1 teaspoon onion powder

1 teaspoon smoked paprika

½ teaspoon ground black pepper

⅛ teaspoon red pepper flakes

½ teaspoon finely ground sea salt

SCRAMBLED EGGS:

8 large eggs

1 tablespoon unsweetened almond milk

½ teaspoon finely ground sea salt

½ teaspoon ground black pepper

1 tablespoon unsalted butter, for the pan

FOR SERVING/GARNISH:

2 cups guacamole, homemade (page 62) or store-bought

6 (5-inch) flour tortillas, charred or toasted (see note, opposite)

2 jalapeño peppers, seeded and sliced into half-moons or finely diced

Condiment or sauce of choice (optional)

Finely chopped fresh cilantro (optional)

Lime wedges (optional)

1. Make the black beans: Heat the olive oil in a 10-inch skillet over medium-high heat. Once hot, add the black beans, spices, and salt, mixing everything together. Cook the beans until they begin to soften and are heated through, 8 to 10 minutes. Remove the pan from the heat and set aside to let the beans cool slightly.

2. Scramble the eggs: In a medium-size bowl, whisk the eggs with the almond milk, salt, and pepper until light in color and well combined. Melt the butter in a large skillet over medium-high heat. Pour in the egg mixture and scramble the eggs with a fork until they are softly cooked and no longer wet, 4 to 5 minutes. Remove the pan from the heat and set aside.

3. To assemble and serve, spread 1 tablespoon of the guacamole in the center of a tortilla, followed by 2 tablespoons of the black beans, 1 to 2 tablespoons of the scrambled eggs, and some jalapeño slices.

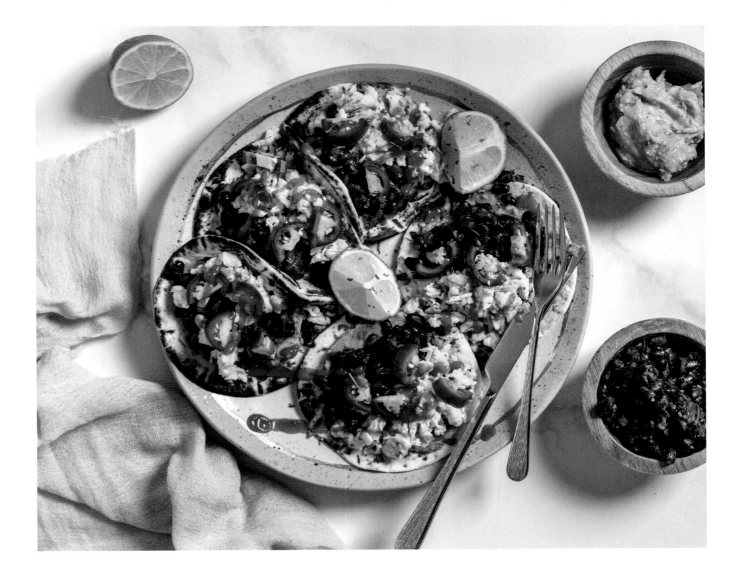

If desired, top with your favorite condiment or sauce and fresh cilantro, and serve with lime wedges. Repeat until all the tortillas and taco fillings and toppings have been used.

HOW TO CHAR OR TOAST TORTILLAS:

To char tortillas, using a tong, hold a tortilla directly over a gas flame on the stovetop until you begin to see a little smoke. Quickly move the tortilla around and flip it over until it becomes darkened and charred on both sides. Repeat until all the tortillas are charred. To toast tortillas, preheat the oven to 425°F and place the tortillas directly on the oven rack. Turn off the oven immediately and let the tortillas warm through for 2 to 3 minutes. You want to lightly toast them; otherwise, you risk making them dry and brittle. You can also toast tortillas in a medium-size skillet over high heat, although, for best results, I prefer using one of the first two methods.

Kam's Superfood
BREAKFAST COOKIES

MAKES
1 dozen

PREP TIME
15 minutes

COOK TIME
18 minutes

These breakfast cookies are ultra-crispy and chewy, yet soft in the middle. In case you were wondering, they are named after my son, Kameron (Kam for short), who absolutely loves cookies and anything with chocolate chips. As a parent, one of my biggest challenges is to ensure that I keep foods interesting enough for him while packing in the nutrients he needs to grow and develop. That's one of the reasons why I love these cookies—they do both! They are a healthy, satisfying, and energizing option for a grab-and-go breakfast for the entire family. I use gluten-free oats, superfood ingredients like chia seeds and flaxseed meal, and banana, peanut butter, chocolate chips, cranberries, pumpkin seeds, and maple syrup as the natural sweetener. These cookies are super easy to make and can be enjoyed for breakfast, as a snack, or for dessert!

2 cups rolled oats (gluten-free)

½ cup dried cranberries

½ cup vegan semi-sweet chocolate chips

¼ cup raw pumpkin seeds

1 tablespoon chia seeds

1 teaspoon ground cinnamon

½ teaspoon finely ground sea salt

1 cup natural peanut butter, softened

1 ripe banana, mashed

2 Flaxseed Eggs (page 38) or Chia Eggs (page 39)

1 teaspoon vanilla extract

¼ cup pure maple syrup, plus more if needed

1. Preheat the oven to 350°F. Line a baking sheet with parchment paper. (*Note:* If your baking sheet is nonstick, you can skip this step.)

2. Put the oats, cranberries, chocolate chips, pumpkin seeds, chia seeds, cinnamon, and salt in a large bowl and mix until combined. Add the peanut butter, mashed banana, flaxseed eggs, vanilla, and maple syrup and stir with a rubber spatula until well combined and the dough is sticky enough to hold together. Add more maple syrup if the dough isn't sticky enough, about 1 tablespoon at a time.

3. Scoop ¼-cup amounts of the dough onto the prepared baking sheet.

4. Bake the cookies for 15 to 18 minutes, or until golden brown around the edges. Remove the pan from the oven, then lightly press down on the cookies using the bottom of a cup to flatten them a bit.

5. Allow the cookies to cool completely on the pan before serving. Store leftover cookies in an airtight container at room temperature for up to 5 days or in the refrigerator for up to 10 days.

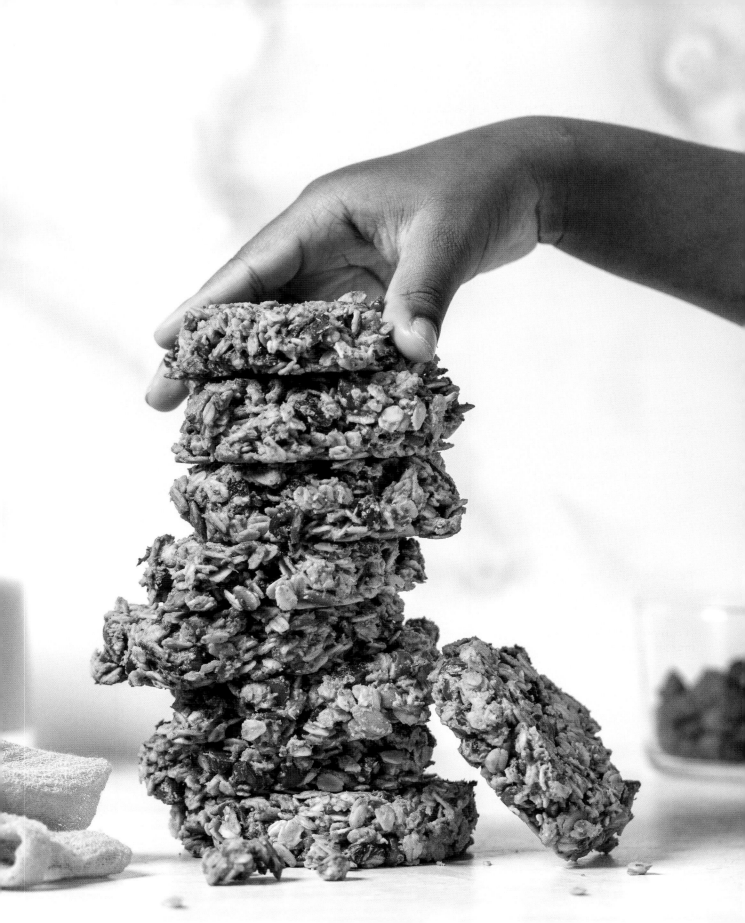

Creamy Cornmeal
PORRIDGE

SERVES
4

PREP TIME
5 minutes

COOK TIME
20 minutes

This creamy cornmeal porridge is a healthier take on the delicious Jamaican cornmeal porridge that I grew up eating. In Jamaican culture, porridge of all kinds (banana, oatmeal, plantain, hominy, etc.) is a breakfast staple whenever you aren't enjoying more savory dishes such as ackee with saltfish, or liver or kidney, both of which are usually served with dumplings and cooked green bananas. Made with sweetened condensed milk, this porridge is boldly sweet and beautifully textured—somewhere between smooth and grainy. To keep things healthier, I top this porridge with fresh berries and toasted pecans, which together create quite the experience in just one bite.

2 cups unsweetened almond milk

2 cups water

1 cup medium-grind yellow cornmeal

1 (14-ounce) can sweetened condensed milk

1 tablespoon lightly packed brown sugar

1 teaspoon vanilla extract

1 teaspoon ground cinnamon

½ teaspoon ground nutmeg

Pinch of ground allspice

Pinch of finely ground sea salt

TOPPINGS (OPTIONAL):

Chopped pecans, toasted (see note, page 107)

Fresh berries of choice

1. Bring the almond milk and water to a boil in a medium-size cocotte or other heavy pot over medium-high heat.

2. While continuously whisking, slowly pour in the cornmeal. Continue whisking until the cornmeal is well incorporated and the mixture is lump-free.

3. Reduce the heat to low, cover the pot, and allow the cornmeal to simmer until thickened and softened, whisking occasionally. This should take about 15 minutes.

4. Remove the lid and whisk in the condensed milk, brown sugar, vanilla extract, spices, and salt until all the ingredients are fully incorporated and the porridge becomes creamy.

5. Remove the pan from the heat and immediately divide the porridge among four bowls. Top with toasted pecans and fresh berries, if desired.

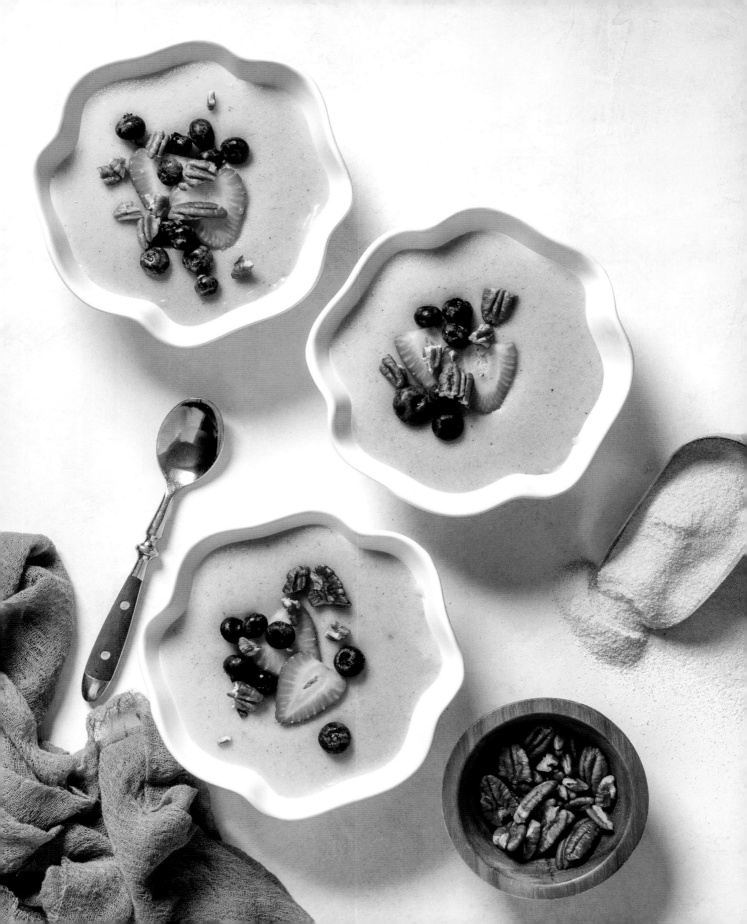

Jamaican-Inspired BANANA OATMEAL PORRIDGE

SERVES
2

PREP TIME
5 minutes

COOK TIME
13 minutes

Oatmeal gives any day a warm and cozy feeling, regardless of the season. This banana oatmeal porridge is no exception. It's one of my favorite versions—I've even gotten my five-year-old son to love it! Traditionally, Jamaican banana porridge is made with a base of green bananas. However, I've never been a fan of green bananas, so I chose to create this spin on the classic Jamaican breakfast. In this recipe, mashed ripe bananas provide a wonderful creamy texture and the perfect amount of sweetness, complemented by the rich flavor of brown sugar. This porridge will keep you filled throughout the morning and can easily be topped with banana slices in addition to your favorite nuts (I like walnuts, but anything goes). When you use certified gluten-free rolled oats, you have a perfect gluten-free breakfast.

1 cup rolled oats (gluten-free)

3 cups unsweetened almond milk

2 teaspoons ground cinnamon

1 teaspoon ground nutmeg

Pinch of finely ground sea salt

2 ripe bananas, mashed

¼ cup lightly packed brown sugar

1 teaspoon vanilla extract

TOPPINGS (OPTIONAL):

Chopped walnuts or other nuts of choice

Sliced bananas

Ground cinnamon

1. Place the oats, milk, cinnamon, nutmeg, and salt in a medium-size saucepan and stir to combine. Bring the mixture to a boil over medium-high heat.

2. Reduce the heat to a simmer and cook, stirring regularly, until the porridge has thickened enough to coat the back of a spoon, about 10 minutes.

3. Add the mashed bananas, brown sugar, and vanilla and stir until well combined and the sugar has fully dissolved, another 2 to 3 minutes.

4. To serve, scoop the oatmeal into two bowls. If desired, top with chopped nuts, sliced bananas, and a sprinkle of cinnamon.

VARIATION: Overnight Jamaican-Inspired Banana Oatmeal Porridge. Put all the ingredients for the porridge in a medium-size bowl and mix until fully combined. With this option, I recommend using a syrup such as agave or maple instead of sugar. Cover the bowl and place in the refrigerator overnight (or for at least 8 hours). To serve cold, divide the porridge between two bowls or jars and top with walnuts, banana slices, and cinnamon, if desired. To heat the porridge before serving, put the porridge in a medium-size saucepan over medium-high heat and cook until warmed through, 5 to 6 minutes. Once ready, divide the porridge between two bowls or jars and add the toppings.

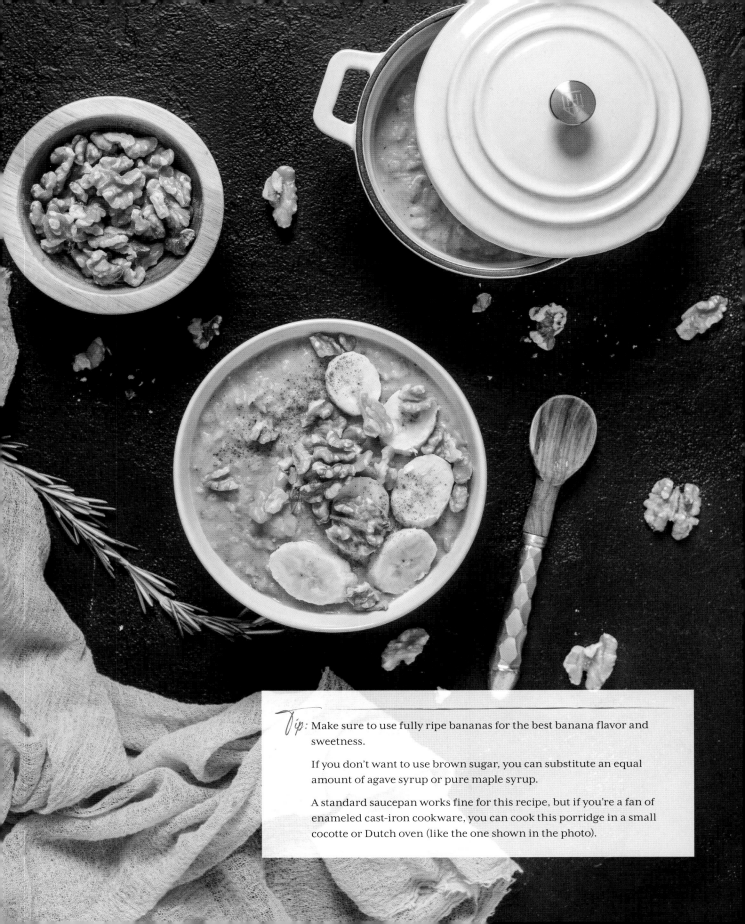

Tip: Make sure to use fully ripe bananas for the best banana flavor and sweetness.

If you don't want to use brown sugar, you can substitute an equal amount of agave syrup or pure maple syrup.

A standard saucepan works fine for this recipe, but if you're a fan of enameled cast-iron cookware, you can cook this porridge in a small cocotte or Dutch oven (like the one shown in the photo).

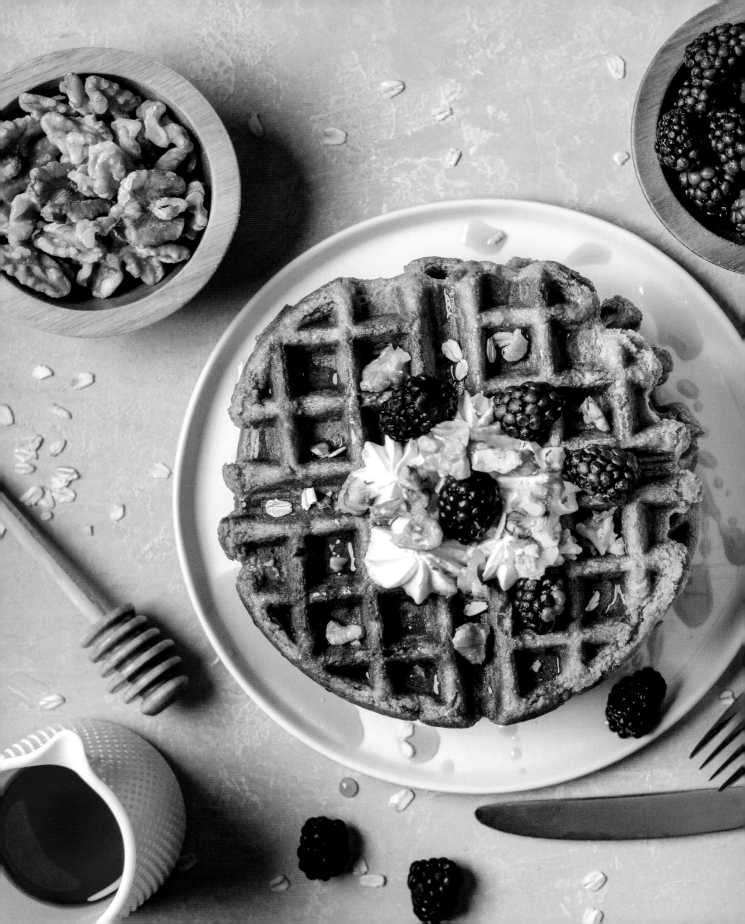

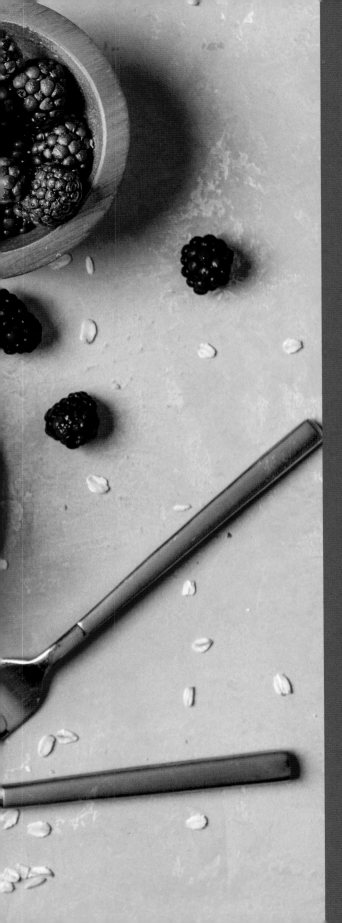

Chapter 5:

BRUNCH GOODNESS

Lemon Raspberry POPPY SEED PANCAKES

SERVES
2

PREP TIME
5 minutes

COOK TIME
4 to 12 minutes
(depending on
size of pan used)

Starting my day with pancakes always makes me feel like the day is bound to be entirely good—almost like a special occasion. While many of my weekday breakfasts consist of an easy bagel, toast, oats, or something of that nature, I'm always happiest when I take the time to make pancakes. These pancakes in particular are perfect for a lazy springtime or summertime brunch. Lemon and poppy seeds is such a great combination, and with the added tartness from the raspberries, you're guaranteed to love this stack!

2 cups all-purpose flour

1½ teaspoons baking powder

½ teaspoon baking soda

½ teaspoon finely ground sea salt

1 tablespoon grated lemon zest

1½ cups unsweetened almond milk

¼ cup plain Greek yogurt (full-fat)

2 tablespoons unsalted butter, melted, plus more for cooking

2 tablespoons freshly squeezed lemon juice

2 large eggs, beaten

3 tablespoons pure maple syrup, plus more for topping if desired

1 cup fresh raspberries, plus more for topping if desired

1½ tablespoons poppy seeds, plus more for topping if desired

TOPPINGS (OPTIONAL):

Whipped cream

Lemon wedges

Fresh rosemary sprigs

1. In a large bowl, whisk together the flour, baking powder, baking soda, salt, and lemon zest.

2. Add the almond milk, yogurt, melted butter, lemon juice, beaten eggs, and maple syrup and stir with a rubber spatula until well combined and thickened. Do not overmix. Fold in the raspberries and poppy seeds until evenly incorporated.

3. Preheat a griddle or a large skillet over medium-high heat, then lightly coat with butter. When hot, scoop ½ cup of the batter onto the griddle (or into the skillet). Repeat, making as many pancakes as you can comfortably fit at once on the griddle (or in the skillet) without crowding them; if using a skillet, I don't recommend cooking more than two at once.

4. Cook the pancakes until the tops begin to bubble, about 2 minutes, then carefully flip over each pancake. Gently press down on the pancakes to ensure that the centers cook through fully and cook for another 1 to 2 minutes, or until golden brown on the undersides.

5. Repeat Steps 3 and 4 with any remaining batter, regreasing the griddle (or skillet) with additional butter after each batch. You should have a total of 6 pancakes.

6. To serve, divide the pancakes between two plates. If desired, top with whipped cream, lemon slices, fresh raspberries, a sprinkle of poppy seeds, rosemary sprigs, and a light drizzle of maple syrup.

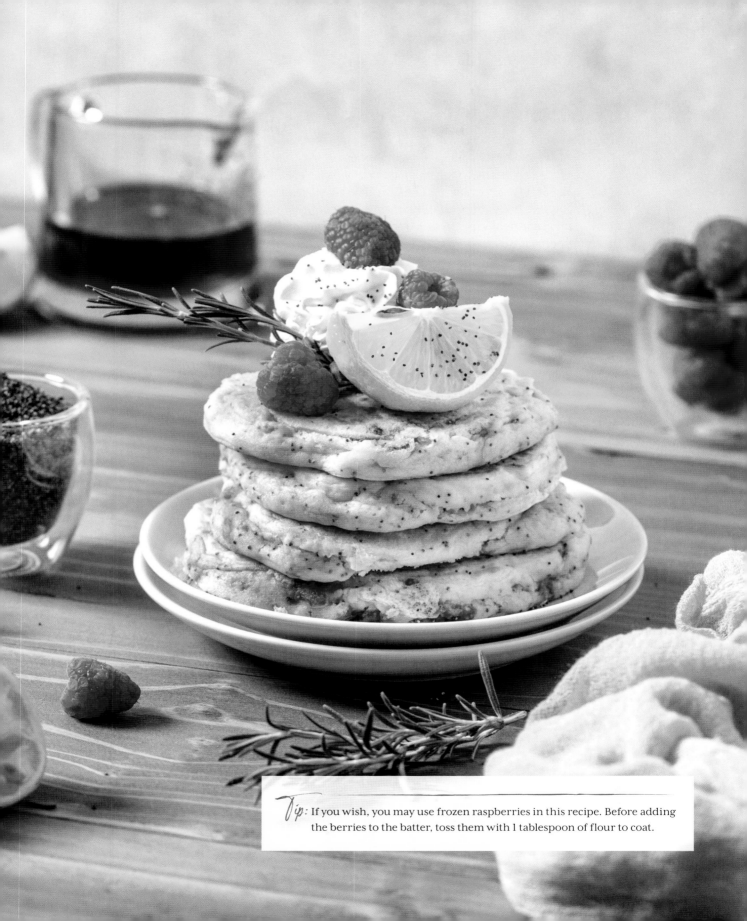

Tip: If you wish, you may use frozen raspberries in this recipe. Before adding the berries to the batter, toss them with 1 tablespoon of flour to coat.

Vegan Peanut Butter
CHOCOLATE CHIP PANCAKES

SERVES
2

PREP TIME
10 minutes

COOK TIME
4 to 12 minutes
(depending on
size of pan used)

Are you staring at these pancakes and jumping for joy on the inside? I know, I have been there too. These pancakes are the epitome of a childhood love affair gone right! They come packaged with two of my favorite things—chocolate chips and peanut butter. Yes, I was the girl who loved all things peanut butter plus chocolate, like Butterfinger, Nutty Buddy, peanut butter chocolate chip cookies, you name it. So, if I'm honest, this flavor marriage is special to me. The best things about these pancakes are that they are dairy-free and a family treat. If you have a peanut allergy, they are just as enjoyable made with peanut butter alternatives like almond butter, cashew butter, sunflower seed butter, tahini, or soy nut butter; if you have a nut allergy, swap out the almond milk for a nut-free, dairy-free milk such as coconut milk, rice milk, or oat milk.

1 cup all-purpose flour

1 tablespoon baking powder

½ teaspoon ground cinnamon

¼ teaspoon finely ground sea salt

1 cup Vegan Buttermilk (page 36)

½ cup creamy natural peanut butter, softened

2 tablespoons vegan butter, melted

1 teaspoon vanilla extract

3 tablespoons pure maple syrup, plus more for topping if desired

1 cup vegan semi-sweet chocolate chips, plus more for topping if desired

Coconut oil, for the pan

Coconut whipped cream, for topping (optional)

1. In a large bowl, whisk together the flour, baking powder, cinnamon, and salt. Set aside.

2. In a medium-size bowl, whisk together the buttermilk, peanut butter, and butter until the mixture thickens. Add the vanilla extract and maple syrup and whisk until just combined.

3. Add the wet ingredients to the dry ingredients and stir with a rubber spatula until just combined. Do not overmix. The batter will be quite thick but still pourable. Fold in the chocolate chips until evenly incorporated.

4. Preheat a griddle or a large skillet over medium-high heat, then lightly coat with oil. When hot, scoop ½ cup of the batter onto the griddle (or into the skillet). Repeat, making as many pancakes at once as you can comfortably fit on the griddle (or in the skillet) without crowding them; if using a skillet, I don't recommend cooking more than two at once.

5. Cook the pancakes until the tops begin to bubble, about 2 minutes, then carefully flip over each pancake. Gently press down on the pancakes to ensure that the centers cook through fully and cook for another 1 to 2 minutes, or until golden brown on the undersides.

6. Repeat Steps 4 and 5 with any remaining batter, regreasing the griddle (or skillet) with additional oil after each batch. You should have a total of 6 pancakes.

7. To serve, divide the pancakes between two plates. If desired, top with coconut whipped cream, extra chocolate chips, and a light drizzle of maple syrup.

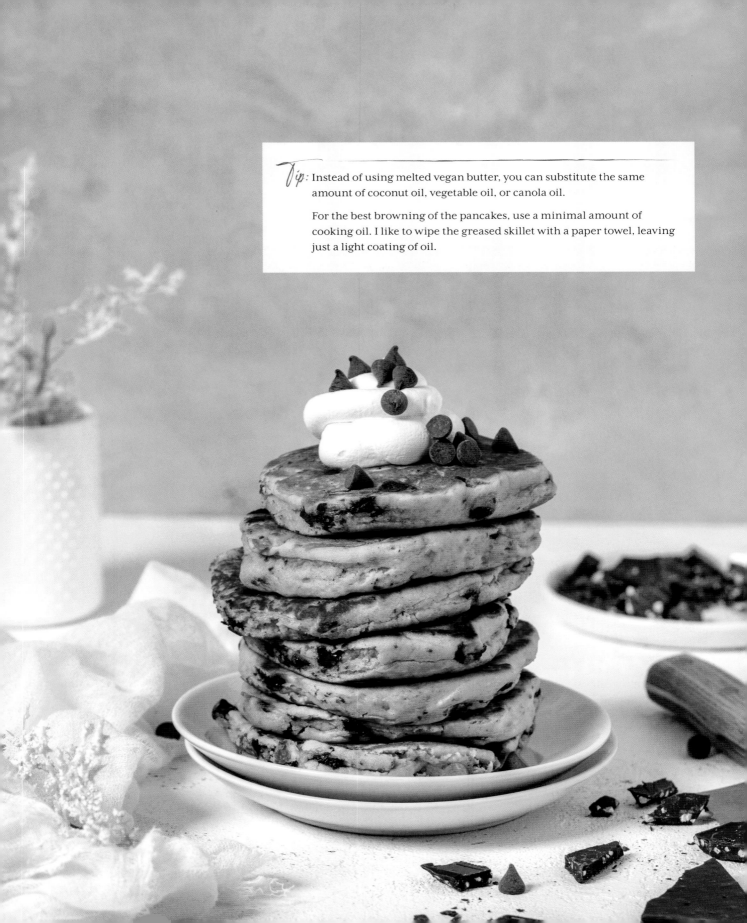

Tip: Instead of using melted vegan butter, you can substitute the same amount of coconut oil, vegetable oil, or canola oil.

For the best browning of the pancakes, use a minimal amount of cooking oil. I like to wipe the greased skillet with a paper towel, leaving just a light coating of oil.

Vegan Blueberry
WHOLE-WHEAT PANCAKES

SERVES
2

PREP TIME
10 minutes

COOK TIME
4 to 12 minutes
(depending on
size of pan used)

When late spring/early summer comes around, I get excited about making all things berry—whether it's blueberries, raspberries, or strawberries. These blueberry pancakes are absolute comfort and fluffiness on a plate and are the best way to kick-start your morning! While I don't often use whole-wheat flour, I enjoy combining it with blueberries to create these deliciously thick pancakes. Plus, I love making most of my pancakes vegan for a nice break from dairy. Instead of using melted vegan butter in the batter, you can substitute the same amount of coconut oil, avocado oil, or grapeseed oil.

1 cup whole-wheat flour

½ cup rolled oats (gluten-free)

2 teaspoons baking powder

1 teaspoon ground cinnamon

½ teaspoon ground nutmeg

¼ teaspoon finely ground sea salt

1 cup Vegan Buttermilk (page 36)

2 tablespoons vegan butter,
melted, plus more for cooking

1 teaspoon vanilla extract

3 tablespoons agave syrup

1 cup fresh blueberries, plus
more for topping if desired

TOPPINGS (OPTIONAL):

Chopped walnuts

Fresh mint leaves

Pure maple syrup

1. In a large bowl, whisk together the flour, oats, baking powder, cinnamon, nutmeg, and salt. Set aside.

2. In a medium-size bowl, whisk together the buttermilk and butter until well combined and the mixture thickens. Add the vanilla extract and agave and whisk until just combined.

3. Add the wet ingredients to the dry ingredients and stir using a rubber spatula until just combined. Do not overmix. The batter will be quite thick but still pourable. Fold in the blueberries until evenly incorporated.

4. Preheat a griddle or a large skillet over medium-high heat, then lightly coat the pan with vegan butter. When hot, scoop ½ cup of the batter onto the griddle (or into the skillet). Repeat, making as many pancakes at once as you can comfortably fit on the griddle (or in the skillet) without crowding them; if using a skillet, I don't recommend cooking more than two at once.

5. Cook the pancakes until the tops begin to bubble, about 2 minutes, then carefully flip over each pancake. Gently press down on the pancakes to ensure that the centers cook through fully and cook for another 1 to 2 minutes, or until golden brown on the undersides.

6. Repeat Steps 4 and 5 with any remaining batter, regreasing the griddle (or skillet) with additional butter after each batch. You should have a total of 6 pancakes.

7. To serve, divide the pancakes between two plates. If desired, top with fresh blueberries, chopped walnuts, mint leaves, and a light drizzle of maple syrup.

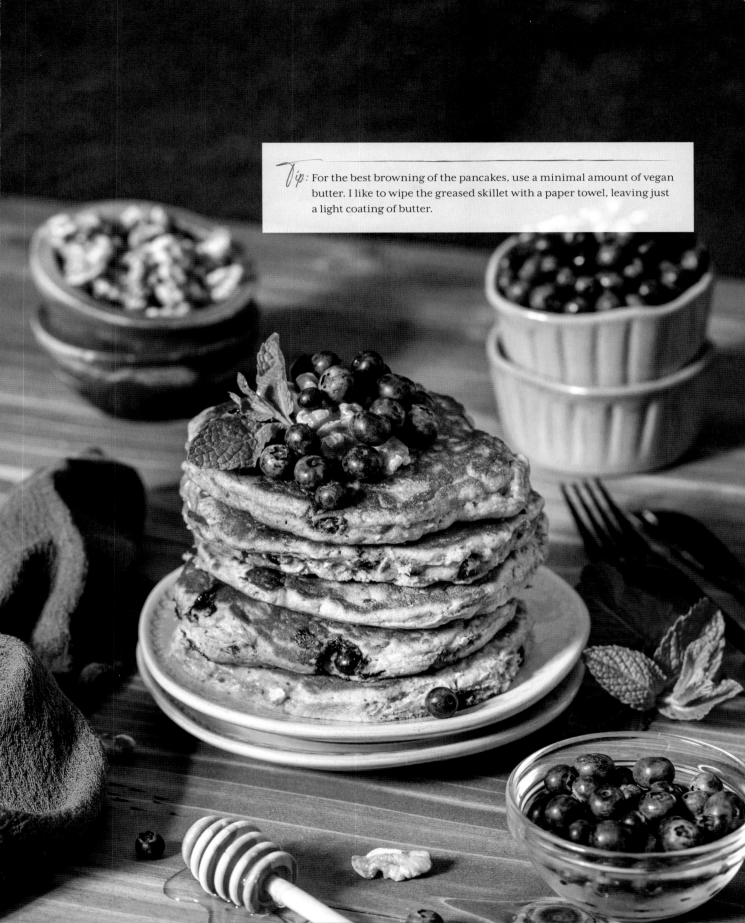

Easy Dairy-Free
PECAN PANCAKES

SERVES
2

PREP TIME
5 minutes

COOK TIME
4 to 12 minutes
(depending on
size of pan used)

These pancakes pay homage to my Southern roots. Pecans are a staple in the South, and I've thoroughly enjoyed them in everything from cheesecakes and breads to waffles, cakes, pies, and so much more. But wait until you add pecans to your pancakes—they become out-of-this-world good! When I was growing up, pancakes were called flapjacks, and while I didn't experiment much with the flavors, I ate them religiously, especially on the weekends. This dairy-free recipe will help you keep things interesting when it comes to pancakes, and it's a nice play on soft and crunchy textures.

2 cups all-purpose flour

1½ teaspoons baking powder

1 tablespoon ground cinnamon

1 teaspoon ground nutmeg

½ teaspoon ginger powder

¼ teaspoon ground allspice

½ teaspoon finely ground sea salt

1½ cups unsweetened almond milk

2 tablespoons vegan butter, melted, plus more for cooking

1 teaspoon vanilla extract

3 tablespoons pure maple syrup, plus more for topping if desired

2 large eggs, beaten

1 cup chopped pecans, toasted (see note, opposite), plus more for topping if desired

Sliced strawberries, for topping (optional)

1. In a large bowl, whisk together the flour, baking powder, cinnamon, nutmeg, ginger, allspice, and salt until combined.

2. Add the almond milk, butter, vanilla extract, maple syrup, and beaten eggs, mixing everything together until combined and you have a mostly smooth batter. Do not overmix. The batter will be quite thick but still pourable. Fold in the toasted pecans until evenly incorporated.

3. Preheat a griddle or a large skillet over medium-high heat, then lightly coat with oil.

4. When hot, scoop ½ cup of the batter onto the griddle (or into the skillet). Repeat, making as many pancakes at once as you can comfortably fit on the griddle (or in the skillet) without crowding them; if using a skillet, I don't recommend cooking more than two at once.

5. Cook the pancakes until the tops begin to bubble, about 2 minutes, then carefully flip over each pancake. Gently press down on the pancakes to ensure that the centers cook through fully and cook for another 1 to 2 minutes, or until golden brown on the undersides.

6. Repeat Steps 4 and 5 with any remaining batter, regreasing the griddle (or skillet) with additional butter after each batch. You should have a total of 6 pancakes.

7. To serve, divide the pancakes between two plates. If desired, top with toasted chopped pecans, strawberry slices, and a light drizzle of maple syrup.

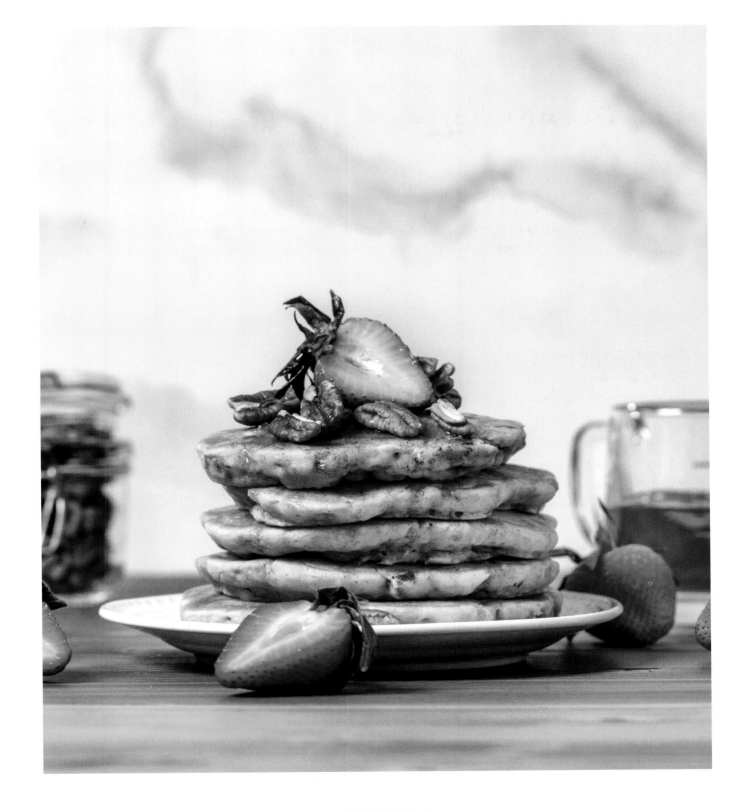

HOW TO TOAST PECANS:

Put the chopped pecans on a sheet pan lined with parchment paper and bake them in a preheated 400°F oven for 10 to 15 minutes, until toasty brown, tossing them halfway through so that the nuts brown evenly on both sides.

Vegan Sweet Potato
PANCAKES

SERVES
2

PREP TIME
10 minutes

COOK TIME
4 to 12 minutes
(depending on
size of pan used)

Sweet potatoes are another beloved Southern staple; therefore, sweet potato pancakes were a given when it came to creating the recipes for this book. Vegan pancakes are one of my favorite things to make for breakfast when I am looking for something comforting and easy to prepare. The sweet potato puree used in this recipe can be stored in the refrigerator for easy additions to other foods, like bread, waffles, tacos, pasta sauce, and burgers.

2 cups all-purpose flour

2 teaspoons baking powder

1 tablespoon ground cinnamon

1 teaspoon ground nutmeg

½ teaspoon ground allspice

¼ teaspoon finely ground sea salt

2 cups Vegan Buttermilk (page 36)

1 cup Simple Sweet Potato Puree
(page 56)

2 tablespoons vegan butter,
melted, plus more for cooking

1 teaspoon vanilla extract

3 tablespoons pure maple syrup,
plus more for topping if desired

TOPPINGS (OPTIONAL):

Fresh blackberries

Chopped pecans, toasted (see
note, page 107)

1. In a large bowl, whisk together the flour, baking powder, spices, and salt. Set aside.

2. In a medium-size bowl, whisk together the buttermilk, sweet potato puree, and butter until well combined and the mixture thickens. Add the vanilla extract and maple syrup and whisk until just combined.

3. Add the wet ingredients to the dry ingredients and stir using a rubber spatula until just combined. Do not overmix.

4. Preheat a griddle or a large skillet over medium-high heat, then lightly coat the pan with vegan butter.

5. When hot, scoop ½ cup of the batter onto the griddle (or into the skillet). Repeat, making as many pancakes as you can comfortably fit on the griddle (or in the skillet) without crowding them; if using a skillet, I don't recommend cooking more than two at once.

6. Cook the pancakes until the tops begin to bubble, about 2 minutes, then carefully flip the pancakes over. Gently press down on the pancakes to ensure that the centers cook through fully and cook for another 1 to 2 minutes, or until golden brown on the undersides.

7. Repeat Steps 5 and 6 with any remaining batter, regreasing the griddle (or skillet) with additional butter after each batch. You should have a total of 6 pancakes.

8. To serve, divide the pancakes between two plates. If desired, top with fresh blackberries, chopped pecans, and a light drizzle of maple syrup.

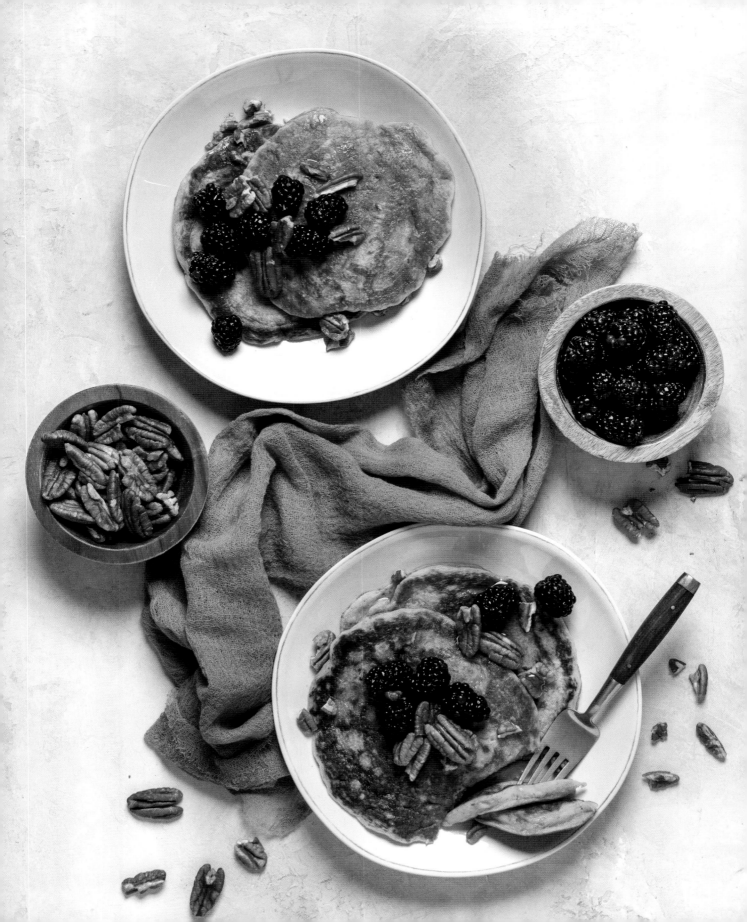

Banana Oat
FLOURLESS BLENDER WAFFLES

MAKES
6 waffles

PREP TIME
5 minutes

COOK TIME
20 minutes

Because I'm a Southern girl at heart, a satisfying breakfast for me consists of either waffles, pancakes, French toast, or grits. Granted, I find myself eating a lot of easy grab-and-go breakfast items such as pastries or bagels; however, if you know me, then you know that they aren't my favorite. While my favorites include all the "loadedness" (yes, I made up this word) that one can think of, like flour and cheese, my newest favorite type of waffle is these flourless ones. The best thing about them is that they are super filling and include a ton of nutrients, especially from the oats. I make these waffles at least once a month because they're a big hit in my house. Who wouldn't want to make their waffle batter in a blender, anyway—right?

WET INGREDIENTS:

2 medium bananas, mashed

1½ cups Vegan Buttermilk (page 46)

3 tablespoons agave syrup

2 tablespoons natural almond butter

2 teaspoons vanilla extract

DRY INGREDIENTS:

4 cups rolled oats (gluten-free)

2 teaspoons baking powder

1 teaspoon baking soda

2 tablespoons ground cinnamon

1 teaspoon ground nutmeg

Pinch of ground allspice

½ teaspoon finely ground sea salt

TOPPINGS (OPTIONAL):

Coconut whipped cream

Fresh fruit, such as berries or sliced banana

Chopped nuts of choice, toasted

Pure maple syrup

1. Preheat a waffle iron. (If you have the option to choose the temperature, select medium-high—that's what works perfectly for me!) Preheat the oven to the lowest setting.

2. Put the wet ingredients in a high-powered blender, then add the dry ingredients. *Note:* Putting the ingredients in the blender in this order—starting with wet and ending with dry—allows everything to blend well and become nice and smooth.

3. Blend on high speed until the batter is smooth—15 to 20 seconds will do it.

4. Grease the preheated waffle iron, then spoon about ½ cup of the batter into the center of the iron. Close the lid and cook according to the manufacturer's instructions until golden brown and crisp.

5. Transfer the completed waffle to a baking sheet and place in the oven to keep warm. Repeat until all the batter is used.

6. To serve, stack the waffles (whole or cut) and, if desired, top with coconut whipped cream, fresh fruit, toasted nuts, and/or a drizzle of maple syrup.

Tip: Once cool, leftover waffles can be stored in a tightly sealed zip-top bag in the refrigerator for a few days. To store them for longer periods, simply put them on a baking sheet lined with parchment paper and place in the freezer for 2 hours. Once fully frozen, remove and store them in a tightly sealed zip-top bag in the freezer for up to 3 months.

To reheat, place the frozen waffles on a baking sheet lined with parchment paper and heat in a preheated 400°F oven for 10 to 15 minutes, or until warmed through.

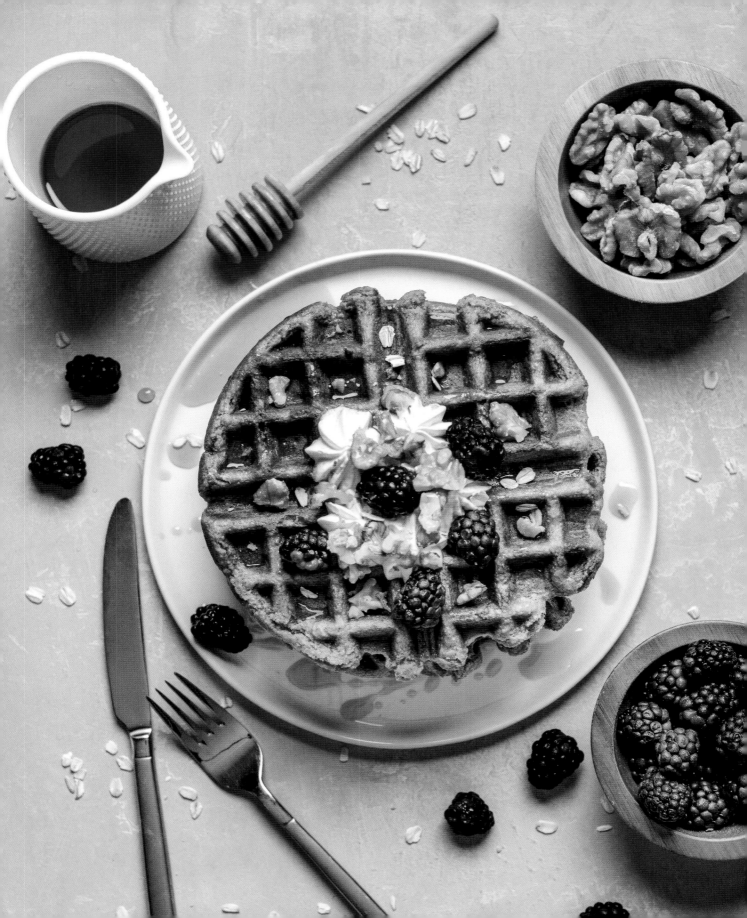

Brown Butter
BLUEBERRY WAFFLES

MAKES
6 waffles

PREP TIME
5 minutes

COOK TIME
20 minutes

Whenever I hear "brown butter," my mouth automatically begins to water. Before it became a trend in the food world, I wasn't even aware that butter in its almost burnt state could taste so good. There have been many times when I've put butter in a very hot skillet to make pancakes or something and it ended up burning, which prompted me to drain the skillet and begin again. Who knew that burnt butter would be the newest rave? Well, it's for good reason, and these waffles are a beautiful balance between nutty and sweet flavors.

¼ cup (½ stick) unsalted butter, plus more for the waffle iron

3 cups all-purpose flour

2 tablespoons baking powder

¼ teaspoon baking soda

1 tablespoon ground cinnamon

1 teaspoon ground nutmeg

¼ teaspoon finely ground sea salt

1 cup plus 1 tablespoon unsweetened almond milk

3 large eggs, beaten

3 tablespoons pure maple syrup

1 tablespoon vanilla extract

1 cup fresh blueberries

TOPPINGS (OPTIONAL):

Whipped cream

Blueberry compote (see note, opposite)

Pure maple syrup

Chopped walnuts

1. Preheat a waffle iron. (If you have the option to choose the temperature, select medium-high—that works perfectly for me!) Preheat the oven to the lowest setting.

2. Make the brown butter: Melt the butter in a medium-size saucepan over medium-high heat, stirring it occasionally and letting it cook until dark bits begin to form and the entire butter becomes fragrant and darker, 3 to 4 minutes. Remove the pan from the heat and set aside to cool for a few minutes.

3. In a large bowl, whisk together the flour, baking powder, baking soda, cinnamon, nutmeg, and salt.

4. Add the almond milk, eggs, maple syrup, vanilla extract, and brown butter to the dry ingredients and stir using a rubber spatula until just combined. Do not overmix. Fold in the blueberries.

5. Grease the preheated waffle iron with butter, then spoon about ½ cup of the batter into the center of the iron. Close the lid and cook according to the manufacturer's instructions until golden brown and crisp.

6. Transfer the completed waffle to a baking sheet and place in the oven to keep warm. Repeat until all the batter is used.

7. To serve, stack the waffles (whole or cut) and, if desired, top with whipped cream, blueberry compote, a drizzle of maple syrup, and/or some chopped walnuts.

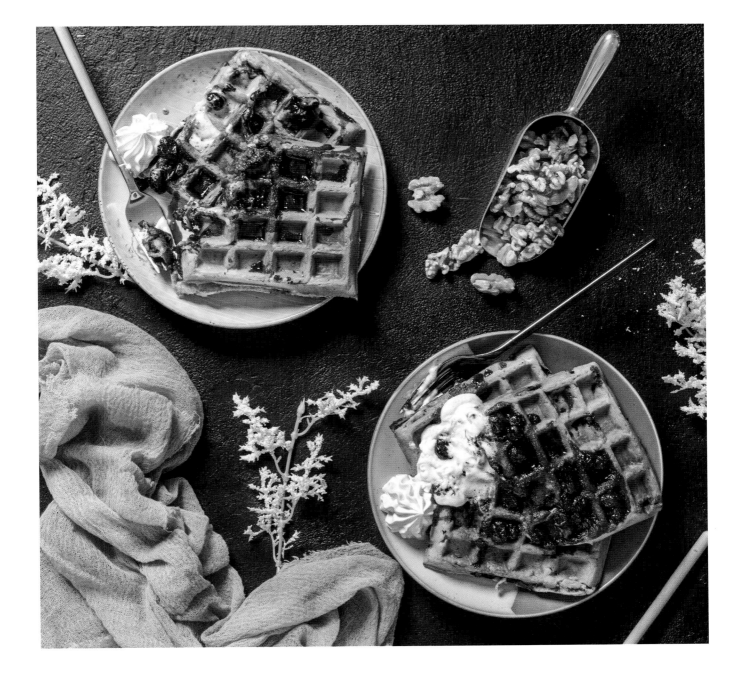

HOW TO MAKE BLUEBERRY COMPOTE:

In a medium-size saucepan over medium-high heat, combine 2 cups of fresh blueberries, ¾ cup of cane sugar, ¼ cup of water, 2 tablespoons of lemon juice, and ½ teaspoon of vanilla extract. Once the mixture comes to a boil, reduce the heat to low and let simmer until the blueberries are soft and begin to burst, about 10 minutes. In a small bowl, stir together ½ teaspoon of arrowroot starch and 2 tablespoons of warm water until it becomes smooth and milky looking. Stir the starch mixture into the blueberry mixture and continue to simmer until the compote begins to thicken slightly. Remove the pan from the heat and let the compote cool for a few minutes before serving. Store any leftover compote in an airtight container or jar in the refrigerator for up to 2 weeks.

Flourless Sweet Potato Waffles &
HOT MAPLE CAULIFLOWER BITES

SERVES
4

PREP TIME
20 minutes

COOK TIME
45 minutes

This dairy-free recipe is a meatless and spicy twist on a Southern classic, chicken and waffles. These flourless sweet potato waffles are the easiest and best-tasting gluten-free waffles that the entire family will love. Made in a blender, the waffles are naturally sweetened, thick yet fluffy and airy, and full of sweet potato and oat flavors that pair perfectly with the "meaty" cauliflower bites. To make this dish entirely gluten-free, see the tip below.

CAULIFLOWER BITES:

1¼ cups water

¾ cup all-purpose flour

1 teaspoon dried parsley

1 teaspoon garlic powder

1 teaspoon smoked paprika

½ teaspoon finely ground sea salt

½ teaspoon ground black pepper

3 cups plain breadcrumbs

1 head cauliflower, chopped into large florets

2 cups pure maple syrup

½ cup Frank's Original hot sauce

1 teaspoon red pepper flakes

1 tablespoon arrowroot starch

3 tablespoons warm water

WAFFLES:

WET INGREDIENTS:

2 cups Simple Sweet Potato Mash (page 56)

1½ cups Vegan Buttermilk (page 46)

3 tablespoons agave syrup

2 tablespoons natural almond butter

2 teaspoons vanilla extract

DRY INGREDIENTS:

4 cups rolled oats (gluten-free)

2 teaspoons baking powder

1 teaspoon baking soda

2 tablespoons ground cinnamon

1 teaspoon ground nutmeg

½ teaspoon finely ground sea salt

Pinch of ground allspice

TOPPINGS (OPTIONAL):

Thinly sliced scallions

Pure maple syrup

MAKE THE CAULIFLOWER BITES:

1. Preheat the oven to 375°F and line a sheet pan with parchment paper.

2. Make the batter: In a large bowl, whisk together the water, flour, parsley, garlic powder, smoked paprika, salt, and black pepper until well combined and the mixture has thickened.

3. Put the breadcrumbs in a medium-size bowl and place it next to the batter.

4. Dip each cauliflower floret into the batter, shaking off any excess, then toss it into the breadcrumbs to coat. Place on the prepared sheet pan. Repeat this step until all the cauliflower florets are breaded.

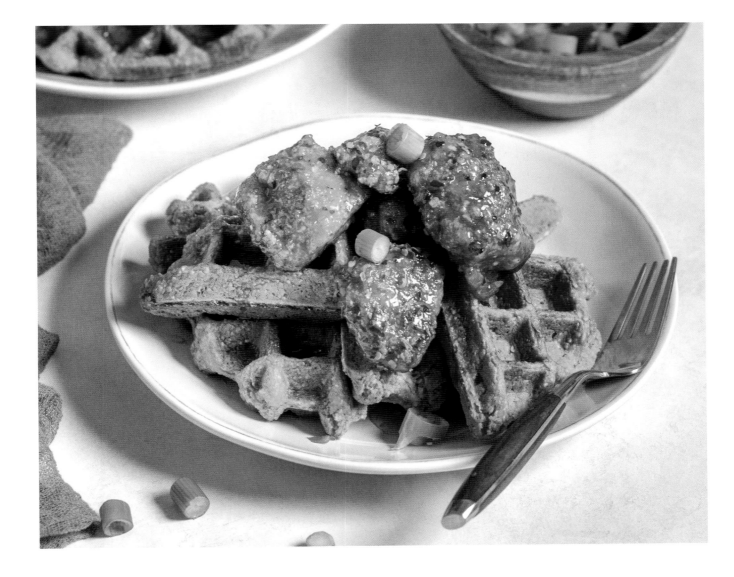

5. Bake the cauliflower bites for 25 to 30 minutes, or until tender and golden brown and crunchy looking.

6. Meanwhile, make the sauce: Put the maple syrup, hot sauce, and red pepper flakes in a medium-size saucepan. Bring to a boil over medium-high heat, whisking continuously. Reduce the heat to low and let it simmer for 2 to 3 minutes. In a small bowl, combine the arrowroot starch and warm water, mixing until the mixture is smooth and milky.

7. Whisk the starch mixture into the sauce until well combined; allow the sauce to simmer for 5 to 6 minutes, or until it becomes thick and sticky.

8. Once the cauliflower bites are crispy, remove them from the oven and let them cool slightly, about 5 minutes. Add the cauliflower bites into the prepared sauce and toss until they are fully coated. Set aside.

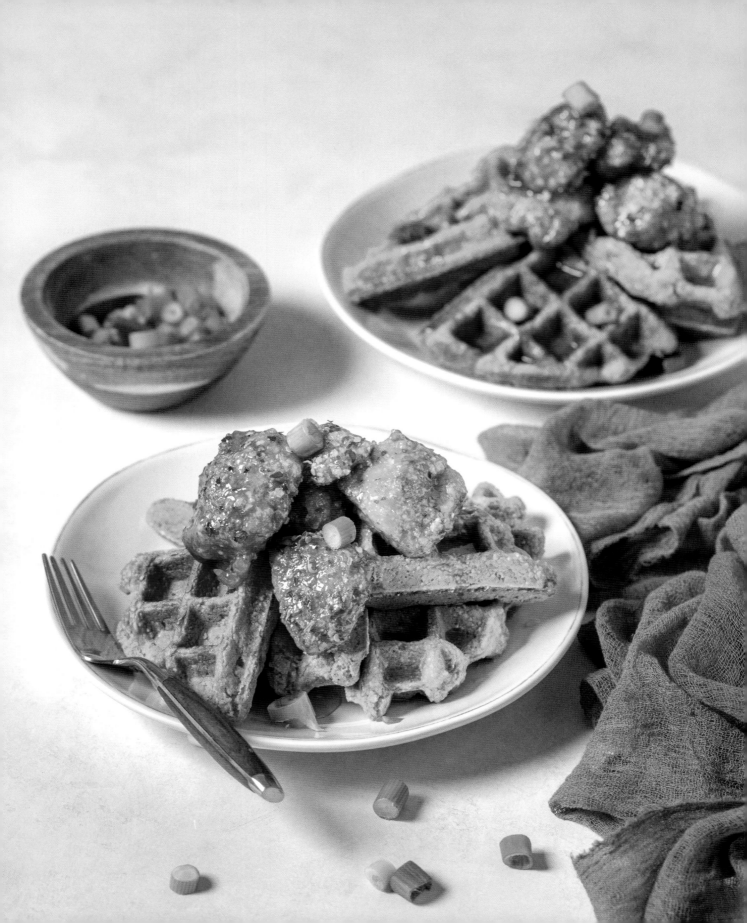

MAKE THE WAFFLES:

1. Preheat a waffle iron. (If you have the option to choose the temperature, select medium-high—that's what works perfectly for me!) Preheat the oven to the lowest setting.

2. Put the wet ingredients in a high-powered blender, then add the dry ingredients. *Note:* Putting the ingredients in the blender in this order—starting with wet and ending with dry—allows everything to blend well and become nice and smooth.

3. Blend on high speed until the batter is smooth—15 to 20 seconds will do it.

4. Grease the preheated waffle iron, then spoon about ½ cup of the batter into the center of the iron. Close the lid and cook according to the manufacturer's instructions until golden brown and crisp.

5. Transfer the completed waffle to a baking sheet and place in the oven to keep warm. Repeat until all the batter is used.

6. To serve, stack the waffles (whole or cut), top with cauliflower bites, and, if desired, top with chopped scallions, and/or a drizzle of maple syrup.

Tip: To make the cauliflower bites gluten-free as well, replace the breadcrumbs with a gluten-free version and replace the all-purpose flour with a gluten-free 1-to-1 baking flour.

Dairy-Free
SPICED BANANA FRENCH TOAST

SERVES
4

PREP TIME
10 minutes

COOK TIME
8 to 24 minutes
(depending on
size of pan used)

If you know me, then you know I love bananas. Growing up, I wasn't the biggest fan of them; however, I've come to love them and honestly would eat anything that includes them. This French toast recipe was inspired by my Jamaican background, and once you take a bite, you're guaranteed to be a fan. In Jamaica, bananas are used in many dishes and come heavily seasoned with warm spices, which is evident in this recipe. This French toast is perfectly thick and fluffy, uses only a handful of ingredients, comes naturally sweetened, and is completely dairy-free. Yum!

CARAMELIZED BANANAS:

2 tablespoons vegan butter

2 ripe bananas, sliced

3 tablespoons pure maple syrup

½ teaspoon vanilla extract

1 teaspoon ground cinnamon

½ teaspoon ground nutmeg

FRENCH TOAST:

1 ripe banana

2½ tablespoons water

1 cup unsweetened almond milk, room temperature

1 teaspoon vanilla extract

2 tablespoons arrowroot starch

1 tablespoon flaxseed meal

1 tablespoon ground cinnamon

½ teaspoon finely ground sea salt

1 loaf challah or vegan brioche bread (about 15 ounces), homemade (page 128) or store-bought

1 tablespoon vegan butter, for cooking

TOPPINGS:

Pure maple syrup

Chopped walnuts (optional)

MAKE THE CARAMELIZED BANANAS:

1. Melt the butter in a medium-size skillet over medium-high heat. Add the sliced bananas and cook until golden brown, 2 to 3 minutes, then turn them and brown the other side, another 2 minutes. Add the maple syrup and vanilla extract, gently stirring them in to ensure that the bananas don't break apart. Season with the spices and let everything bubble for 20 to 30 seconds before removing the pan from the heat. Set the bananas aside.

MAKE THE FRENCH TOAST:

2. Put the banana and water in a high-powered blender and blend until fully broken down and smooth. Transfer the pureed banana to a large bowl.

3. To the banana, add the almond milk, vanilla extract, arrowroot starch, flaxseed meal, cinnamon, and salt and whisk to combine; set the batter aside to thicken slightly, about 5 minutes.

4. Preheat a griddle or large skillet over medium-high heat. Meanwhile, cut the loaf of bread into 8 slices, ¾ to 1 inch thick, depending on loaf size. Once the pan is hot, drop the butter onto the griddle (or in the skillet) and let it melt completely.

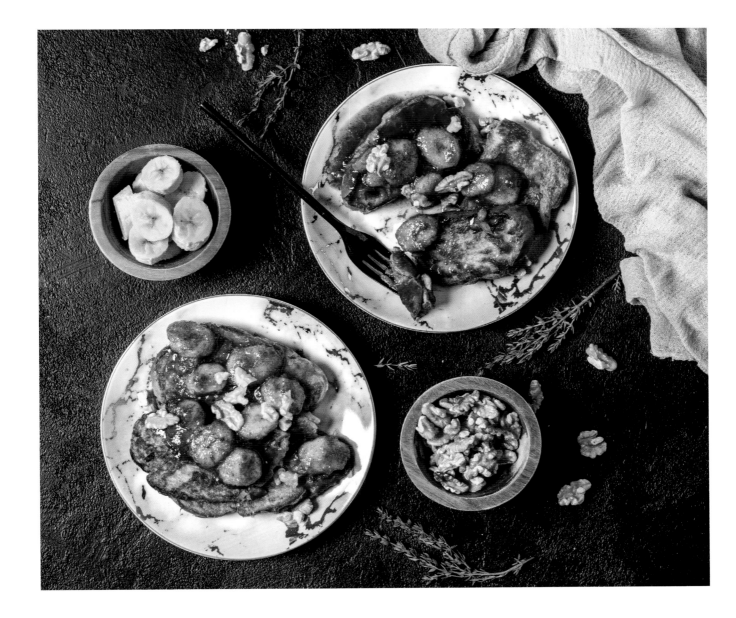

5. Dip a slice of bread into the batter, rotating it around on both sides and letting it soak for 1 to 2 seconds. Lay the soaked slice on the greased griddle (or in the skillet) and cook until it's golden brown with crisp edges and fully cooked through, 3 to 4 minutes on each side. Continue to dip, soak, and cook each slice until all the bread slices are made. Cook as many slices as you can comfortably fit on the griddle (or in the skillet) at once without crowding them.

6. To serve, stack two pieces of French toast on a plate and top with the caramelized bananas, a drizzle of maple syrup, and some chopped walnuts, if desired.

Tip: If you don't have arrowroot starch on hand, you can use cornstarch or tapioca flour.

Apple Blackberry Brioche
FRENCH TOAST

SERVES
4

PREP TIME
15 minutes

COOK TIME
8 to 24 minutes
(depending on
size of pan used)

I love French toast for breakfast, especially on the weekends. But it can't be any French toast! Texture has always been my biggest deal breaker when it comes to food, which is why I love using brioche bread to make French toast. I adore the way brioche soaks up the batter without becoming overly soggy, and it works beautifully in this recipe. Unlike the traditional version, this French toast uses flaxseed meal and arrowroot starch in place of regular eggs as binders and almond milk in place of regular milk in the batter, minimizing the amount of eggs and dairy. Yet the results are equally good! It also means that making this French toast vegan is fairly easy; see the tip below. My favorite parts of this recipe are the apple slices that are sandwiched between the pieces of French toast and the fresh blackberry topping. You can use your favorite type of apple in place of Granny Smith if you aren't in the mood for anything tart. Gala, Honeycrisp, and Fuji apples are great options for this recipe as well.

FRENCH TOAST:

1 cup unsweetened almond milk, room temperature

1 teaspoon vanilla extract

2 tablespoons arrowroot starch

1 tablespoon flaxseed meal

1 teaspoon ground cinnamon

Pinch of finely ground sea salt

1 loaf brioche bread (about 15 ounces)

1 tablespoon unsalted butter, for cooking

1 Granny Smith apple, thinly sliced

TOPPINGS:

Fresh blackberries

Maple syrup

Fresh rosemary leaves (optional)

1. In a large bowl, whisk together the almond milk, vanilla extract, arrowroot starch, flaxseed meal, cinnamon, and salt; set the batter aside to thicken slightly, about 5 minutes.

2. Cut the loaf of bread into 8 slices, ¾ to 1 inch thick, depending on loaf size.

3. Preheat a griddle or a large skillet over medium-high heat. Once hot, drop the butter onto the griddle (or in the skillet) and let it melt completely.

4. Dip a slice of bread into the batter, rotating it around on both sides and letting it soak for 1 to 2 seconds. Lay the soaked slice on the greased griddle or skillet and cook until it's golden brown with crisp edges and fully cooked through, 3 to 4 minutes on each side. Continue to dip, soak, and cook each slice until all the bread slices are made. Cook as many slices as you can comfortably fit on the griddle (or in the skillet) at once without crowding them.

5. To serve, stack two pieces of French toast on a plate, layering 1 or 2 slices of apples between them. Top each stack with blackberries, a drizzle of maple syrup, and, if desired, fresh rosemary.

Tip: If you don't have arrowroot starch on hand, you can use cornstarch or tapioca flour.

To make this recipe vegan, simply use vegan butter in place of the regular butter and change out the brioche, which traditionally contains eggs and butter, for a vegan version or another vegan bread option. If you'd like to stay with the brioche theme, you can make my Easy Vegan Brioche Bread (page 128); if you prefer a store-bought option, use any loaf of vegan bread you like. I find that the best options are light wheat and whole wheat.

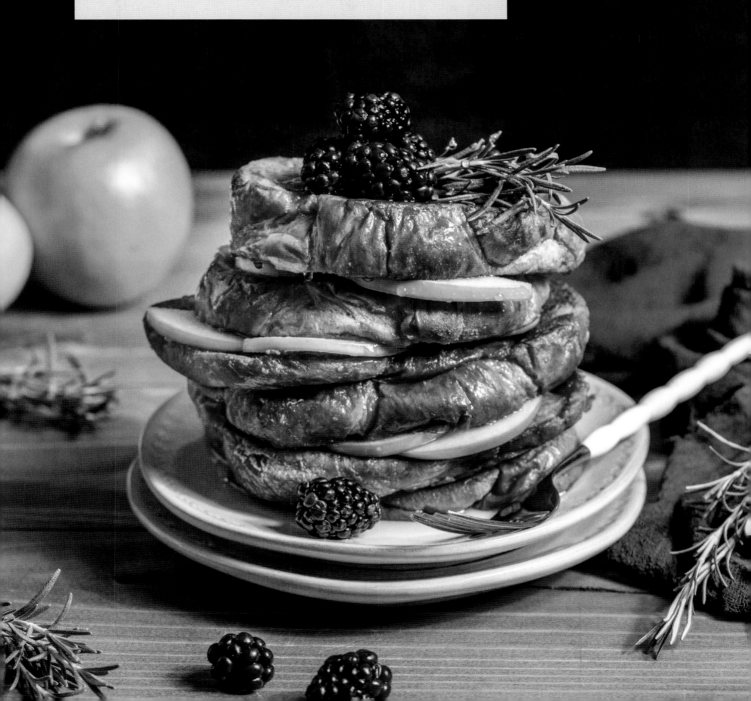

Dairy-Free Strawberry Pecan
FRENCH TOAST CASSEROLE

SERVES
4

PREP TIME
15 minutes

COOK TIME
45 minutes

This recipe takes French toast to a whole other level! Everyone needs a good French toast casserole recipe in their back pocket, and this one, made with fresh strawberries, pecans, and a brown sugar pecan streusel, is just the thing. When it comes to dairy-free breakfast casseroles, I love using challah bread because, like brioche, it has a nice pillowy texture, which soaks up the batter perfectly; vegan brioche (find my recipe on page 128) and sourdough bread are also good choices. If you have time on the weekend to whip together something over-the-top, bake up this casserole! You will love the balance of sweetness and nuttiness. Be sure to toast the pecans to get that full nutty flavor!

1 loaf challah, vegan brioche, or sourdough bread (about 15 ounces)

1 cup sliced strawberries

1 cup chopped pecans, toasted (see note, page 107)

BATTER:

8 large eggs

2 cups unsweetened almond milk

1 tablespoon vanilla extract

1 cup lightly packed brown sugar

1 tablespoon ground cinnamon

1 teaspoon ground nutmeg

BROWN SUGAR PECAN STREUSEL:

½ cup lightly packed brown sugar

½ cup all-purpose flour

½ cup chopped pecans, toasted (see note, page 107)

⅓ cup vegan butter, room temperature, plus more for the pan

2 teaspoons ground cinnamon

TOPPINGS (OPTIONAL):

Coconut whipped cream

Sliced strawberries

Fresh mint leaves

Pure maple syrup

1. Preheat the oven to 350°F. Grease a 9 by 13-inch baking pan with butter and set aside.

2. Cut the loaf of bread into 1-inch cubes. Put the cubed bread in the prepared baking pan, spreading it out evenly, then top evenly with the strawberries and pecans. Set aside.

3. Make the batter: In a large bowl, whisk together the eggs, almond milk, vanilla extract, brown sugar, cinnamon, and nutmeg until everything is well combined and no brown sugar lumps remain, 1 to 2 minutes. Pour the mixture over the cubed bread in the baking pan.

4. Make the streusel: In a medium-size bowl, mix the brown sugar, flour, pecans, butter, and cinnamon with your fingers or a rubber spatula until well combined and the mixture has the appearance of damp sand. Generously sprinkle the streusel topping over the bread until evenly covered.

5. Bake the casserole for 40 to 45 minutes, or until golden brown on the top and a butter knife comes out clean when inserted in the center. Once done, remove the casserole from the oven and let it cool slightly, about 5 minutes, before slicing.

6. To serve, cut the casserole into squares and stack two pieces on a plate, topping each stack with whipped cream, strawberry slices, mint leaves, and a drizzle of maple syrup, if desired.

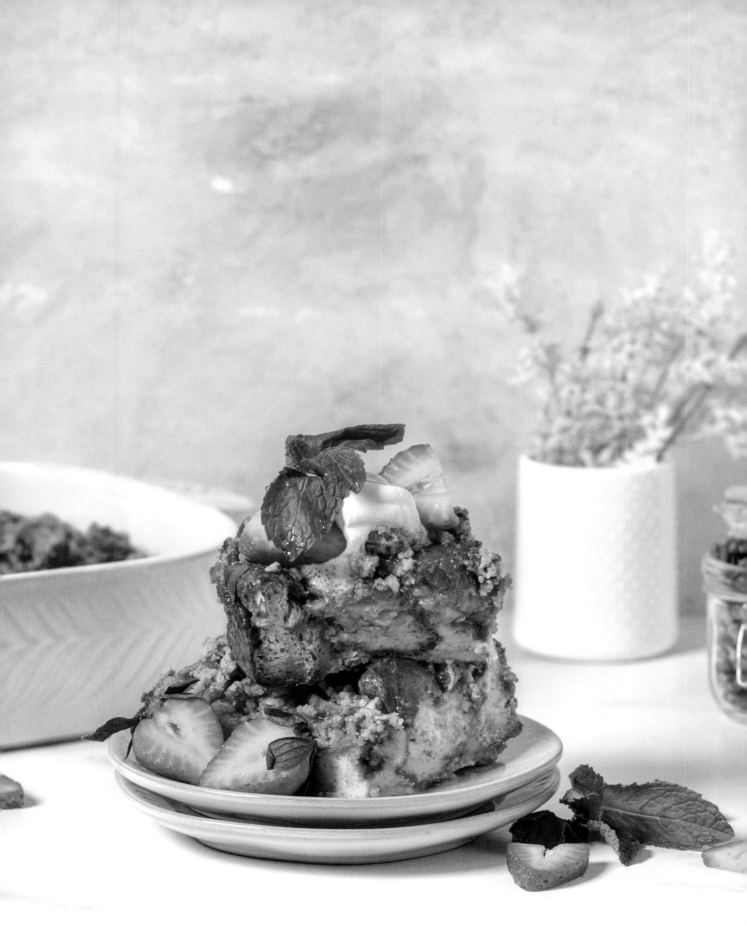

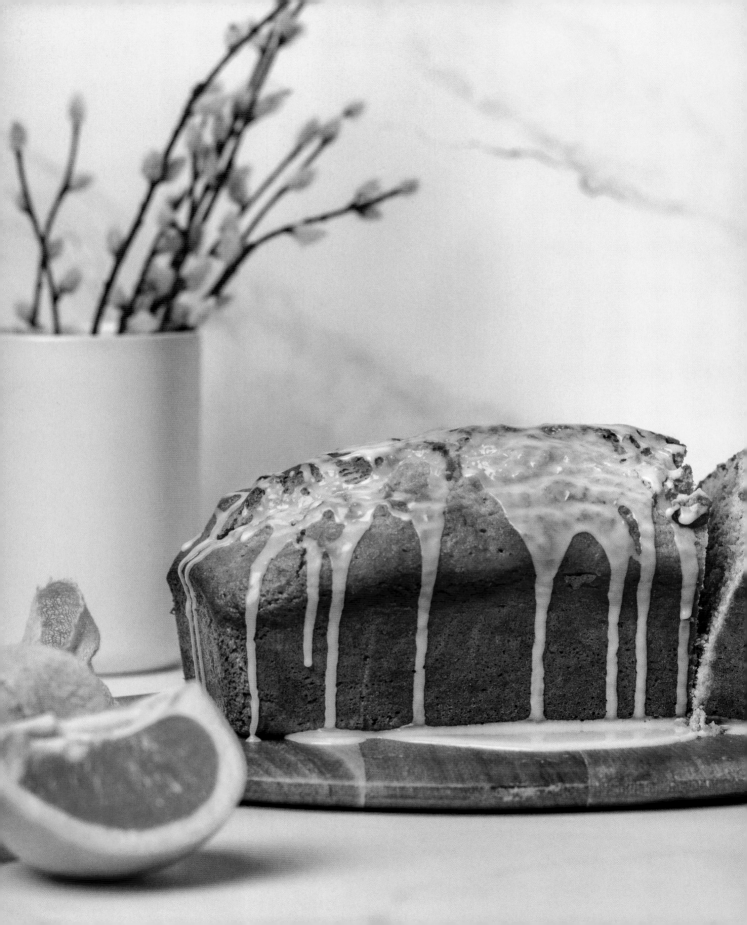

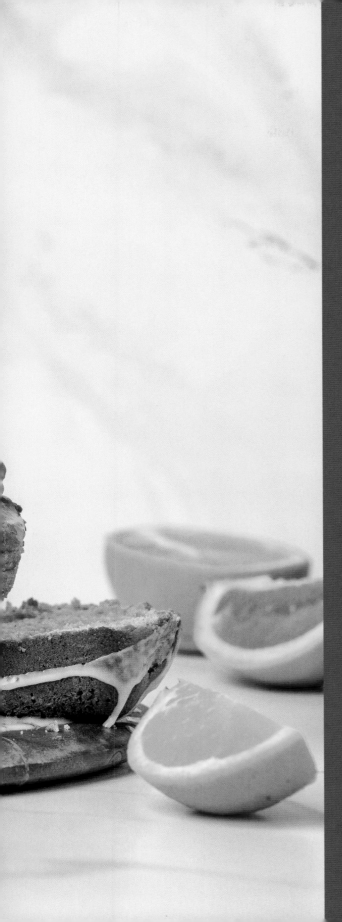

Chapter 6:
BREADS, MUFFINS & SCONES

Easy Vegan
BRIOCHE BREAD

MAKES
two 15- to
17-ounce loaves

PREP TIME
20 minutes,
plus 2 to 3
hours to rise
and proof and
4 hours to chill

COOK TIME
35 minutes

I pride myself in making homemade bread. I don't always have the time to make yeast bread from scratch, so naturally I have my favorite go-to brands; however, homemade bread has a very special place in my heart. This vegan brioche is incredibly soft and fluffy and has so many uses. While it might be hard to find vegan brioche at your nearest grocer, making your own has never been so easy. This recipe makes two loaves, which means that you can easily store one to use for French toast, regular toast, breakfast casseroles, and so on.

½ cup unsweetened, unflavored almond milk

½ cup vegan butter, melted, plus more for the pan and for brushing

¼ cup cane sugar

¾ cup aquafaba (see Tip, page 131)

2¼ teaspoons instant yeast

3½ cups bread flour, preferably artisan, plus more if needed

1 teaspoon finely ground sea salt

1 tablespoon extra-virgin olive oil, for greasing the bowl

Dried parsley, for topping (optional)

1. Fit a stand mixer with the whisk attachment. Pour the almond milk, melted butter, sugar, and aquafaba into the mixer bowl and whisk on medium speed until combined. Add the yeast, flour, and salt and mix until just combined.

2. Replace the whisk attachment with the dough hook and continue mixing on high speed until the dough is thoroughly kneaded, 10 to 15 minutes. When sufficiently kneaded, the dough should look shiny and feel elastic. If the dough feels too sticky and sticks easily to the bowl, add additional flour to the dough, about ⅓ cup at a time, and continue to knead until it no longer sticks.

3. Lightly grease a large bowl with the olive oil, then remove the kneaded dough from the mixer to the prepared bowl, gently turning it around so that it is coated with the oil. Cover the bowl and let the bread rise at room temperature until doubled in size, about 1 hour.

4. After the initial rise, place the bowl of dough in the refrigerator and let it chill for a minimum of 4 hours or overnight.

5. Remove the chilled dough from the refrigerator and cut it into 6 even pieces, then roll each piece into a ball.

6. Lightly grease two 9 by 5-inch loaf pans with melted butter and line them with parchment paper, leaving some paper overhanging the sides for easy removal.

(Recipe continues on page 131)

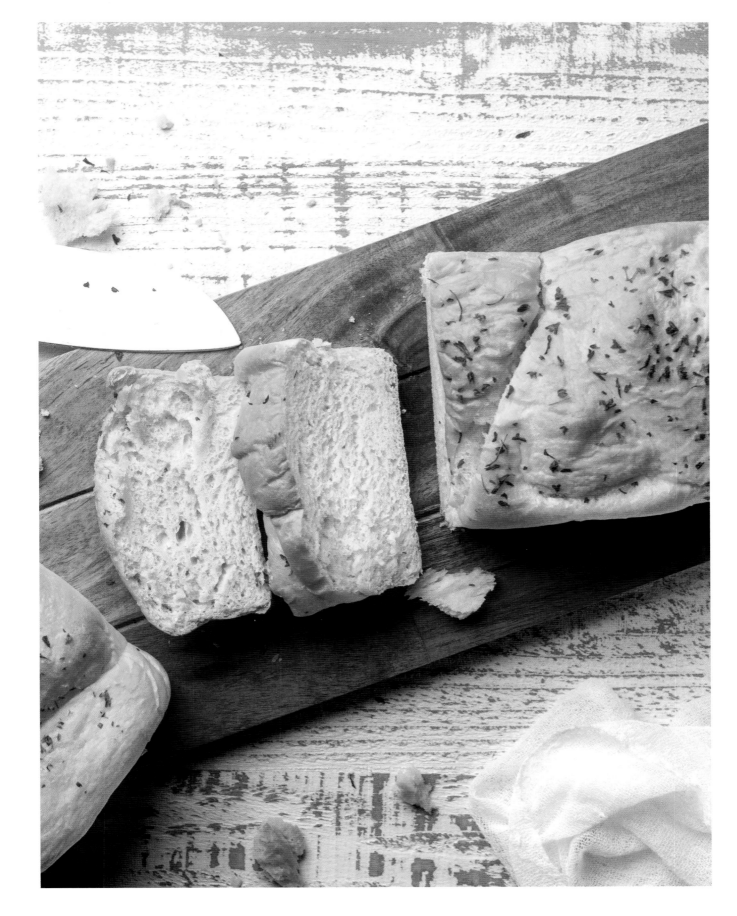

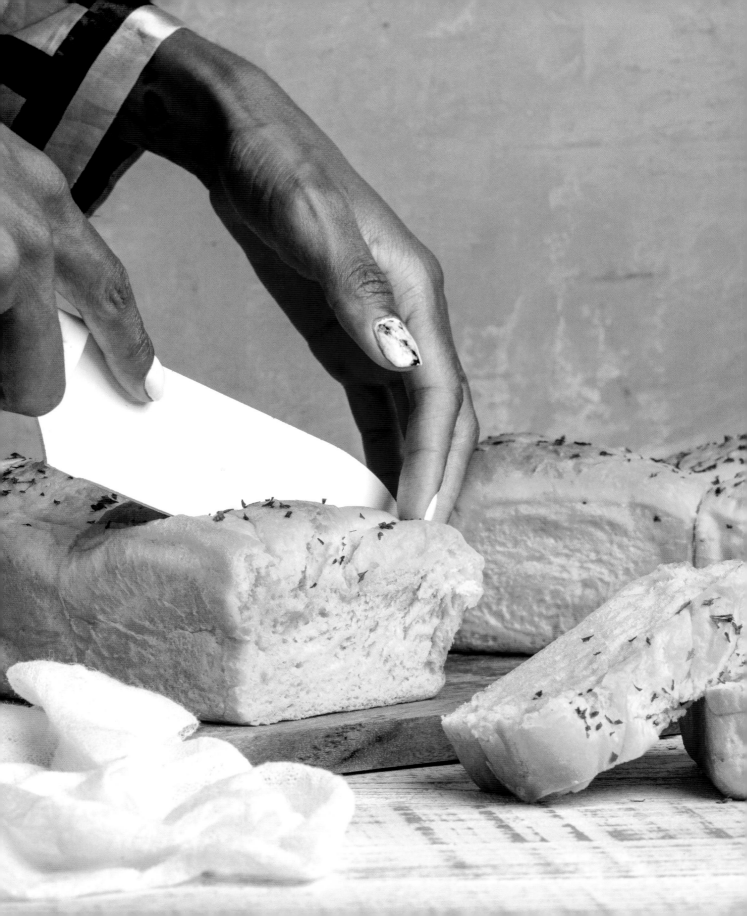

7. Place the dough balls in the prepared pans, offsetting them slightly to create a staggered lineup. Cover the pans with a kitchen towel and let the dough balls rise for another 1 to 2 hours, until doubled in size.

8. About 15 minutes before the dough balls are done rising, preheat the oven to 350°F. Brush the tops of the breads with about 1 tablespoon of melted vegan butter and bake for 30 to 35 minutes, or until the tops are golden brown and a toothpick or cake tester inserted in the center of a loaf comes out clean.

9. Remove the breads from the oven and let them cool for 15 to 20 minutes, then use the sides of the parchment paper to gently lift the breads from their pans and transfer them to a cooling rack. Allow to cool completely before slicing. If desired, lightly sprinkle the tops with dried parsley before serving.

10. Leftover bread can be stored in an airtight container, foil, or plastic wrap for 3 to 5 days at room temperature. To freeze, tightly wrap any leftovers in foil and place in a freezer bag; the bread will keep in the freezer for up to 2 months.

Tip: Aquafaba is the liquid that comes in a can of chickpeas. Simply drain the chickpeas over a bowl, reserving the liquid for use in this recipe. For the amount needed here, you will need one 15-ounce can of chickpeas. Save the chickpeas for one of the recipes in this book that calls for them; you have three to choose from!

Be sure your oven is fully preheated before placing the pans in the oven; this helps ensure that the bread bakes well and rises correctly.

Citrus Whole-Wheat
BREAKFAST LOAF

MAKES
1 loaf

PREP TIME
10 minutes

COOK TIME
1 hour

I'm always excited when I have an excuse to eat anything close to cake or cookies for breakfast. This bread is the epitome of sunshine in loaf form. I don't often get a chance to use citrus in my baking; however, once citrus season hits, I try to use it at least once. In this recipe, I call for a mixture of grapefruit and orange juice as well as lemon zest, which gives the bread an incredible burst of citrus flavor and a nice balance of sweetness and tartness. This early-morning treat goes especially well with a nice cup of tea or coffee.

3 cups whole-wheat flour

2 teaspoons baking powder

½ teaspoon baking soda

1 tablespoon ground cinnamon

Pinch of ground cardamom

½ teaspoon finely ground sea salt

1 tablespoon grated lemon zest

5 tablespoons unsalted butter, melted, plus more for the pan

1 cup cane sugar

¾ cup freshly squeezed orange juice, plus more if needed

½ cup freshly squeezed grapefruit juice

2 large eggs, room temperature

½ cup plain Greek yogurt (full-fat)

1 teaspoon vanilla extract

GRAPEFRUIT GLAZE:

2 cups powdered sugar, sifted, plus more if needed

¼ cup freshly squeezed grapefruit juice, plus more if needed

1 tablespoon unsweetened almond milk

1. Preheat the oven to 375°F. Grease a 9 by 5-inch loaf pan with butter and line it with parchment paper, leaving some paper overhanging the sides for easy removal.

2. In a medium-size bowl, whisk together the flour, baking powder, baking soda, cinnamon, cardamom, salt, and lemon zest.

3. In a large bowl, whisk the melted butter and sugar until the mixture becomes like wet sand. Add the orange juice, grapefruit juice, eggs, yogurt, and vanilla extract, whisking to combine.

4. Add the dry ingredients to the bowl with the wet ingredients and mix with a rubber spatula or wooden spoon just until fully combined. The batter should be smooth and thick yet easy to mix. If too thick, add 2 tablespoons of additional orange juice.

5. Scrape the batter into the prepared loaf pan and spread it out evenly. Bake for 55 to 60 minutes, or until a toothpick inserted in the center comes out mostly clean.

6. Remove from the oven and let cool in the pan for 30 minutes, then lift the bread from the pan and transfer to a cooling rack. Allow to cool completely before glazing.

7. To make the glaze, whisk together the powdered sugar, grapefruit juice, and milk in a medium-size bowl until smooth and silky. When at the right consistency, the glaze should slowly run off the whisk. Adjust the consistency with more juice or powdered sugar if needed.

8. Drizzle the glaze over the cooled loaf. Slice and enjoy!

9. Store any leftover bread in an airtight container at room temperature for up to 4 days or in the refrigerator for up to 5 days. To freeze, wrap in foil, then place in a freezer bag; the bread will keep in the freezer for up to 3 months.

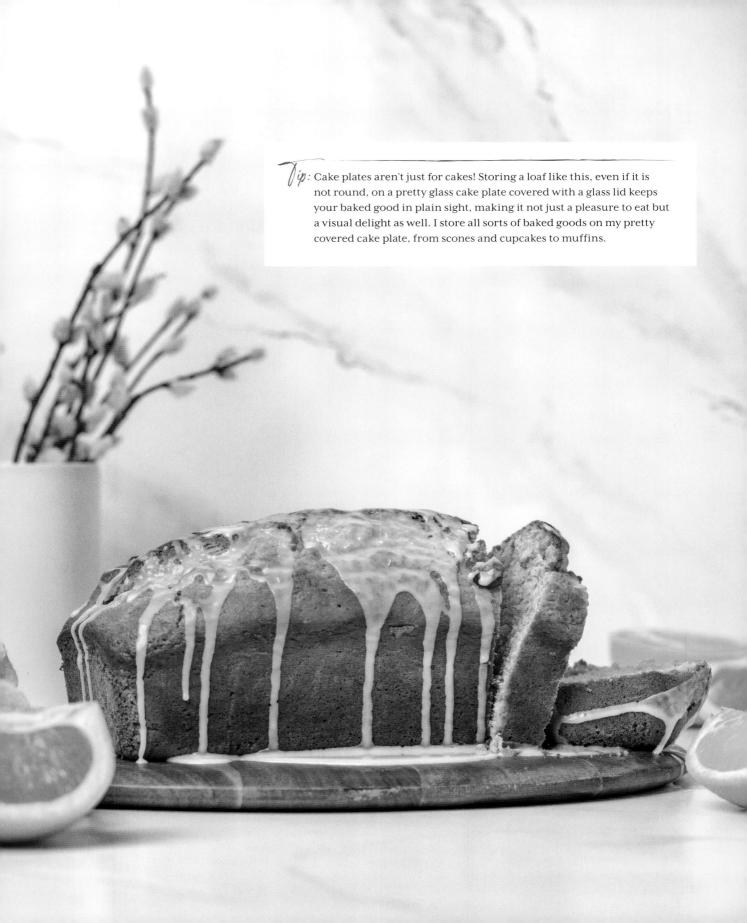

Tip: Cake plates aren't just for cakes! Storing a loaf like this, even if it is not round, on a pretty glass cake plate covered with a glass lid keeps your baked good in plain sight, making it not just a pleasure to eat but a visual delight as well. I store all sorts of baked goods on my pretty covered cake plate, from scones and cupcakes to muffins.

Vegan Pecan Chia
BANANA BREAD

MAKES
1 loaf

PREP TIME
15 minutes

COOK TIME
1 hour

I've probably eaten my millionth slice of banana bread since learning to whip quick breads together; however, I still get a thrill every time I slide a loaf into the oven to bake. The sweet aroma of banana, nuts, and warm spices wafting from the oven is just as exciting as my first attempt at banana bread. Laden with pecans, this particular loaf was inspired by my Southern roots. When incorporating pecans into a recipe, I often toast them to add a bold nutty flavor. Chia seeds are one of my favorite superfoods to incorporate into baked goods, especially vegan ones, because they not only add great nutritional value but also work as a binder, much like bananas. Once you make this bread, you won't look at banana bread the same way again!

1½ cups all-purpose flour

2 teaspoons baking powder

½ teaspoon baking soda

1 tablespoon ground cinnamon

1 teaspoon ground nutmeg

Pinch of finely ground sea salt

5 ripe bananas, divided

½ cup lightly packed brown sugar

½ cup Vegan Buttermilk (page 46)

¼ cup vegan butter, melted, plus more for the pan

¼ cup pure maple syrup

1 teaspoon vanilla extract

½ cup chia seeds

¾ cup chopped pecans, toasted (see note, page 107), divided

Pure maple syrup, for serving (optional)

1. Preheat the oven to 375°F. Grease a 9 by 5-inch loaf pan with butter and line it with parchment paper, leaving some paper overhanging the sides.

2. In a medium-size bowl, whisk together the flour, baking powder, baking soda, cinnamon, nutmeg, and salt.

3. Mash four of the bananas and place in a large bowl. Add the brown sugar, buttermilk, melted butter, maple syrup, vanilla extract, and chia seeds and stir until combined and the mixture becomes thick and somewhat fluffy.

4. Add the dry ingredients to the bowl with the wet ingredients, mixing with a rubber spatula or wooden spoon just until fully combined. The batter will be smooth and thick yet easy to stir. Fold in ½ cup of the toasted pecans until well incorporated.

5. Scrape the batter into the prepared loaf pan and spread it out evenly. Slice the remaining banana and place the slices atop the batter followed by the remaining ¼ cup of toasted pecans, gently pressing them in (just a little) to ensure that they bake into the bread and won't fall off later.

6. Bake for 55 to 60 minutes, or until a toothpick inserted in the center comes out mostly clean.

7. Remove the bread from the oven and let it cool for about 20 minutes, then lift it out of the pan and place on a cooling rack to cool completely.

8. Once cool, slice and serve, drizzling a little maple syrup on each slice, if desired.

9. Store any leftover bread in an airtight container at room temperature for up to 4 days, in the refrigerator for up to 5 days, or in the freezer for up to 3 months.

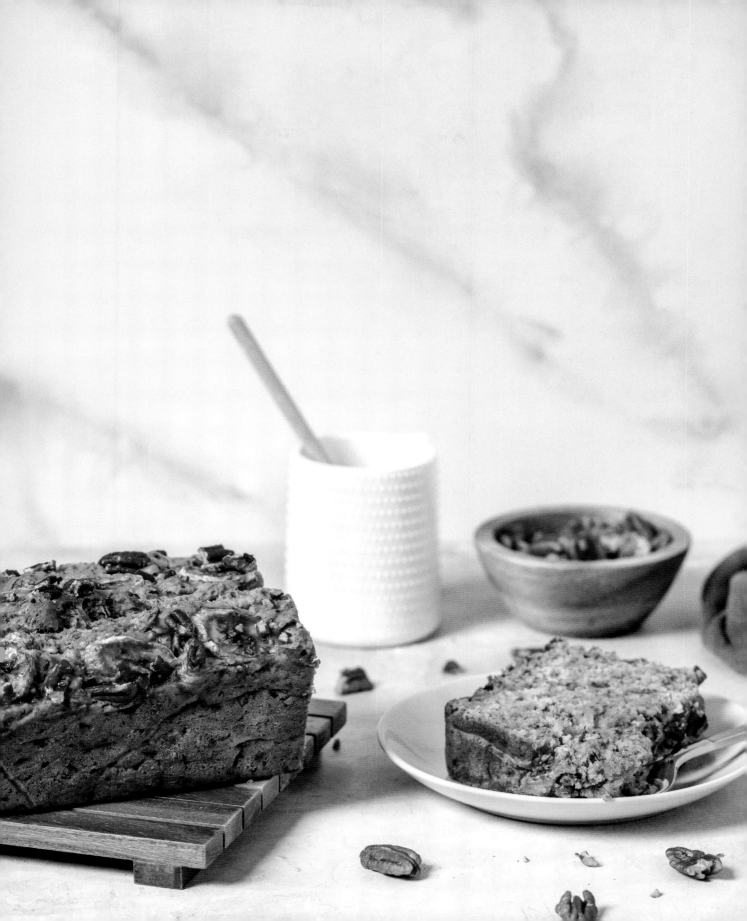

Garlic Cheese Herb
ZUCCHINI BREAD

MAKES
1 loaf

PREP TIME
15 minutes

COOK TIME
1 hour

This bread tops my list of favorites. I tend to make a lot more sweet breads than savory ones, but this loaf wins me over every time. Filled with garlic and herb flavors, it will remind you of a delicious pull-apart bread, but you don't actually have to pull it apart. I like to use bread flour to create that chewy yet airy breadlike texture; however, all-purpose flour works just fine. This bread lasted only two days in my house—it is that good! I enjoy it as a quick savory breakfast option with a cup of tea or juice and even as a midday snack.

3 cups bread flour, preferably artisan

1 tablespoon baking powder

1 teaspoon ground dried oregano

1 teaspoon dried parsley

½ teaspoon ground dried thyme

½ teaspoon smoked paprika

1 teaspoon finely ground sea salt

1 large egg

1½ cups Vegan Buttermilk (page 46), made with lemon juice

3 tablespoons unsalted butter, melted, plus more for the pan

1 medium zucchini, grated (about 1 cup)

8 cloves garlic, minced

1 cup shredded mild cheddar cheese

EGG WASH:

1 large egg, beaten

1 teaspoon unsweetened, unflavored almond milk

1. Preheat the oven to 375°F. Grease a 9 by 5-inch loaf pan with butter and line it with parchment paper, leaving some paper overhanging the sides.

2. In a medium-size bowl, whisk together the flour, baking powder, oregano, parsley, thyme, paprika, and salt.

3. In a large bowl, stir the egg, buttermilk, melted butter, zucchini, garlic, and cheese until combined.

4. Add the dry ingredients to the bowl with the wet ingredients, mixing everything together using a rubber spatula or wooden spoon just until fully combined. The batter will be thick yet easy to stir.

5. Scrape the batter into the prepared loaf pan and spread it out evenly.

6. In a small bowl, beat the egg and almond milk until well combined, then lightly brush the top of the batter with the egg wash.

7. Bake for 55 to 60 minutes, or until a toothpick inserted in the center comes out mostly clean.

8. Remove the bread from the oven and let cool for about 20 minutes, then lift it out of the pan and put it on a cooling rack. Allow the bread to cool completely before slicing.

9. Store any leftover bread tightly wrapped in foil or an airtight container in the refrigerator for up to 4 days or in the freezer for up to 6 months.

Tip: Instead of using fresh garlic cloves, you can substitute 1 to 1½ teaspoons of garlic powder, depending on how much garlic flavor you prefer, adding the garlic powder in Step 2 with the other dried seasonings.

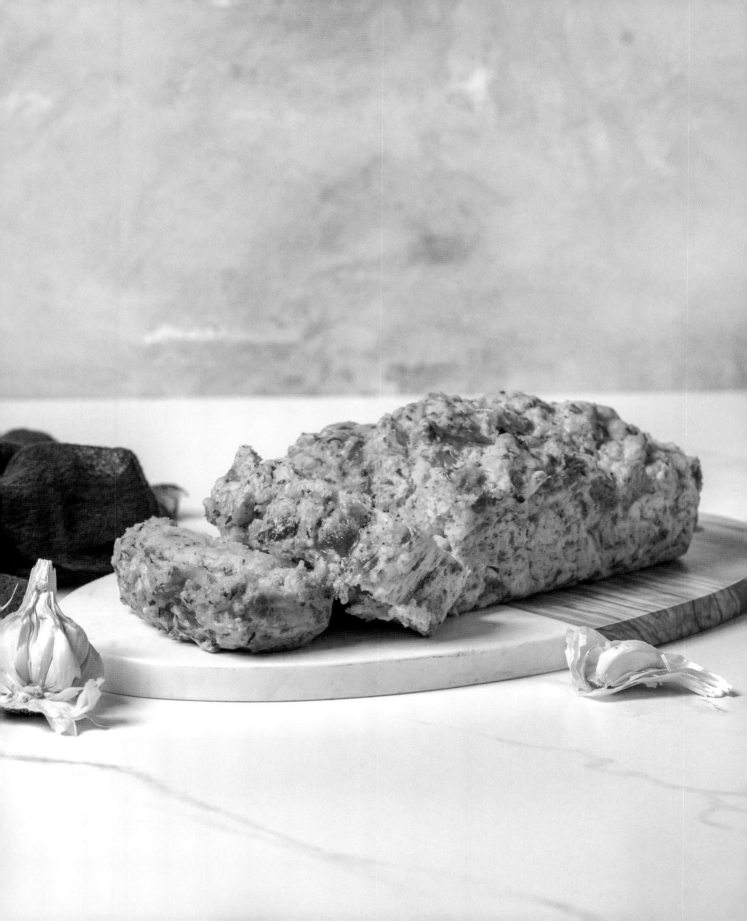

Gluten-Free
DOUBLE CHOCOLATE MUFFINS

MAKES
12 muffins

PREP TIME
10 minutes

COOK TIME
25 minutes

There's nothing like a great grab-and-go breakfast that packs chocolate flavor! These gluten-free double chocolate muffins are so decadent, my son loves them just as much as I do. I purposefully added extra chocolate chips so that they are loaded, and it was the best decision ever! I don't often eat muffins, but when I do, I enjoy them with a tall glass of milk or a cup of hot tea if it's early in the morning. This recipe is made in just one bowl and comes together really quickly.

1½ cups gluten-free 1-to-1 baking flour

¾ cup cane sugar

½ cup cacao powder

2 teaspoons baking powder

½ teaspoon finely ground sea salt

Pinch of ground cinnamon

1 cup Vegan Buttermilk (page 46)

¼ cup virgin coconut oil, melted

1 cup vegan semi-sweet chocolate chips, plus more for topping

1. Preheat the oven to 375°F. Line a 12-cavity muffin pan with cupcake liners.

2. In a large bowl, whisk together the flour, sugar, cacao powder, baking powder, salt, and cinnamon until combined. Add the buttermilk and coconut oil and mix until the batter is evenly wet and thick. Fold in the chocolate chips.

3. Divide the batter evenly among the cavities of the prepared muffin pan, using about 3 tablespoons of batter for each muffin. Sprinkle the tops with additional chocolate chips.

4. Bake for 20 to 25 minutes, or until a toothpick inserted in the center of a muffin comes out clean. Remove the pan from the oven and let the muffins cool in the pan for 10 minutes, then transfer to a cooling rack to cool completely, about 45 minutes.

5. Store leftover muffins in an airtight container at room temperature for up to 1 week. They can also be placed in a freezer bag and frozen for up to 2 months.

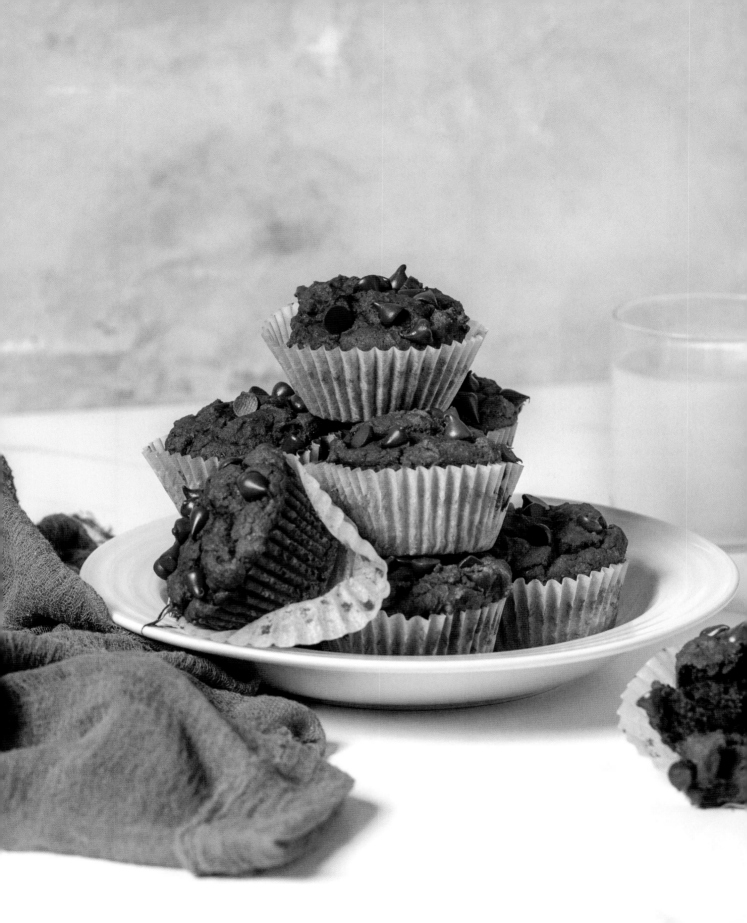

Jumbo Blueberry WALNUT MUFFINS

MAKES
6 jumbo
muffins

PREP TIME
10 minutes

COOK TIME
25 minutes

They say that the best things come in small packages, but I disagree when it comes to these muffins. I sometimes enjoy making my muffins jumbo because there's more to love in one sitting, and there's lots to love here. Blueberries, one of my favorite fruits, make these muffins the perfect sweet treat. Plus, walnuts work really well with blueberries and the combination of savory and buttery (from the walnuts) and sweetness (from the blueberries) just works! These muffins are already vegan, but if you want to make them gluten-free as well, you can substitute 1-to-1 baking flour for the all-purpose flour. If you'd like to substitute almond or oat flour, you'll need to add 1 teaspoon of xanthan gum to ensure that the muffins come out fluffy and airy.

2 cups all-purpose flour

2 teaspoons baking powder

1 teaspoon ground cinnamon

½ teaspoon finely ground sea salt

1 cup Vegan Buttermilk (page 46)

¼ cup pure maple syrup

¼ cup vegan butter, melted, plus more for the pan

1 cup fresh blueberries

½ cup chopped raw walnuts

1. Preheat the oven to 375°F. Grease a 6-cavity jumbo muffin pan with butter.

2. In a large bowl, whisk together the flour, baking powder, cinnamon, and salt until combined. Add the buttermilk, maple syrup, and melted butter and mix until the batter is evenly wet and thick. Fold in the blueberries and walnuts.

3. Divide the batter evenly among the cavities of the prepared muffin pan, using about ⅓ cup of batter for each muffin.

4. Bake for 20 to 25 minutes, or until a toothpick inserted in the center of a muffin comes out clean. Remove the pan from the oven and let the muffins cool in the pan for 20 minutes, then remove from the pan and place on a cooling rack to cool completely, another 20 to 25 minutes.

5. Store leftover muffins in an airtight container at room temperature for up to 1 week. They can also be placed in a freezer bag and frozen for up to 2 months.

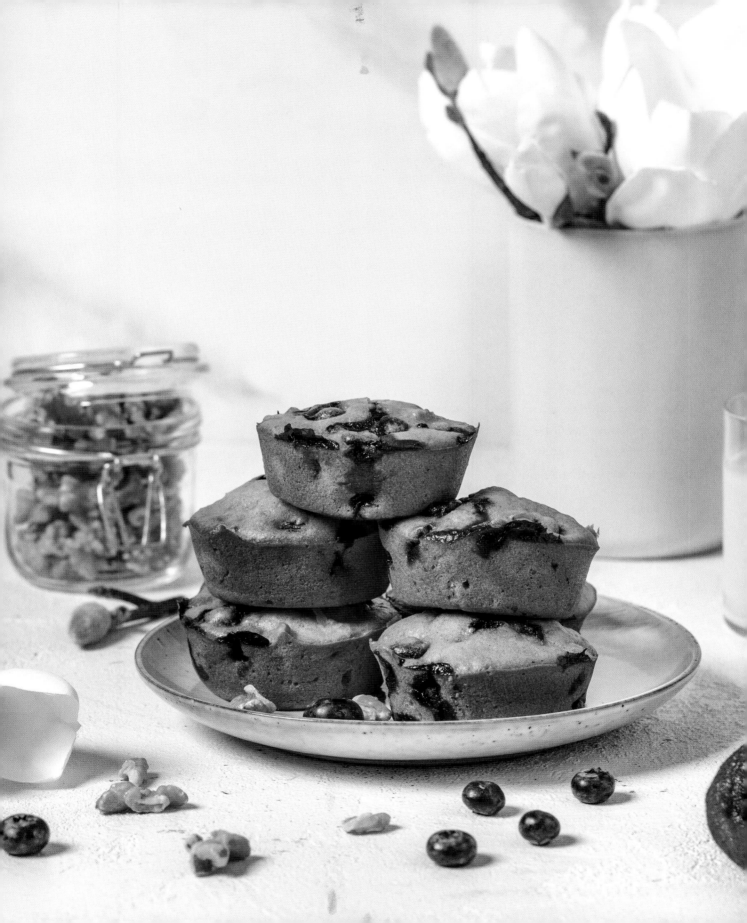

Sweet Cornmeal
RUM MUFFINS

MAKES
12 muffins

PREP TIME
10 minutes

COOK TIME
17 minutes

Cornmeal is a staple in Jamaican cuisine. While I enjoy Jamaican cornmeal porridge the most, these cornmeal rum muffins are a close second. Trust me; once you try these muffins, you'll be hooked! I don't drink alcohol; therefore, I use rum extract in these muffins; however, you can always substitute actual white rum if you like.

1 cup medium-grind yellow cornmeal

1 cup all-purpose flour

½ cup cane sugar

2 tablespoons baking powder

1 teaspoon ground cinnamon

½ teaspoon finely ground sea salt

1 large egg, room temperature

1 cup unsweetened, unflavored almond milk

¼ cup (½ stick) unsalted butter, melted

1 teaspoon rum extract

1. Preheat the oven to 400°F. Line a 12-cavity muffin pan with cupcake liners.

2. In a large bowl, whisk together the cornmeal, flour, sugar, baking powder, cinnamon, and salt until combined and lump-free.

3. In a separate bowl, whisk together the egg, milk, melted butter, and rum extract until just combined. Add the wet ingredients to the dry ingredients and mix them together using a rubber spatula or wooden spoon until the batter becomes evenly wet and thick.

4. Divide the batter evenly among the prepared cavities of the muffin pan, using about 3 tablespoons of batter for each muffin.

5. Bake for 13 to 17 minutes, or until a toothpick inserted in the center of a muffin comes out clean. Remove the muffins from the oven and let them cool slightly in the pan for 5 to 10 minutes, then remove them from the pan and serve while still warm.

6. Store leftover muffins in an airtight container at room temperature for up to 1 week. They can also be placed in a freezer bag and frozen for up to 2 months. For the best texture and flavor, reheat the muffins in a preheated 350°F oven for 10 minutes, or until warmed through.

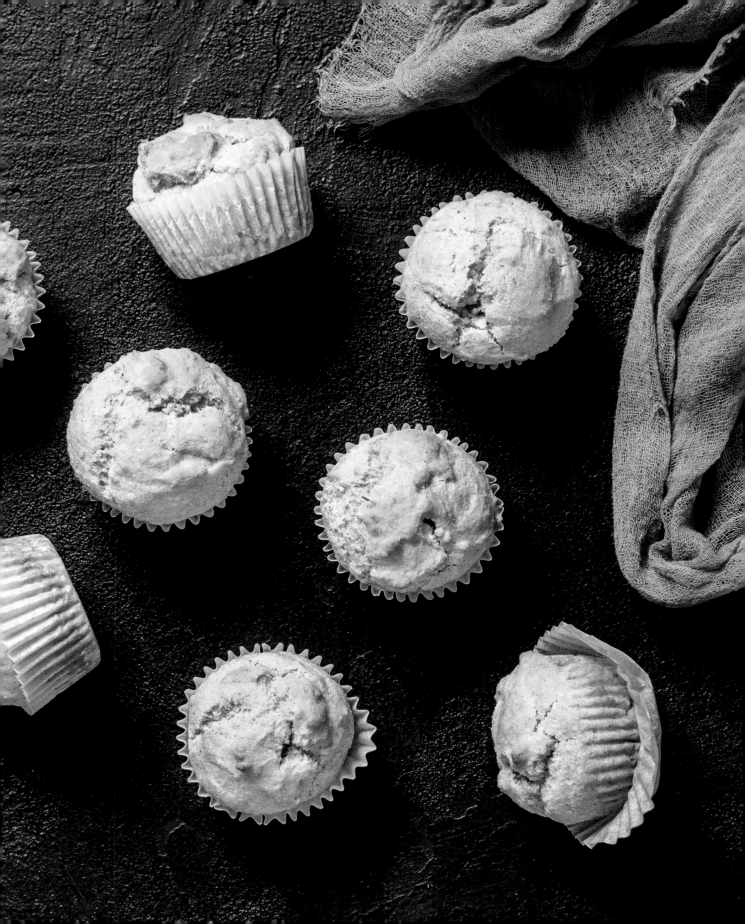

Jerk Chicken
WHITE CHEDDAR SCALLION SCONES

MAKES
8 scones

PREP TIME
10 minutes

COOK TIME
18 minutes

Enjoying tender, buttery scones is one of my favorite pastimes these days. My husband introduced scones to me, and I remember being mind-blown by how delicious they were. Now that I make homemade scones, I love experimenting with both sweet and savory versions, depending on my taste buds' preferences and what I have on hand. This particular recipe was inspired by my love for Jamaican jerk chicken and wanting to find a creative way to use up leftovers. Believe me, spicy jerk chicken paired with creamy white cheddar cheese and fresh scallions creates a divine eating experience in every bite!

2¼ cups all-purpose flour, plus more for the work surface

2 teaspoons baking powder

1 teaspoon dried parsley

1 teaspoon garlic powder

1 teaspoon smoked paprika

½ teaspoon finely ground sea salt

½ cup (1 stick) cold unsalted butter, cubed

1 cup unsweetened, unflavored almond milk

1 large egg

1 cup Shredded Jerk Chicken (page 60)

1 cup shredded mild cheddar cheese

⅓ cup thinly sliced scallions, plus more for garnish if desired

EGG WASH:

1 large egg, beaten

1 tablespoon unsweetened, unflavored almond milk

1. Preheat the oven to 425°F. Line a baking sheet with parchment paper.

2. In a large bowl, whisk together the flour, baking powder, parsley, garlic powder, smoked paprika, and salt until well combined.

3. Add the cubed butter to the dry ingredients and, using a pastry blender or two forks, cut in the butter until it is broken down into pieces the size of peas. Create a well in the center of the dry ingredients.

4. In a medium-size bowl, whisk together the almond milk and egg until smooth and well combined, then pour the wet mixture into the well of the dry ingredients. Add the chicken, cheese, and scallions and mix together using a rubber spatula until just combined and the dough is evenly moistened.

5. Lightly flour a clean work surface, then scrape the dough onto the work surface. Dust your hands with flour, then knead the dough for 1 to 2 minutes, or until it no longer sticks to the surface.

6. Pat and shape the dough into an 8-inch circle. Using a very sharp knife or a pastry cutter, slice the dough into 8 equal wedges, dusting the knife or pastry cutter with flour if the dough is sticky.

7. In a small bowl, whisk together the egg and milk for the egg wash.

8. Place the scones on the prepared baking sheet and brush the tops with the egg wash. Bake for 15 to 18 minutes, or until the tops are golden brown and a toothpick inserted in the center of a scone comes out clean.

9. Remove the pan from the oven and let the scones cool on the pan for 2 to 3 minutes before serving. Enjoy warm or at room temperature, garnished with sliced scallions, if desired.

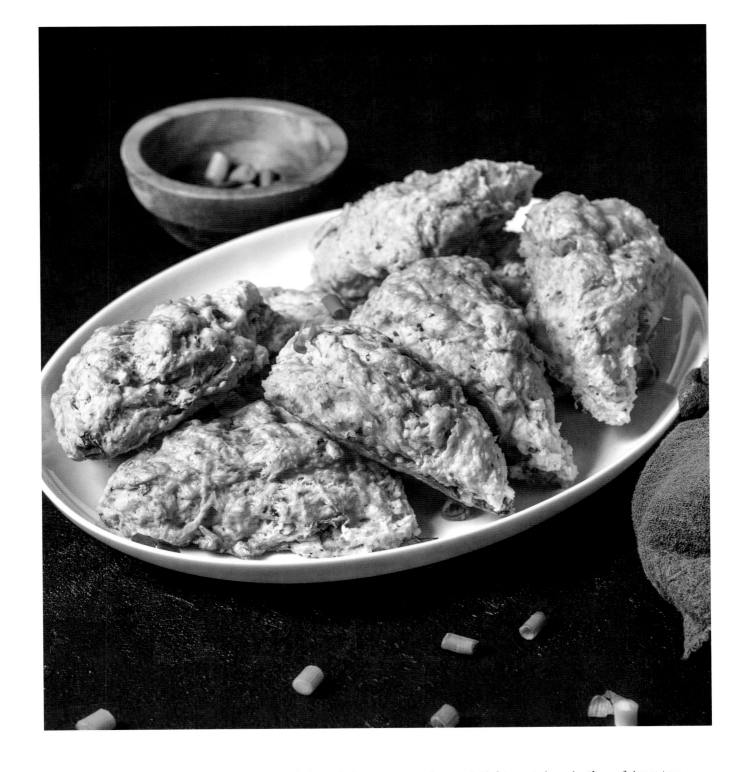

10. Store leftover scones in an airtight container in the refrigerator for up to 1 week. They can also be frozen for up to 3 months in a freezer bag or airtight container with parchment paper layered between them to prevent sticking. For the best texture and flavor, reheat the scones in a preheated 400°F oven for 10 to 15 minutes, or until warmed through.

Brown Butter Apple Pie Scones
WITH CARAMELIZED APPLES

MAKES
8 scones

PREP TIME
15 minutes

COOK TIME
22 minutes

There's nothing like a slice of warm, sweet apple pie. But can you image having the same incredible experience for breakfast or brunch? Well, these scones are something special, and they come loaded with many sweet notes, including warm spices that are so comforting. I love extra flavor, so topping these tender buttery scones with some caramelized apples and toasted pecans only made sense. If you're an apple lover, then these apple pie scones are for you!

BROWN BUTTER:

¼ cup (½ stick) unsalted butter

SCONES:

2¼ cups all-purpose flour, plus more for the work surface

2 teaspoons baking powder

¼ teaspoon baking soda

⅓ cup cane sugar

1 tablespoon ground cinnamon

1 teaspoon ground nutmeg

¼ teaspoon ground allspice

⅛ teaspoon ground cloves

½ teaspoon finely ground sea salt

½ cup (1 stick) cold unsalted butter, cubed

½ cup unsweetened almond milk

1 large egg

1 Granny Smith apple, cut into small dice

EGG WASH:

1 large egg, beaten

1 tablespoon unsweetened almond milk

CARAMELIZED APPLE TOPPING:

2 tablespoons unsalted butter

½ cup lightly packed brown sugar

1 teaspoon ground cinnamon

Pinch of finely ground sea salt

1 Granny Smith apple, peeled and cut into small dice

1 cup chopped pecans, toasted (see note, page 107)

Fresh mint leaves (optional)

1. Preheat the oven to 425°F. Line a baking sheet with parchment paper.

2. Make the brown butter: Melt the butter in a medium-size saucepan over medium-high heat, stirring occasionally. Continue to cook the butter, stirring occasionally, until dark flecks begin to form, the butter becomes fragrant (the aroma will be sweet and slightly nutty), and the color darkens, 3 to 4 minutes. Remove the pan from the heat and set aside to cool for a few minutes.

3. In a large bowl, whisk together the flour, baking powder, baking soda, sugar, spices, and salt until well combined.

4. Add the cubed butter to the dry ingredients and, using a pastry blender or two forks, cut in the butter until it is broken down into pieces the size of peas. Create a well in the center of the dry ingredients.

(Recipe continues on page 149)

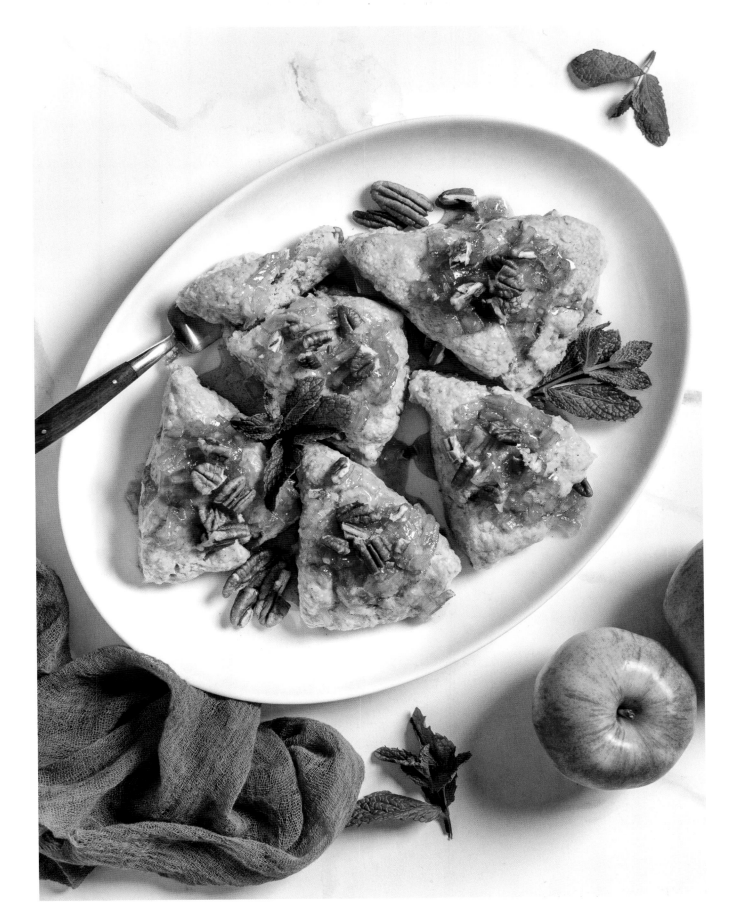

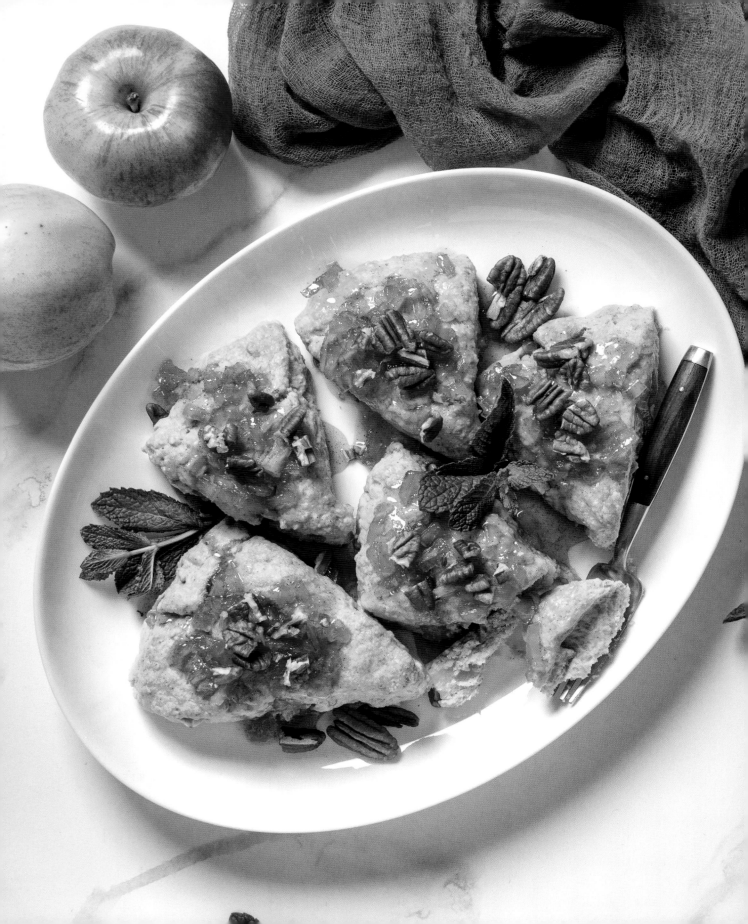

5. In a medium-size bowl, whisk the almond milk, brown butter, and egg until smooth and well combined. Pour the wet ingredients into the well of the dry ingredients, then add the diced apples and mix everything together using a rubber spatula until just combined and the dough is evenly moistened.

6. Lightly flour a clean work surface, then scrape the dough onto the work surface. Dust your hands with flour, then knead the dough for 1 to 2 minutes, or until it no longer sticks to the surface.

7. Pat and shape the dough into an 8-inch circle. Using a very sharp knife or pastry cutter, slice the dough into 8 equal wedges, dusting the knife or pastry cutter with flour if the dough is sticky.

8. In a small bowl, whisk together the egg and milk for the egg wash.

9. Place the sliced scones on the prepared baking sheet and brush the tops with the egg wash. Bake the scones for 15 to 18 minutes, or until the tops are golden brown and a toothpick inserted in the center of a scone comes out clean.

10. While the scones are baking, make the caramelized apple topping: Melt the butter in a medium-size saucepan over high heat. Add the brown sugar, cinnamon, and salt and stir everything together until combined and it begins to bubble, 2 to 3 minutes. Add the diced apple and toss everything together until the apple is well coated. Cook, stirring occasionally, until the apple becomes tender and the sauce has thickened, 8 to 10 minutes. Remove the pan from the heat and set aside until ready to use.

11. When the scones are done, remove them from the oven and let cool on the pan for 2 to 3 minutes before serving. Enjoy warm or at room temperature topped with the caramelized apples, toasted pecans, and, if desired, mint leaves.

12. Store leftover scones at room temperature for 1 day or in an airtight container in the refrigerator for up to 1 week. They can also be frozen for up to 3 months in a freezer bag or airtight container with parchment paper layered between them to prevent sticking. For the best texture and flavor, reheat the scones in a preheated 400°F oven for 10 to 15 minutes, or until warmed through.

Maple
BLUEBERRY SCONES

MAKES
6 scones

PREP TIME
15 minutes

COOK TIME
18 minutes

There's something about maple and blueberries—they just go together! Maple syrup is one of my favorite things to add to scones, and with good reason. It's a great natural sweetener and it adds a bold flavor, particularly when you use a darker syrup. These scones are so easy to whip together, and the blueberry-maple combo is a classic that will never get old.

2¼ cups all-purpose flour

2 teaspoons baking powder

¼ teaspoon baking soda

1 tablespoon ground cinnamon

1 teaspoon ground nutmeg

½ teaspoon finely ground sea salt

½ cup (1 stick) unsalted butter, cubed

¾ cup unsweetened almond milk

⅓ cup pure maple syrup, plus more for topping if desired

1 large egg

1 cup fresh blueberries, plus more for topping if desired

EGG WASH:

1 large egg, beaten

1 tablespoon unsweetened almond milk

1. Preheat the oven to 425°F. Line a baking sheet with parchment paper.

2. In a large bowl, whisk together the flour, baking powder, baking soda, cinnamon, nutmeg, and salt until well combined.

3. Add the cubed butter to the dry ingredients and, using a pastry blender or two forks, cut in the butter until it is broken down into pieces the size of peas. Create a well in the center of the dry ingredients.

4. In a medium-size bowl, whisk the almond milk, maple syrup, and egg until smooth and well combined. Pour the wet ingredients into the well in the dry ingredients, then mix everything together using a rubber spatula until just combined and the dough is evenly moistened. Fold in the blueberries.

5. Lightly flour a clean work surface, then scrape the dough onto the work surface. Dust your hands with flour, then knead the dough for 1 to 2 minutes, or until it no longer sticks to the surface.

6. Pat and shape the dough into an 8-inch circle. Using a very sharp knife or pastry cutter, slice the dough into 8 equal wedges, dusting the knife or pastry cutter with flour if the dough is sticky.

7. In a small bowl, whisk together the egg and milk for the egg wash.

8. Place the scones on the prepared baking sheet and brush the tops with the egg wash. Bake for 15 to 18 minutes, or until the tops are golden brown and a toothpick inserted in the center of a scone comes out clean.

9. Remove the pan from the oven and let the scones cool on the pan for 2 to 3 minutes before serving. Enjoy warm or at room temperature, topped with additional blueberries and a drizzle of maple syrup, if desired.

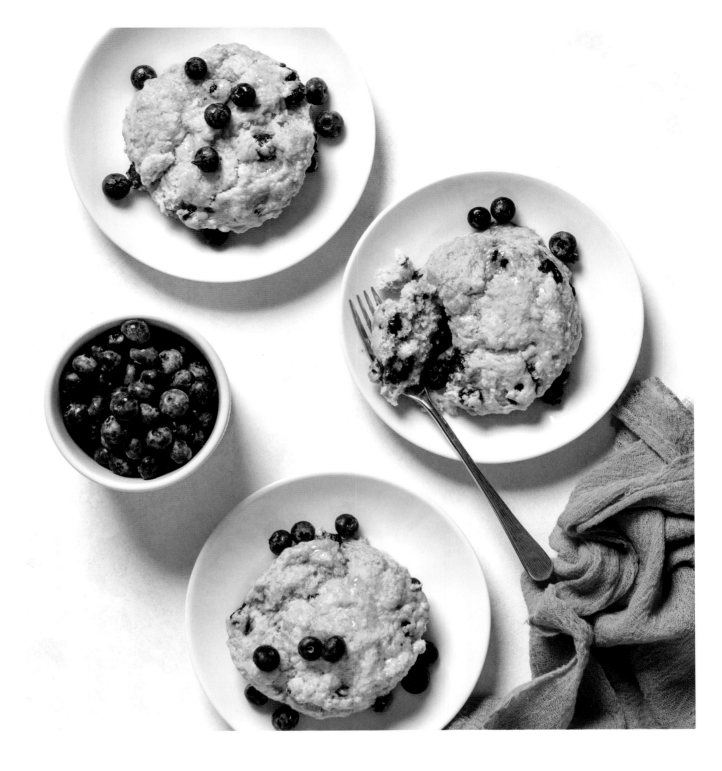

10. Store leftover scones at room temperature for 1 day or in an airtight container in the refrigerator for up to 1 week. They can also be frozen for up to 3 months in a freezer bag or airtight container with parchment paper layered between them to prevent sticking. For the best texture and flavor, reheat the scones in a preheated 400°F oven for 10 to 15 minutes, or until warmed through.

Rum Raisin Bread

MAKES
1 loaf

PREP TIME
10 minutes

COOK TIME
1 hour

This rum raisin bread was inspired by one of my later childhood favorites, often made around the holidays or for special gatherings. I'm so happy to share it with you. (If this recipe is your introduction to Jamaican cuisine, it's a great place to start!) In Jamaican culture, one of the most coveted cakes is rum cake, aka "black cake," which is jam-packed with white rum flavor. This bread is a mash-up of that cake and the traditional Jamaican spice bun cake, creating a decadent and irresistible flavor of rum and aromatic spices. The best parts about this bread are that it uses all vegan ingredients and takes only 10 minutes to whip together in one bowl. Although using bread flour creates a chewier texture more like that of traditional bread, you can use all-purpose flour instead—either way, your bread is guaranteed to come out soft and fluffy. If you use white rum instead of extract, increase the quantity to 2 tablespoons. This is the perfect breakfast, snack, or dessert option!

1 cup raisins

2 cups bread flour, preferably artisan

2 teaspoons baking powder

2 tablespoons ground cinnamon

½ teaspoon ground allspice

Pinch of finely ground sea salt

2 Flaxseed Eggs (page 38) or Chia Eggs (page 39)

¼ cup plus 1 tablespoon unflavored almond milk, plus more if needed

¼ cup vegan butter, melted, plus more for the pan

¼ cup agave syrup

1 teaspoon rum extract

1. Preheat the oven to 375°F. Grease a 9 by 5-inch loaf pan with butter and line it with parchment paper, leaving some paper overhanging the sides.

2. Put the raisins in a small heatproof bowl or a 2-cup measuring cup, then completely cover with boiling water. Allow to soak until the raisins are slightly softened and swollen, 5 to 10 minutes. Drain, rinse, and set aside.

3. In a medium-size bowl, whisk together the flour, baking powder, cinnamon, allspice, and salt. Add the flaxseed/chia eggs, milk, melted butter, agave, and rum extract to the dry ingredients and stir using a rubber spatula until just combined and evenly moist, yet thick. If the batter is too dry and isn't coming together, add more milk, 1 tablespoon at a time. Fold in the raisins.

4. Scrape the batter into the prepared loaf pan and spread it out evenly. Bake for 55 to 60 minutes, or until a toothpick inserted in the center comes out mostly clean.

5. Remove the bread from the oven and let it cool in the pan for about 20 minutes, then lift the bread from the pan and place on a cutting board. Slice and serve while still warm!

6. Store any leftover bread in an airtight container at room temperature for up to 4 days, in the refrigerator for up to 5 days, or in the freezer for up to 3 months.

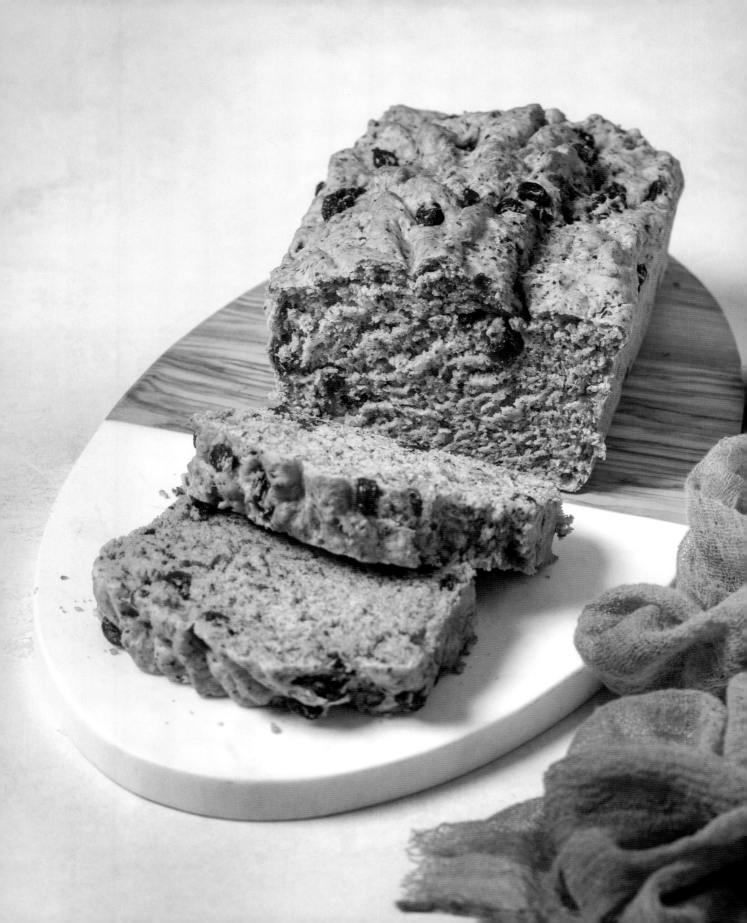

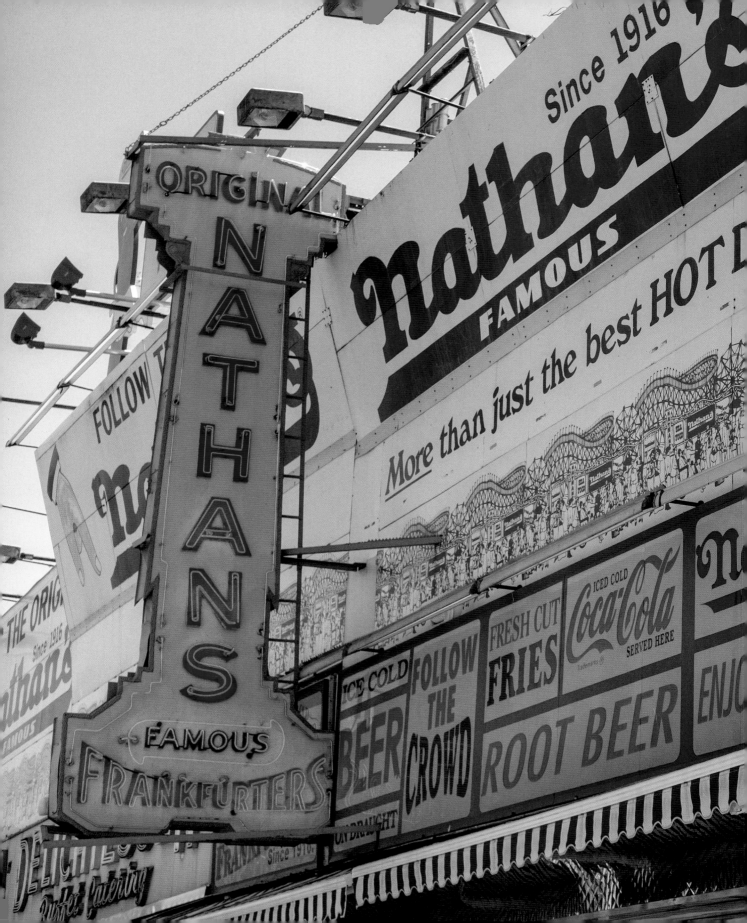

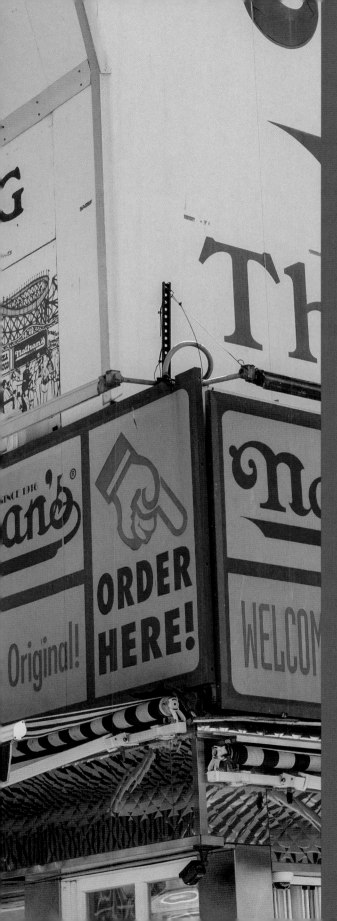

Chapter 7:

BITS & PIECES

Spicy Avocado
DEVILED EGGS

MAKES
24 deviled eggs

PREP TIME
15 minutes

COOK TIME
20 minutes

Deviled eggs were one of the first things I learned to make. I was in the fifth grade, and every day after school my best friend and I would go to my house and make deviled eggs for a quick snack before hanging out and doing homework. Of course, back then, I made them so simple and literally threw together mayonnaise with egg yolk and a big sprinkle of salt and pepper. Now, I like to experiment with deviled eggs and have come to enjoy them in so many ways, including this healthier version with avocado. These deviled eggs are a great reminder that not all foods associated with the South have to be unhealthy. Make these as a quick snack, as a way to change things up for breakfast, or as appetizers for your next gathering.

12 large eggs

Finely ground sea salt and ground black pepper

2 Hass avocados, pitted

3 tablespoons freshly squeezed lemon juice

2 cloves garlic, minced

1 tablespoon mayonnaise

1 tablespoon red pepper flakes, plus more for topping

½ teaspoon cayenne pepper

½ teaspoon hot sauce

Sliced scallions, for topping

1. Place the eggs in a pot large enough to fit them in a single layer. Add just enough water to cover the eggs, then add a dash of salt. Turn the heat to high and bring the water to a rolling boil. Boil for 8 to 10 minutes, then drain the eggs and place them in a large bowl with cold water and ice. Once the eggs are cool enough to handle, peel them.

2. Cut each egg in half lengthwise, then carefully remove the yolks and place them in a food processor; set the whites aside. Scoop the avocado flesh into the food processor, then add 1 teaspoon each of salt and pepper, the lemon juice, garlic, mayonnaise, red pepper flakes, cayenne, and hot sauce. Pulse until the yolk mixture is smooth.

3. Using a spoon, scoop the yolk mixture into the hard-boiled egg whites. (For a pretty presentation, pipe the mixture into the egg whites using a pastry bag fitted with a star tip.) Top with red pepper flakes and chopped scallions and serve. Leftovers can be stored in an airtight container in the refrigerator for up to 2 days.

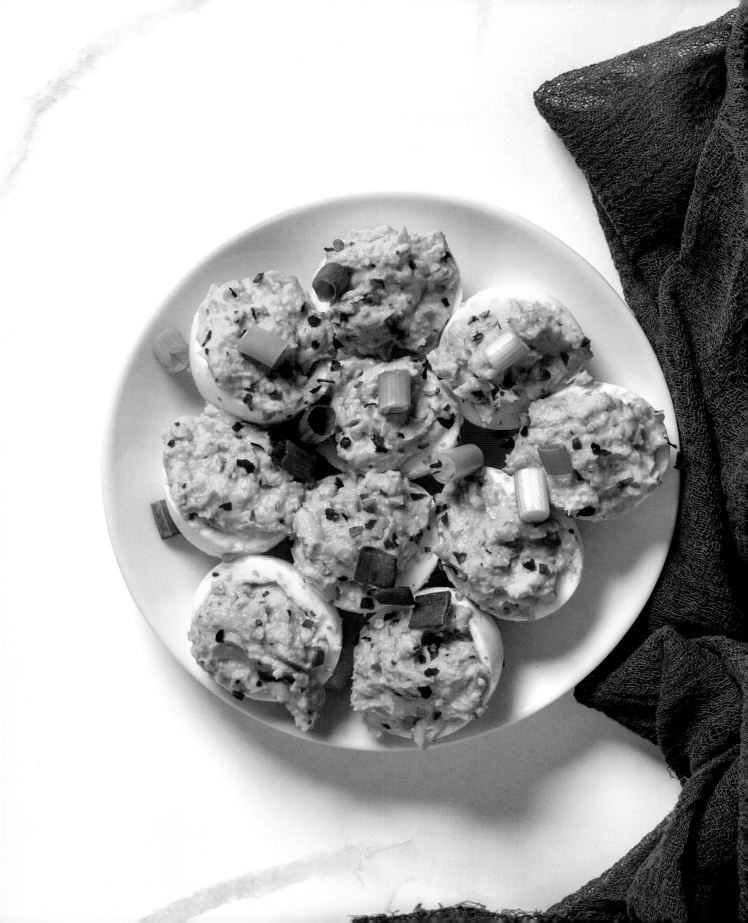

Dairy-Free
CRISPY BUFFALO CAULIFLOWER BITES

SERVES
4

PREP TIME
15 minutes

COOK TIME
40 minutes

I must admit that I am the one to take the first bite of this recipe as soon as it's finished, even in the middle of a photo shoot! I absolutely love spice, and this dish has a nice kick, so it's only right—right? As you may know, I eat meatless and dairy-free dishes a few times a week, and this recipe works perfectly for those days. The amazing thing about these bites is that you can substitute ingredients to modify them for your needs. To keep things simple, I use water as the base for the batter along with flour, seasonings, and Buffalo sauce; however, you can make the batter a little richer by substituting unsweetened almond milk for the water. To make the bites vegan, use the vegan version of my homemade BBQ sauce or a store-bought equivalent and either omit the honey used in the sauce or replace it with maple syrup or agave.

1¼ cups water

¾ cup all-purpose flour

1 cup plus 2 tablespoons dairy-free Buffalo wing sauce, divided (see Tip, opposite)

1 to 3 teaspoons red pepper flakes (see Tip, opposite)

1 teaspoon dried parsley, plus more for garnish if desired

1 teaspoon garlic powder

1 teaspoon smoked paprika

½ teaspoon finely ground sea salt

½ teaspoon ground black pepper

3 cups plain breadcrumbs

1 head cauliflower, chopped into medium-size florets

¼ cup raw honey

3 tablespoons BBQ sauce, homemade (page 50) or store-bought

1 tablespoon Sriracha sauce

FOR SERVING (OPTIONAL):

Vegan ranch dressing

Lemon wedges

1. Place an oven rack in the lower third of the oven and preheat the oven to 375°F. Line a sheet pan with parchment paper.

2. Make the batter: In a large bowl, whisk together the water, flour, 2 tablespoons of the Buffalo sauce, the red pepper flakes, parsley, garlic powder, smoked paprika, salt, and black pepper until fully combined. Set aside. Put the breadcrumbs in a medium-size bowl and set aside.

3. Dip a cauliflower floret into the batter, then shake off any excess and toss it into the breadcrumbs until well coated. Place on the prepared pan. Repeat until all the cauliflower florets are breaded, spacing them about an inch apart on the pan.

4. Bake on the lower rack of the oven for 25 to 30 minutes, or until golden brown and crunchy looking. If not crispy enough, turn the oven to the broil setting and broil for 5 to 10 minutes.

5. About 10 minutes before the cauliflower bites are done, make the sauce: Combine the remaining 1 cup of Buffalo sauce, the honey, BBQ sauce, and Sriracha in a medium-size saucepan over medium-high heat. Bring to a simmer, then lower the heat and continue to simmer for 2 to 3 minutes, until the sauce begins to thicken slightly. Remove the pan from the heat and let the sauce cool for 2 to 3 minutes.

6. Toss the cauliflower pieces in the sauce until fully coated. Turn the oven to the low broil setting and place the cauliflower back on the pan. Return the bites to the oven, placing the pan on the lower rack, until the sauce is fully baked onto the bites, 5 to 6 minutes.

7. To serve, garnish with more parsley and serve with ranch dressing and/or lemon wedges, if desired.

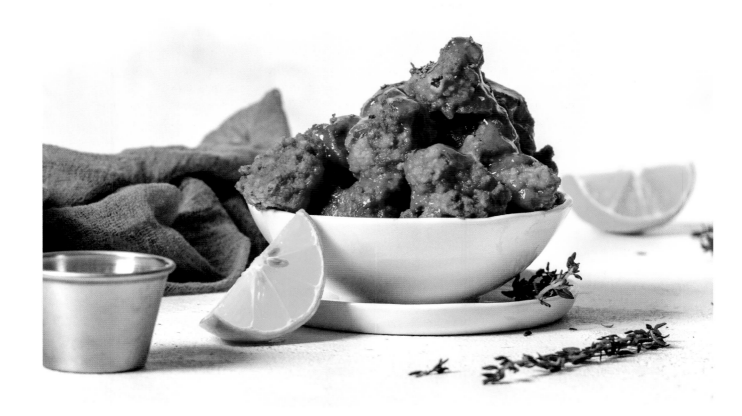

Tip: If you do not require this dish to be dairy-free, use any Buffalo sauce you like; my homemade version on page 54 works beautifully here.

Don't skip the step of lining the pan in Step 1; it's crucial in this recipe to prevent sticking.

To achieve maximum crispiness, add 1 cup of crushed cornflakes to the breadcrumbs and lightly spray the tops of the cauliflower bites with cooking oil before baking.

To make these bites vegan, use a vegan Buffalo sauce, such as Frank's RedHot Buffalo Wings Sauce, or the vegan version of my homemade BBQ sauce or a store-bought equivalent, and omit the honey or replace it with maple syrup or agave syrup.

As you've probably realized by now, I like my food with a lot of heat, so I typically use a full 3 teaspoons of red pepper flakes. Use 1 or 2 teaspoons if you don't like super spicy foods.

These bites are delicious on their own as an appetizer or side but are also great served atop salad, pasta, pizza, quinoa, or rice.

Jerk Sweet Potato Wedges

SERVES
8

PREP TIME
20 minutes,
plus 1 hour to
soak (optional)

COOK TIME
30 minutes

Growing up, I remember watching my grandfather whip together traditional Jamaican meals. He never forgot to add the pepper, and I mean the whole Scotch bonnet pepper. It brought such heat to his dishes, but it was always perfect—never too much. This simple recipe is sure to give your taste buds the same balance of flavors with a spicy kick that doesn't overwhelm, making it the perfect side dish for any gathering, whether it's a summertime BBQ, the weekly family meal, or anything in between. To ensure that these wedges are as crispy as possible, I suggest you soak them in water before roasting them. However, if you're in a rush, you can skip this optional step; the wedges will still be delicious, just not quite as crispy.

2 large sweet potatoes (about 1 pound), scrubbed and cut lengthwise into wedges

2 tablespoons arrowroot starch

2 tablespoons extra-virgin olive oil, plus more for the pans

2 tablespoons jerk seasoning, homemade (page 42) or store-bought

Dried parsley, for topping (optional)

1. Optional: To create the crispiest wedges possible, soak the sweet potato wedges in a bowl of cold water for 1 hour, then drain and rinse.

2. Place two oven racks in the upper part of the oven and preheat the oven to 450°F. Lightly grease two sheet pans with olive oil and place the pans in the oven until they are nice and hot.

3. Put the arrowroot starch in a large zip-top bag, then pat the sweet potato wedges dry and add them to the bag. Seal the bag and shake vigorously to evenly coat.

4. Remove the wedges from the bag, shaking off any excess starch, and transfer them to the preheated pans. Drizzle with the olive oil, then season with the jerk seasoning and toss to evenly coat. Spread the wedges out, leaving at least a ½-inch gap between them.

5. Bake the wedges for 20 minutes, then remove the pans from the oven and test the wedges with a fork. If they have started to become tender, flip them and then bake for another 5 to 10 minutes, or until fully tender and crisp. If they haven't become tender just yet, return the wedges to the oven for another 10 minutes before flipping them. Turn the oven off and leave the pans in the oven with the oven door slightly ajar for about 5 minutes, allowing the wedges to dry slightly.

6. Remove the wedges from the oven, sprinkle with parsley, if desired, and serve immediately.

Tip: The secret to getting the sweet potatoes super crispy is soaking the wedges in water for an hour. Soaking them draws out the excess starch and guarantees crispy edges. You can use this same technique for white potatoes, too.

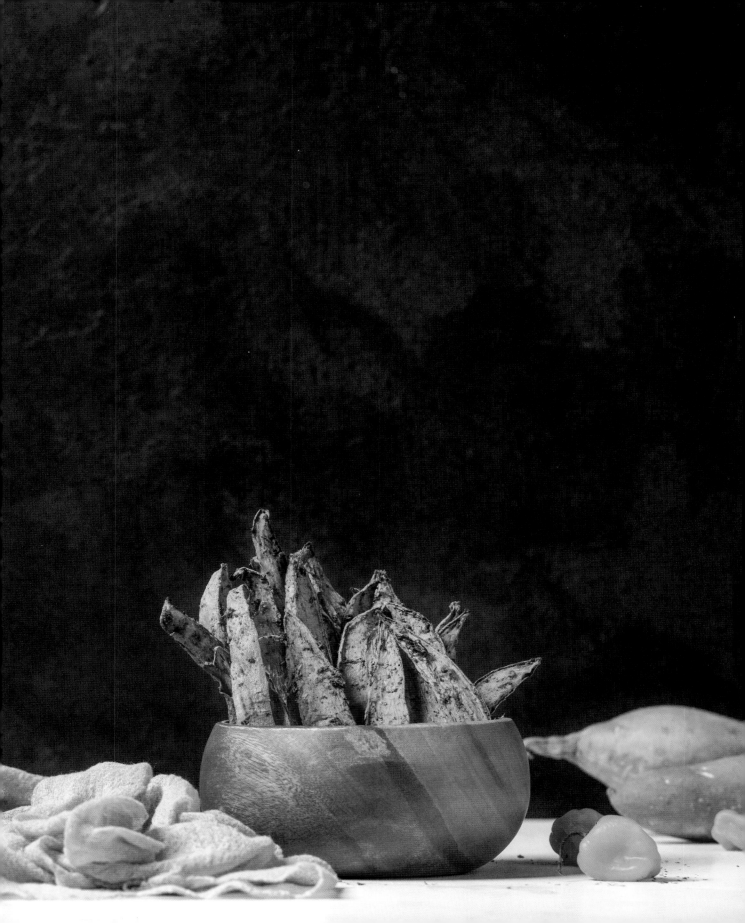

Crispy Lemon Pepper
SMASHED POTATOES WITH PESTO

SERVES
6

PREP TIME
15 minutes

COOK TIME
40 minutes

If I had a chance to choose my favorite potato recipe, it would have to be this one. I'm such a fan of lemon and black pepper together, so adding them to these potatoes was the best decision I've ever made. Whoever invented the method of smashing potatoes was a genius in my opinion because it creates the perfect texture—that sweet spot between mashed and whole potatoes. Smashing them also allows the edges to get ultra-crispy while the insides remain tender. To ensure that my potatoes are perfectly smashed and not too messy, I use baby potatoes, which makes them easier to eat. The flattened surface of baby potatoes is the perfect conveyor for all sorts of toppings, and they're small enough to be handheld. Top these potatoes with a delicious, easy pesto sauce, for example, and you have the perfect finger food! For a complete meal, add your favorite roasted veggies or a side of chicken or salmon and voilà!

SMASHED POTATOES:

1½ pounds baby red potatoes

1 tablespoon dried parsley

1 teaspoon finely ground sea salt

1½ teaspoons ground black pepper

¼ cup extra-virgin olive oil

1 tablespoon plus 1 teaspoon freshly squeezed lemon juice, divided

PESTO:

1 cup fresh basil leaves

¼ cup destemmed and chopped kale

3 tablespoons toasted pine nuts

1 clove garlic, peeled

¼ cup plus 2 tablespoons extra-virgin olive oil

3 teaspoons freshly squeezed lemon juice

Finely ground sea salt and ground black pepper, to taste

FOR GARNISH/SERVING (OPTIONAL):

Fresh thyme sprigs

Dried parsley

Lemon wedges or slices

1. Place an oven rack in the bottom position and preheat the oven to 425°F. Line a sheet pan with parchment paper.

2. Pour ½ inch of water into a large microwave-safe bowl. Add the potatoes to the bowl and cover with plastic wrap, poking the wrap a few times to vent. Microwave the potatoes until they are cooked through and tender, about 10 minutes.

3. Remove the wrap and drain the potatoes. Let cool slightly. Put the potatoes on the prepared pan, then season them with the parsley, salt, and pepper and drizzle with the olive oil and 1 tablespoon of the lemon juice. Toss to evenly coat. Spread the potatoes out on the pan and use the heel of your hand to smash them into flat rounds.

4. Place the pan on the bottom oven rack and roast the potatoes for 20 to 25 minutes, or until the bottoms have begun to crisp. Remove the pan from the oven, flip the potatoes, and roast for another 10 to 15 minutes, until both sides are crispy. Drizzle with the remaining teaspoon of lemon juice and set aside.

5. Make the pesto: Put all the ingredients in a food processor and blend until nearly smooth.

6. To serve, divide the smashed potatoes among six plates and top with the pesto. Garnish with thyme and parsley and serve with lemon wedges, if desired.

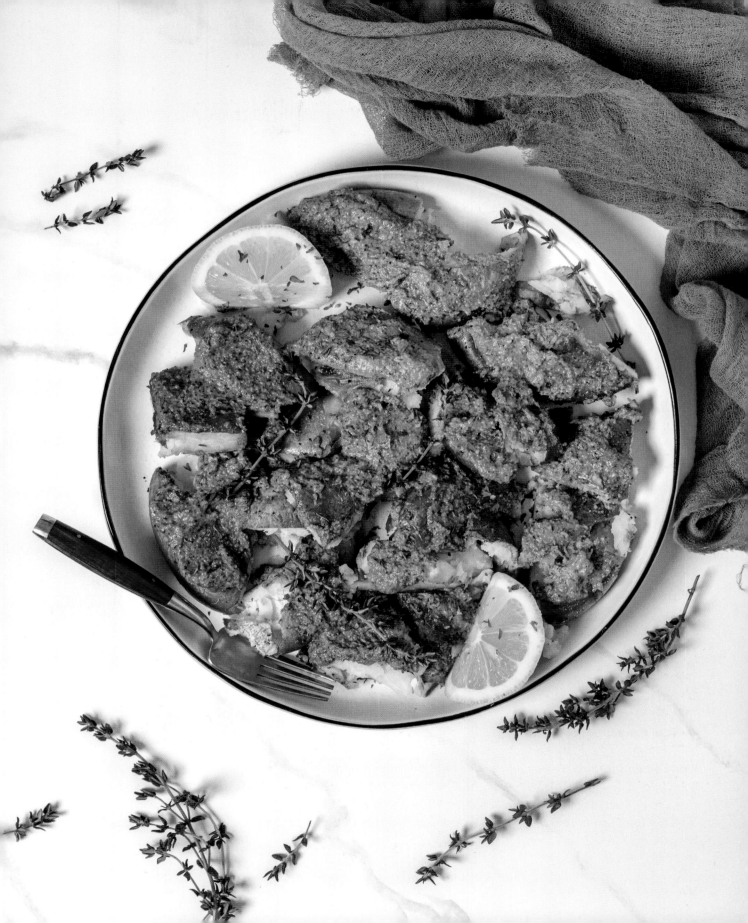

Spicy Vegan
JERK BBQ MEATBALLS

MAKES
12 meatballs

PREP TIME
10 minutes

COOK TIME
30 minutes

If you think spaghetti and meatballs is the only way to enjoy meatballs, then you are absolutely wrong. These little jerk BBQ bites are by far the most savory form of veggie meatballs I've made. I enjoy them as is or with a little dipping sauce, such as vegan garlic aioli or vegan ranch. Using a base of chickpeas, cooked quinoa, breadcrumbs, and a flaxseed egg, this flexible meatball recipe can be customized to suit your needs. A modified version makes an appearance in my Meatball Po' Boys on page 230.

MEATBALLS:

1 tablespoon extra-virgin olive oil

½ red onion, chopped

3 cloves garlic, minced

1 (15-ounce) can chickpeas, drained and rinsed

1 cup cooked red or tri-color quinoa (see page 58)

1 Flaxseed Egg (page 38)

½ cup plain breadcrumbs

¼ cup nutritional yeast

½ cup chopped pecans, toasted (see note, page 107)

1 teaspoon dried basil

1 teaspoon dried oregano leaves

1 teaspoon dried parsley

1 teaspoon red pepper flakes, plus more for garnish if desired

1 teaspoon smoked paprika

½ teaspoon finely ground sea salt

Pinch of ground black pepper

SPICY JERK BBQ SAUCE:

2 cups vegan jerk BBQ sauce, homemade (page 52) or store-bought

2 teaspoons red pepper flakes, plus more for garnish if desired

Sliced scallions, for topping (optional)

1. Preheat the oven to 400°F. Line a sheet pan with parchment paper.

2. Make the meatballs: Heat the olive oil in a medium-size skillet over medium-high heat. Once hot, add the onion and sauté for 3 minutes, or until translucent. Then add the garlic and sauté for an additional 30 seconds to 1 minute, until the garlic begins to become fragrant. Transfer the onion and garlic to a food processor.

3. To the food processor, add the remaining meatball ingredients and pulse until everything is broken down and well combined and holds together when pinched between your fingers. Taste and adjust the seasoning as you see fit.

4. Working with about 2 tablespoons of the meatball mixture at a time, use your hands to roll it into balls and place the meatballs on the prepared pan.

5. Bake the meatballs for 25 to 30 minutes, or until golden brown. Remove from the oven and set aside to cool for 2 to 3 minutes.

6. When the meatballs are nearly done, warm the jerk BBQ sauce and red pepper flakes in a medium-size saucepan over medium-high heat.

7. In a large heatproof bowl, toss the meatballs in the sauce until evenly coated. Serve immediately garnished with red pepper flakes and sliced scallions, if desired.

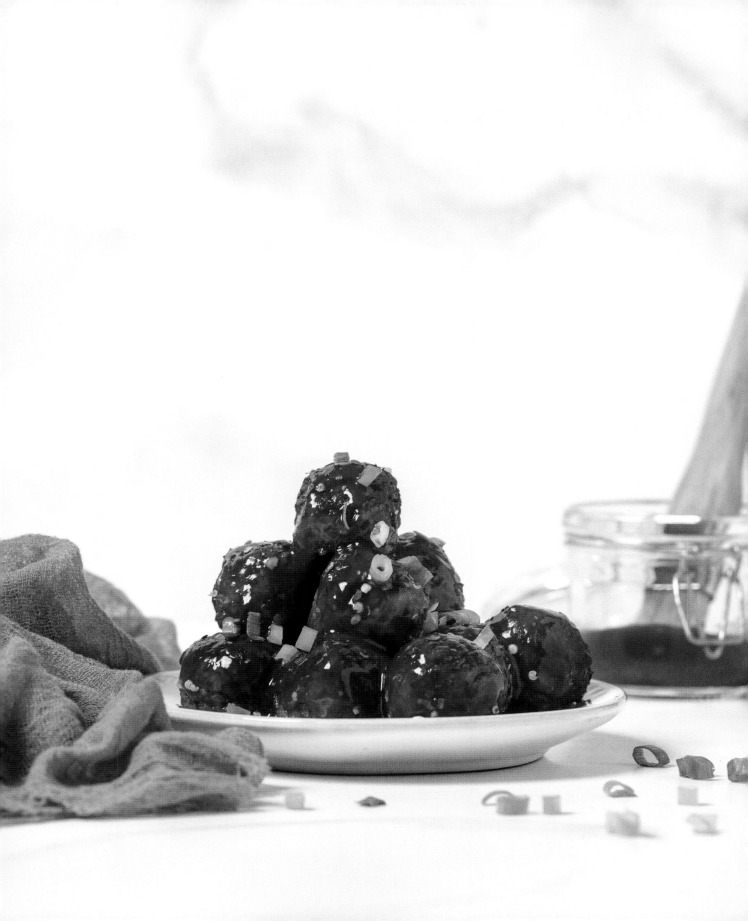

Baked Cajun
CARROT CHIPS

SERVES
4 to 6

PREP TIME
10 minutes

COOK TIME
20 minutes

These easy-to-make Cajun carrot chips are so delicious, and they are the perfect add-ins to so many meals. I love sprinkling them atop a salad in place of the usual roasted carrots, and I even enjoy them alongside a veggie burger or as a burger topping if I'm feeling fancy. For the best results, I purchase extra-large carrots to compensate for the inevitable shrinkage that will occur during baking—that way, I always end up with a nice-size chip! You'd be surprised at what a little extra seasoning can do to something as simple as sliced carrots.

4 extra-large carrots, peeled and thinly sliced

¼ cup extra-virgin olive oil

2 tablespoons Cajun seasoning, homemade (page 43) or store-bought

Dried parsley, for topping (optional)

1. Preheat the oven to 425°F. Line a sheet pan with parchment paper.

2. Put the carrot chips on the pan, then drizzle with the olive oil and season with the Cajun seasoning. Toss to coat. Arrange the chips in a single layer and bake for 12 to 15 minutes, until the edges begin to crisp. Remove the pan from the oven and flip the carrot chips. Return to the oven and continue to bake for another 5 to 8 minutes, until both sides are crisp.

3. Remove the carrot chips from the oven and allow to cool for 1 to 2 minutes. Top with parsley, if desired, and serve.

Tip: For crispy chips, the carrots have to be cut very thin. The best way to do this is to use a mandoline (which gives them a nice waffle cut, depending on the blade used), but you can also use a sharp knife. You can cut the chips on the diagonal to get a larger surface area.

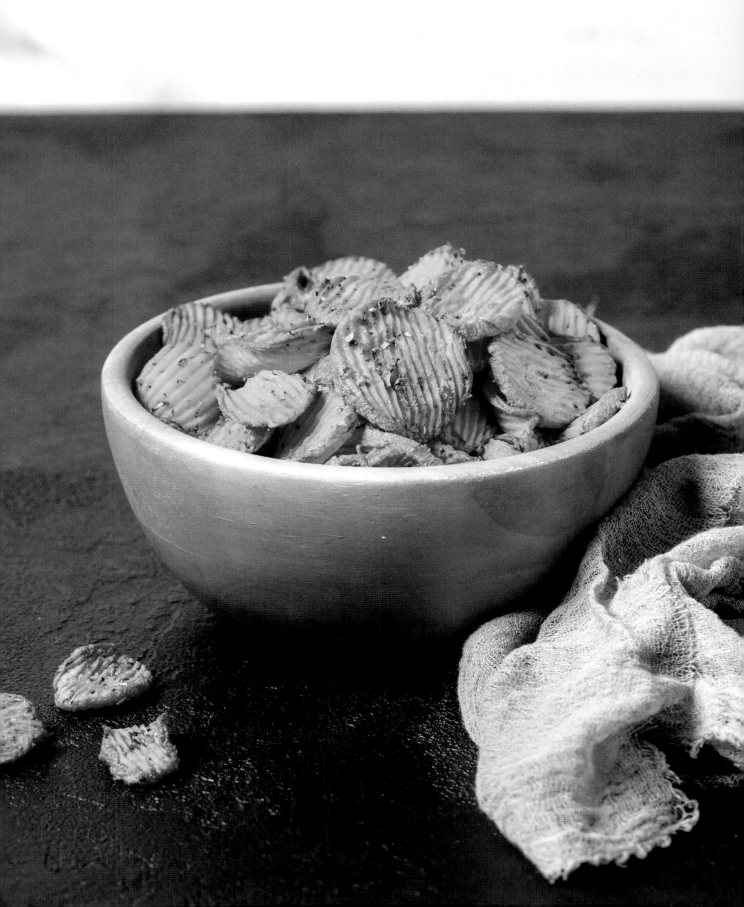

Mini Garlic-Herb
TOMATO GALETTES

MAKES
6 mini galettes

PREP TIME
20 minutes

COOK TIME
35 minutes

When it comes to mini handheld pies, galettes are my go-to. Typically, I enjoy making sweet pies; however, this savory garlic-herb-tomato recipe is incredible. These galettes can be topped with additional veggies to make them heartier and more plant-forward, such as broccoli, asparagus, kale, spinach, or Brussels sprouts. The best part is that this recipe uses my easy-to-make Everyday Pie Crust recipe on page 46 as the base; to make the process easier for yourself, you can even make the dough the day before.

2 cups grape tomatoes, halved

1 tablespoon extra-virgin olive oil

1 tablespoon dried parsley, plus more for sprinkling if desired

2 teaspoons garlic powder

1 teaspoon dried basil

1 teaspoon dried oregano leaves

1 teaspoon red pepper flakes

1 teaspoon smoked paprika

½ teaspoon finely ground sea salt, plus more for the tomatoes

½ teaspoon ground black pepper

1 recipe Everyday Pie Crust (page 46), made without cinnamon

Sesame seeds, for sprinkling (optional)

Fresh thyme sprigs, for topping (optional)

1. Preheat the oven to 425°F. Line a sheet pan with parchment paper.

2. Place the tomatoes cut side up on a sheet pan lined with paper towels. Sprinkle with salt and allow to sit for 15 minutes. This will draw out the excess moisture and keep your galettes crisp.

3. In a large mixing bowl, toss the tomatoes in the olive oil and seasonings until well coated. Let sit while you prepare the galettes.

4. Divide the pie crust dough into 6 equal parts and roll them out on a lightly floured surface. Aim for ½ inch thick and the best circle you can manage, though they don't have to be perfect! Transfer the dough circles to the prepared baking sheet, leaving at least 1 inch of space between them.

5. From the tomatoes, drain any liquid that has accumulated. Then scoop the tomatoes into the centers of the dough circles, leaving a 2- to 3-inch border. Fold the edges of the dough toward the center, overlapping if needed to create pleats, slightly covering the tomato filling. Make sure to leave the center of the filling exposed. Press the overlaps gently to seal the dough. If desired, sprinkle sesame seeds and parsley over the crusts.

6. Bake the galettes until the crusts are golden brown and the tomatoes are wilted, about 35 minutes. Remove from the oven and allow to cool for about 10 minutes before serving. Top with fresh thyme, if desired.

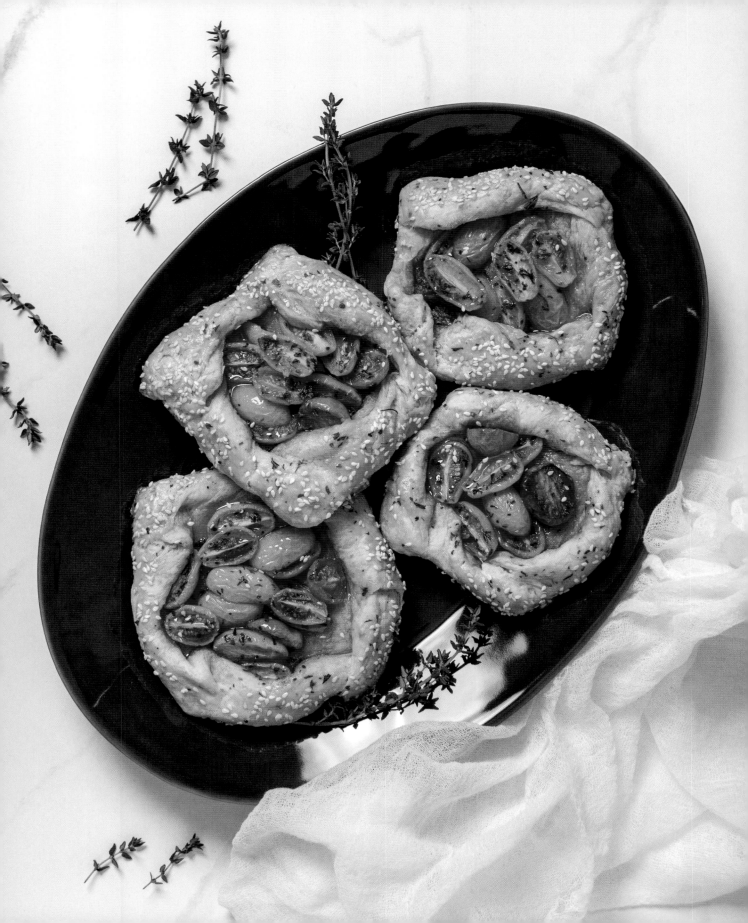

Creamy Cajun Pumpkin
MAC & "CHEESE"

SERVES
6

PREP TIME
10 minutes

COOK TIME
15 minutes

Growing up, I loved mac and cheese. Eating an entire bowl of the stuff was nothing for me. I remember going grocery shopping with my mom, pointing to that blue box of Kraft mac & cheese, especially the one with the broccoli, and always feeling lucky when she added it to our cart. In the South, mac and cheese is a staple at nearly every cookout or gathering, so how could I not be obsessed, right? This Cajun version is even more amazing, and while this recipe includes absolutely no dairy, it's just as creamy and melt-in-your-mouth good! But have you ever tried your mac and cheese with pumpkin flavor? It's truly the best combo and deserves to be your next bowl.

1 (8-ounce) box elbow macaroni

2 tablespoons vegan butter

2 cloves garlic, minced

¼ cup all-purpose flour

1¾ cups unsweetened, unflavored almond milk

1 cup canned pumpkin puree

1½ cups Vegan Cream Cheese Sauce (page 48)

2 tablespoons nutritional yeast

1 tablespoon Cajun seasoning, homemade (page 43) or store-bought

½ teaspoon mustard powder

1 teaspoon freshly squeezed lemon juice

TOPPINGS (OPTIONAL):

Chopped fresh cilantro or parsley

Toasted plain breadcrumbs

1. Bring a large pot of salted water to a boil. Add the macaroni and cook according to the package directions. When done, drain the macaroni well and set aside. Meanwhile, make the cheese sauce.

2. Heat the butter in a medium-size saucepan over medium-high heat. Once hot, add the garlic and sauté for 30 seconds to 1 minute, until the garlic begins to become fragrant. While constantly whisking, slowly add the flour until well incorporated and bubbly.

3. Reduce the heat to medium and slowly pour in the almond milk, whisking constantly to avoid clumps. Whisk in the pumpkin puree and allow the mixture to simmer for a bit until it becomes thick. Whisk in the cream cheese sauce, then add the nutritional yeast, Cajun seasoning, mustard powder, and lemon juice, whisking until combined.

4. Add the cooked macaroni to the sauce and stir to coat evenly. Remove the pan from the heat and spoon the mac and "cheese" into bowls. Top with fresh cilantro and toasted breadcrumbs, if desired. Serve immediately.

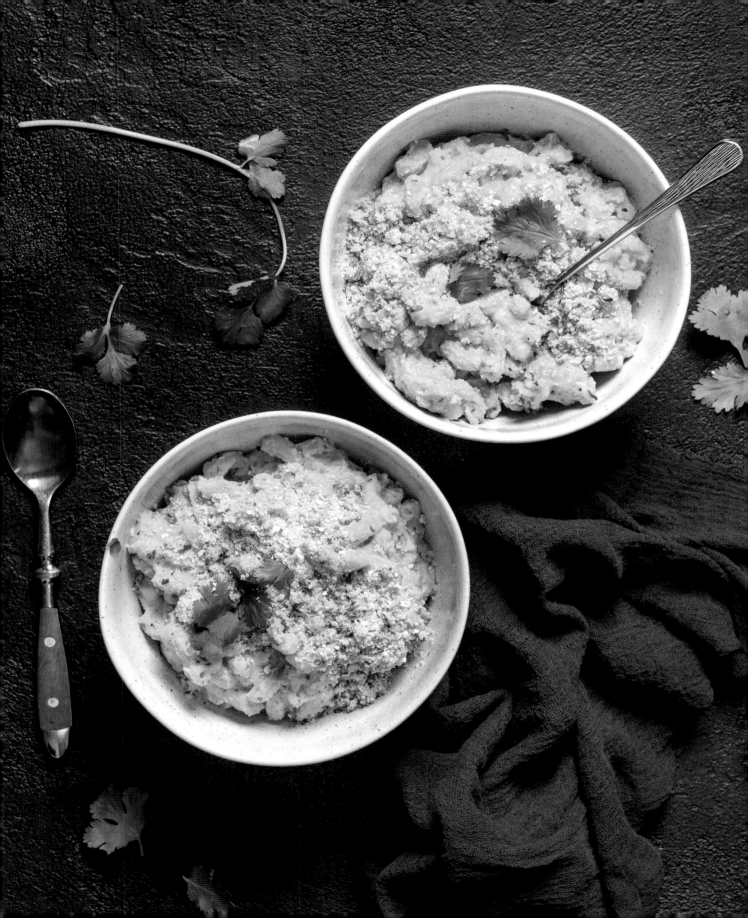

Hot Honey
SKILLET CORNBREAD

SERVES
12

PREP TIME
15 minutes

COOK TIME
30 minutes

At first glance, you might assume that this cornbread is spicy; however, it's not, or only barely so. If you aren't familiar with the flavor of hot honey, it's actually more honey sweet than spicy heat; therefore, it's a great option for the entire family. When I was growing up, it was unheard of for cornbread not to be on the menu for Sunday meals and holiday gatherings; you simply couldn't have a gathering of any sort without mac & cheese, collard greens, potato salad, mashed potatoes, and cornbread. My grandparents would make cornbread using Jiffy brand boxed corn muffin mix, which comes presweetened. That cornbread was one of only a handful of foods that I enjoyed as a picky eater. Some kids snack on cookies; I snacked on sweet cornbread! Not much has changed since then; however, I've grown to love making cornbread from scratch and adding different flavors to keep things interesting for my family. This hot honey version is definitely at the top of our list.

1½ cups medium-grind yellow cornmeal

1½ cups all-purpose flour

1 tablespoon baking powder

1 teaspoon finely ground sea salt

1 teaspoon dried parsley

½ teaspoon dried thyme leaves

½ teaspoon ground cinnamon

½ teaspoon smoked paprika

1½ cups unsweetened, unflavored almond milk

½ cup hot honey (see Tip)

6 tablespoons (¾ stick) unsalted butter, melted but not hot

2 large eggs, room temperature, beaten

TOPPINGS (OPTIONAL):

Sliced scallions

Hot honey

1. Preheat the oven to 400°F. Generously grease a 10-inch cast-iron or other ovenproof skillet and line the bottom with parchment paper. Set aside.

2. In a large mixing bowl, whisk together the cornmeal, flour, baking powder, salt, herbs, and spices until well combined.

3. Add the almond milk, hot honey, melted butter, and beaten eggs and stir with a rubber spatula until well incorporated and the batter becomes thick yet easy to stir. Pour the batter into the prepared skillet and spread it out evenly.

4. Bake for 25 to 30 minutes, or until a paring knife comes out clean when inserted in the middle. Remove the cornbread from the oven and let it cool for 10 to 15 minutes before slicing and serving. Top with scallions and hot honey, if desired.

VARIATION: Vegan Skillet Cornbread.
To make this bread vegan, substitute the same amount of agave syrup for the honey and add 2 to 3 tablespoons of Tabasco. In addition, use vegan butter in place of the dairy butter and replace the eggs with 1 Flaxseed Egg (page 38) or Chia Egg (page 39).

Tip: When it comes to hot honey, I am talking about spicy-hot honey, not temperature-hot honey. My favorite brand is Mike's Hot Honey, although there are other store-bought brands available. If you prefer making your own hot honey, you can simply mix together ½ cup of honey and 2 to 3 tablespoons of Tabasco, depending on the amount of heat (spiciness) preferred.

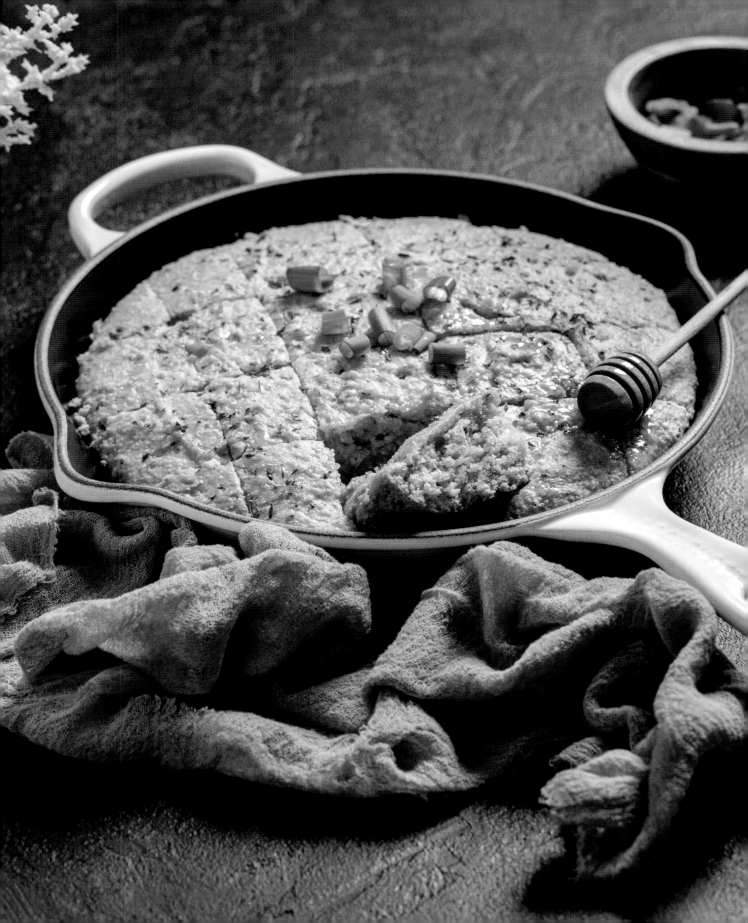

Southern
COLLARD GREENS

SERVES
8 to 10

PREP TIME
30 minutes

COOK TIME
about 3 hours

I've been a fan of collard greens for as long as I can remember. That's lucky for me because this dish is a Southern staple, and my Southern card would probably be revoked if I felt otherwise. This rendition is tender and silky and has a great balance of spicy and sweet—it's just delicious. Traditionally, collard greens are made with smoked turkey (usually necks) or smoked pork, such as ham hock or bacon. Using bacon gives you the option to lessen the amount of meat, slice by slice, and make the dish more plant-forward. Trust me, greens aren't hard to make; most of the work goes into the prepping. I love cooking these greens the old-school Southern way, simmering them for a few hours in a Dutch oven. A few stirs every 30 minutes or so is all it takes.

3 to 4 large bunches collard greens (about 6 pounds)

3 teaspoons apple cider vinegar, divided

1 tablespoon extra-virgin olive oil

1 pound bacon

½ medium red onion, chopped

2 cloves garlic, minced

1 teaspoon finely ground sea salt

1 teaspoon ground black pepper

1 teaspoon garlic powder

1 teaspoon red pepper flakes

1 teaspoon smoked paprika

¼ teaspoon ground mustard

2 cups low-sodium chicken stock

1 cup water

2 tablespoons firmly packed brown sugar

2 teaspoons Worcestershire sauce

1. Soak the collard greens in a large bowl of water with 1 teaspoon of the vinegar for 10 minutes to loosen the dirt and ensure that the greens are thoroughly clean, then rinse well. Roll the leaves tightly into cigar shapes—you can stack a couple of leaves to cut down on prep time—and, using a sharp chef's knife, cut them crosswise into ribbons; if desired, finely slice the remaining stems to be cooked along with the leaves. Alternatively, tear the leafy part away from the central rib into small to medium-size pieces, then finely chop some of the remaining stems/ribs or discard them. You should have 12 to 14 cups of sliced or torn collards. Set the greens aside.

2. Heat the olive oil in a 4-quart soup pot or Dutch oven over medium-high heat. Add the bacon, laying the slices flat across the bottom of the pot, and cook until slightly crisp, 2 to 3 minutes per side. Remove the bacon to a plate and set aside to cool a bit.

3. In the pot with the rendered bacon grease, sauté the onion and garlic until translucent and fragrant, 2 to 3 minutes. Add the salt and spices and stir until they are well distributed.

4. Roughly chop the bacon, then add it to the pot along with the collards, the remaining 2 teaspoons of vinegar, and the rest of the ingredients. Stir until fully combined and the greens begin to shrink and wilt. Cover and cook over medium-high heat until the liquid begins to boil, 4 to 5 minutes.

5. Reduce the heat to low and simmer, covered, for 2½ to 3 hours, stirring every 30 minutes or so. The greens are done once they are completely tender and most of the liquid has evaporated. Remove from the heat and add additional salt to taste if needed. Serve in bowls with some of the cooking liquid.

6. Store leftovers in an airtight container in the refrigerator for up to 5 days.

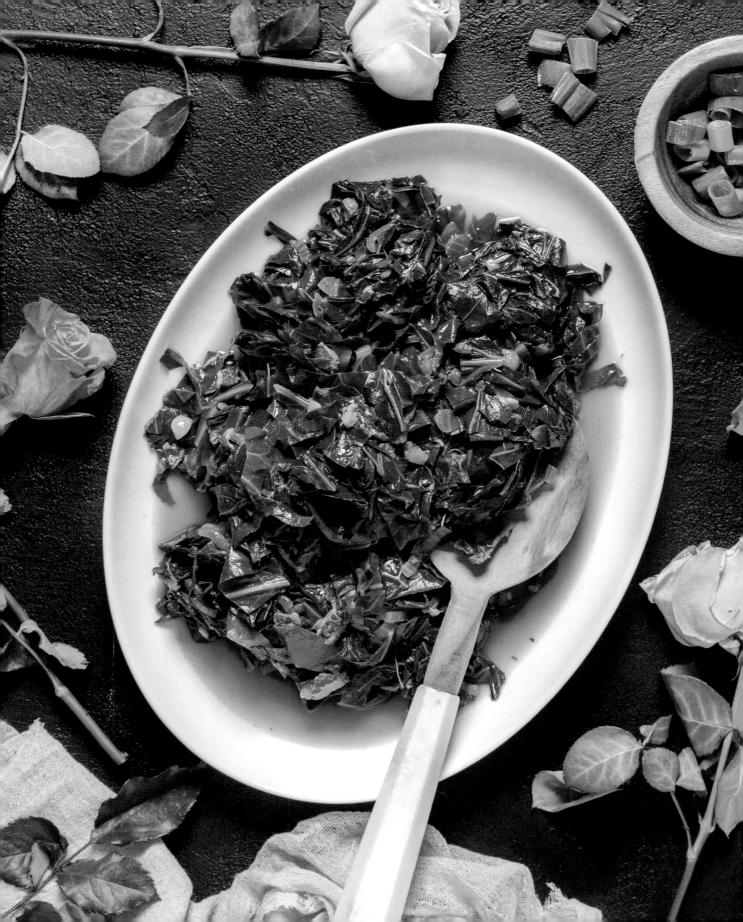

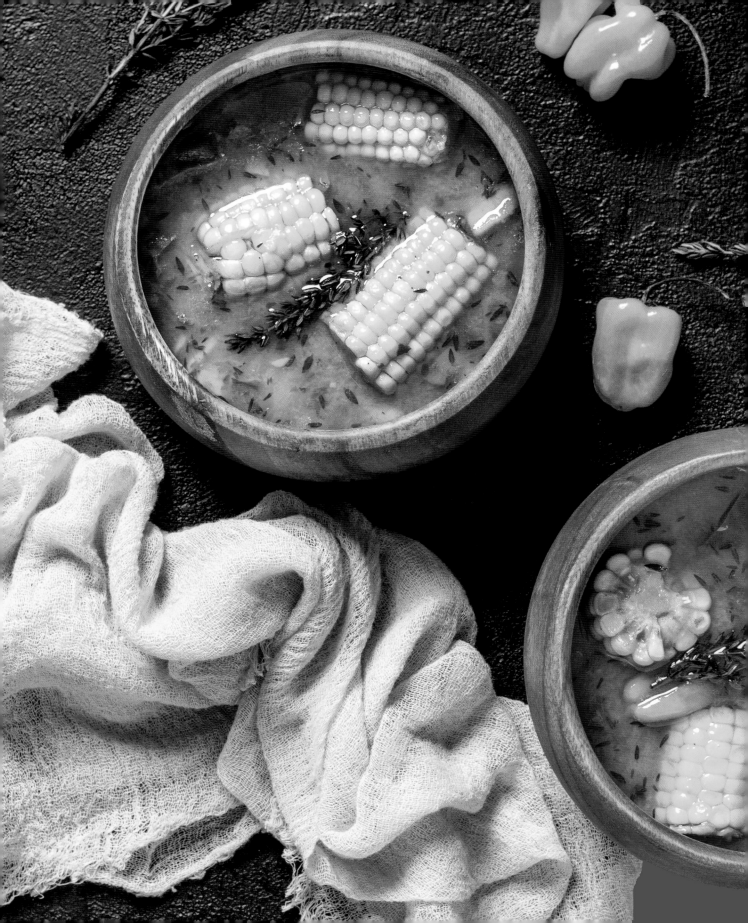

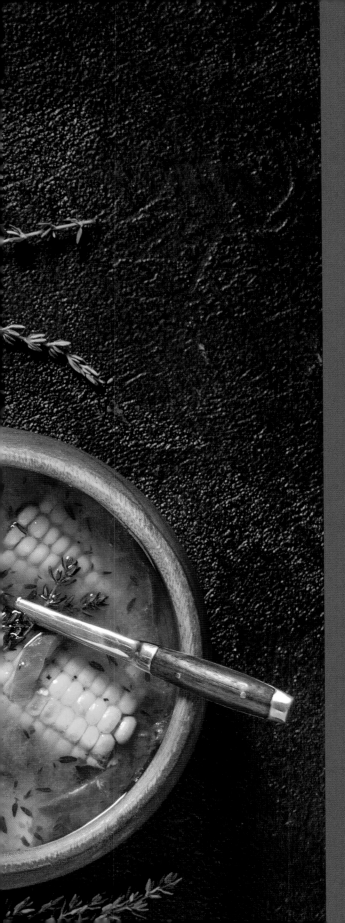

Chapter 8:

SOUPS & SALADS

Plant-Based
JAMAICAN "PEPPERPOT" SOUP

SERVES
4

PREP TIME
20 minutes

COOK TIME
30 minutes

Soup is a major part of Jamaican culture, and pepperpot soup in particular is a classic. Traditionally, Jamaican pepperpot soup consists of cooked callaloo, an ancient green leafy vegetable also known as amaranth, and dumplings, which can be found in many other Jamaican soups. Similar to spinach, callaloo has a strong flavor profile and is known for being a valuable source of iron, calcium, folate, vitamin C, and the list goes on. Traditional versions of the soup often include yellow yam, pig's tail, and shrimp; however, I chose to change things up by omitting the meat and using kale as a substitute for that beautiful green color of callaloo and Yukon Gold potatoes instead of yellow yams. I love a good spicy flavor, so the spice profile stays the same. I think you'll find this comforting, zesty soup is a great way to enjoy your greens.

DUMPLINGS:

2 cups all-purpose flour

1 teaspoon finely ground sea salt

1 teaspoon ground black pepper

1½ cups water

4 cups low-sodium vegetable stock

3 cups destemmed and chopped kale

2 celery stalks, chopped

2 large Yukon Gold potatoes, peeled and cubed

1 tablespoon red pepper flakes

1 teaspoon finely ground sea salt

1 teaspoon ground black pepper

1 Scotch bonnet or habanero pepper

1 cup canned full-fat coconut milk

1 bunch scallions, chopped

Fresh thyme sprigs, for garnish (optional)

MAKE THE DUMPLINGS:

1. Whisk together the flour, salt, and pepper in a large mixing bowl. Make a well in the center and pour in the water. Using a small metal spoon, work the water into the flour mixture until a stiff dough forms.

2. Divide the dough into 8 to 10 pieces, then roll each piece between your hands to create a long, thin dumpling between ¼ and ½ inch thick. Cover the dumplings with a damp cloth or paper towel and set aside.

MAKE THE SOUP:

3. Place the vegetable stock, kale, celery, potatoes, red pepper flakes, salt, and black pepper in a 4-quart soup pot or Dutch oven. Bring to a boil over medium-high heat, then cover and reduce the heat to a simmer; continue to simmer for 15 minutes, stirring occasionally, or until the potatoes are slightly tender.

4. Remove the lid and stir in the dumplings. Then place the Scotch bonnet pepper on top of the soup and cover the pot. Simmer for an additional 10 to 15 minutes, or until all the vegetables are tender and a toothpick or knife inserted in the center of a dumpling comes out clean. Remove and discard the Scotch bonnet.

5. Turn off the heat and stir in the coconut milk until completely incorporated, then stir in the scallions. Serve immediately in bowls and garnish with thyme sprigs, if desired.

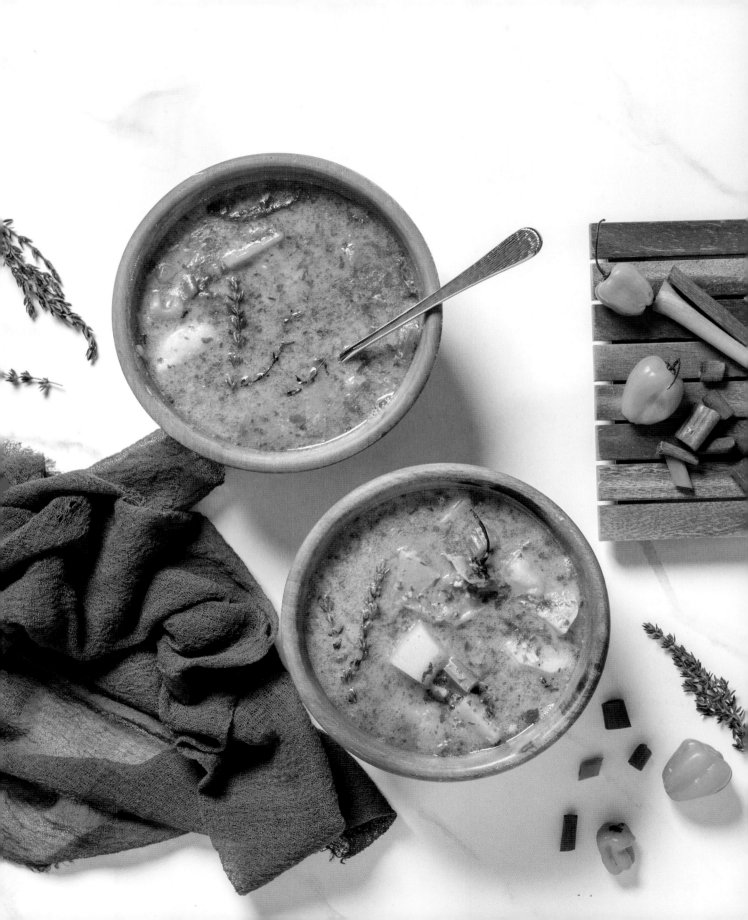

Hearty Quinoa
VEGGIE SOUP

SERVES
6

PREP TIME
10 minutes

COOK TIME
25 to 35 minutes

When it comes to soup, I'm a fan of loaded versions with a variety of veggies and spices. This quinoa soup is definitely one of my favorites to make for my family, right next to my popular Vegan Tuscan Kale Chickpea Soup (you can find the recipe on my blog, Orchids + Sweet Tea*). If you've never tried quinoa in soup, then you're missing out. It's so good! Just know that a small amount of quinoa goes a long way in this recipe, unless you want the consistency to be thicker. In just a half hour, you'll be enjoying a nice warm bowl of this soup, and you'll walk away filled and satisfied because of the burst of flavors. So grab a spoon and dig in!*

1 tablespoon extra-virgin olive oil

1 red onion, diced

1 yellow bell pepper, chopped

1 red bell pepper, chopped

1 carrot, sliced

1 celery stalk, chopped

2 cloves garlic, minced

1 teaspoon finely ground sea salt

2 teaspoons dried basil

1 teaspoon dried thyme leaves

1 tablespoon red pepper flakes

½ teaspoon ground black pepper

½ teaspoon turmeric powder (optional)

1 cup red or tri-color quinoa

4 cups low-sodium vegetable stock, plus more if needed

2 cups water

1 tablespoon freshly squeezed lemon juice

1 (15-ounce) can lima beans (aka butter beans) or Great Northern beans, drained and rinsed

1 cup destemmed and chopped kale

1. Heat the olive oil in a 4-quart soup pot or Dutch oven over medium-high heat. Once hot, add the vegetables and garlic and sauté until tender and translucent, 2 to 3 minutes, reducing the heat as needed so that the vegetables and garlic don't burn.

2. Once the vegetables are translucent, add the salt, herbs, and spices. Stir and sauté for an additional 30 seconds to heighten the flavor of the seasonings.

3. Stir in the quinoa, vegetable stock, water, lemon juice, beans, and kale. Bring to a boil, then cover, reduce the heat to a simmer, and cook for 20 to 30 minutes, stirring occasionally. After about 20 minutes, begin checking the thickness of the soup: if the quinoa is sufficiently tender and the soup is thickened to your liking, pull the pot off the heat; to allow the quinoa to swell further and create a thick soup, continue cooking for the full 30 minutes.

4. Taste the soup and add additional seasonings, if desired, or more stock if the soup has become thicker than you prefer. Ladle into bowls and enjoy!

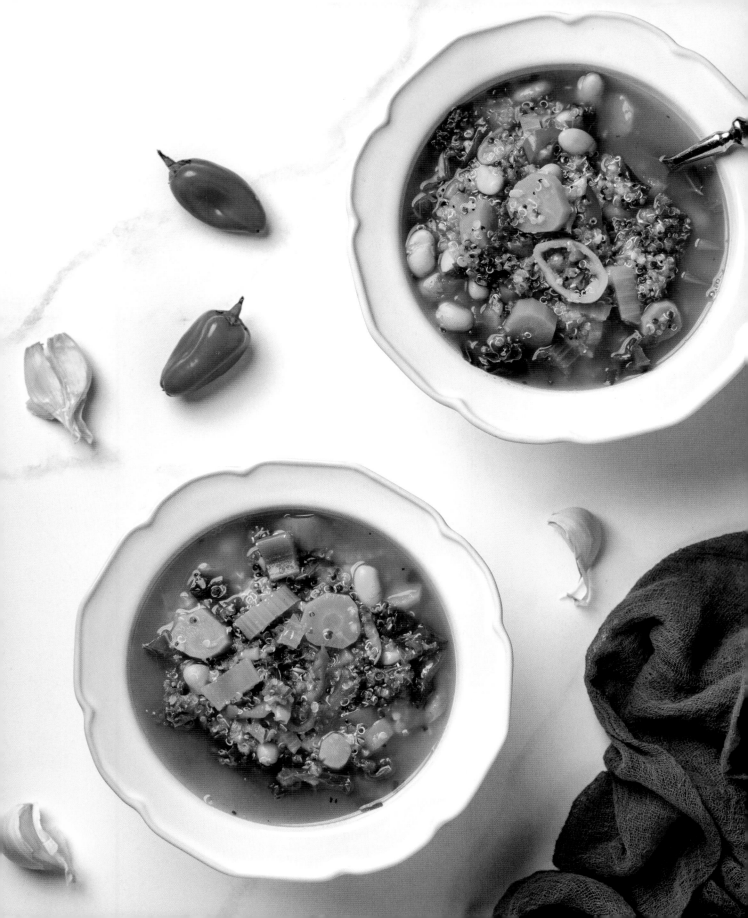

Jamaican Spiced CORN SOUP

SERVES
6

PREP TIME
10 minutes

COOK TIME
35 minutes

I have a great love for soups. Perhaps it stems from watching my Jamaican grandfather enjoy soup almost on a daily basis. Today, I often enjoy traditional Jamaican soups featuring goat, red kidney beans (called "peas" in Jamaican culture), pig's tails, chicken, chicken feet, beef, and, most recently, corn. Corn soup has become my "every-chance-I-get" bowl of goodness, especially when eating at my local Jamaican restaurant. This spicy corn soup is so easy to make, and you can adjust the heat level. Traditional recipes for Jamaican corn soup call for white potatoes (known as "Irish potatoes" in Jamaica), but my version uses sweet potatoes to offset the spicy flavor. If you prefer, you can mix and match your potatoes; substitute other veggies, like okra; or add dumplings (see page 180 for a recipe).

1 tablespoon extra-virgin olive oil

1 red onion, diced

1 green bell pepper, chopped

2 cloves garlic, minced

1 teaspoon cayenne pepper

½ teaspoon red pepper flakes

1 teaspoon dried parsley

1 teaspoon dried thyme leaves

1 teaspoon finely ground sea salt

2 sweet potatoes (about 12 ounces), peeled and cubed (see Tip)

2 ears of corn, cut into 2-inch pieces

4 cups low-sodium vegetable stock

2 cups water

2 Scotch bonnet or habanero peppers, slit on either side (see Tip)

1 (13.5-ounce) can full-fat coconut milk

Fresh thyme sprigs, for garnish (optional)

1. Heat the olive oil in a 4-quart soup pot or Dutch oven over medium-high heat, then add the red onion and bell pepper. Sauté, stirring occasionally, for 2 to 3 minutes, or until the onion is translucent. Reduce the heat if needed to prevent the vegetables from burning. Add the garlic, cayenne, red pepper flakes, parsley, thyme, and salt and sauté for an additional 30 seconds.

2. Put the sweet potatoes and corn in the pot, then pour in the vegetable stock and water and give the soup a quick stir. Bring the soup to a rolling boil, then reduce the heat to a simmer and add the Scotch bonnet peppers. Cover with a lid and simmer, stirring occasionally, for 30 minutes, or until the sweet potatoes and corn are tender.

3. Turn off the heat. To serve the soup rustic-style, leave the large pieces of corn on the cob in the soup for people to fish out and eat with their hands; otherwise, scoop out the pieces, cut the kernels off the cob, and return the kernels to the soup for added texture and sweetness in each spoonful! Stir in the coconut milk until the soup is creamy. Serve immediately in bowls and garnish with a sprig of thyme, if desired.

Tip: I usually add *whole* Scotch bonnet (or habanero) peppers, slit once or twice on both sides, to this soup to control the amount of heat distributed throughout. If you prefer your soup a bit less spicy, remove the seeds and pith from the peppers before adding them to the pot.

My preferred sweet potato for this recipe is the Japanese sweet potato. Its white flesh turns a pale yellow color when cooked and more closely mimics the white potatoes traditionally used in this soup while providing a touch of sweetness. But easy-to-find sweet potatoes with orange flesh are fine to use here as well.

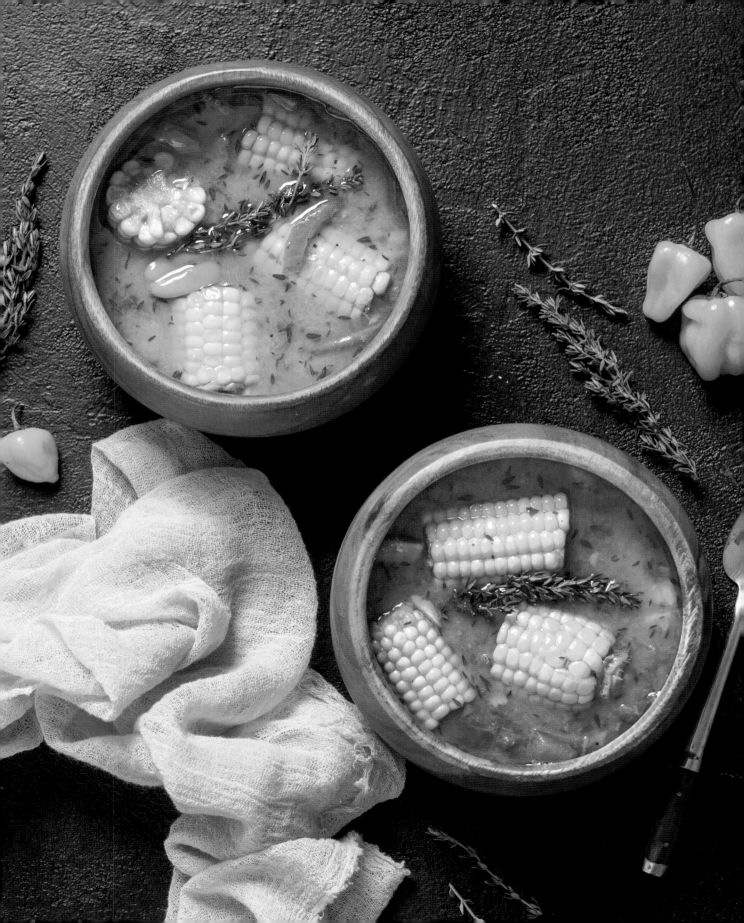

Creamy Tortellini Soup
WITH KALE & ROASTED GARLIC

SERVES
4

PREP TIME
15 minutes

COOK TIME
1 hour 5 minutes

Anytime I have an excuse to add pasta to my soup, I take it. I love hearty soups like this one that include a pasta of some sort and have a creamy base. And I'm not alone; most people find this sort of soup incredibly satisfying and irresistible, even the ones who say they aren't soup lovers. While I love all kinds of soup, whether creamy or broth-based, my husband is more of a fan of creamy ones. Therefore, this recipe is heavily influenced by his love for anything that includes Parmesan cheese and comes creamy with great bold flavor. And while this soup doesn't include meat, you really won't miss it.

ROASTED GARLIC:

3 heads garlic

1 teaspoon extra-virgin olive oil

Finely ground sea salt and ground black pepper

1 tablespoon extra-virgin olive oil

1 onion, chopped

1 tablespoon dried basil

1 tablespoon dried thyme leaves

½ teaspoon finely ground sea salt

½ teaspoon ground black pepper

4 cups low-sodium chicken stock

2 cups destemmed and chopped kale

1 (9-ounce) package four-cheese tortellini

1 cup grated Parmesan cheese

1 cup heavy cream

TOPPINGS (OPTIONAL):

Sliced scallions

Chopped fresh parsley or dried parsley

Grated Parmesan cheese

MAKE THE ROASTED GARLIC:

1. Preheat the oven to 350°F.

2. Place the heads of garlic on a cutting board and, using a sharp knife, slice the very top off of each head, just enough to expose the cloves. Place all 3 heads, cut side up, on a sheet of aluminum foil and pour 1 teaspoon of olive oil over the tops. Sprinkle with salt and pepper. Wrap the foil over the garlic heads, making a sealed pouch, and place on a sheet pan or in a small casserole dish.

3. Roast the garlic heads in the oven for 45 minutes, then remove and allow to cool completely. Once cooled, squeeze the roasted cloves from each head of garlic.

MAKE THE SOUP:

4. Heat 1 tablespoon of olive oil in a 4-quart soup pot or Dutch oven over medium-high heat. Add the onion and sauté, stirring frequently, until it begins to caramelize, about 10 minutes. Reduce the heat to medium-low, add the basil, thyme, salt, and pepper, and sauté for another 30 seconds to 1 minute. Turn off the heat.

5. If you have an immersion blender, add the chicken stock and roasted garlic cloves to the pot and use the immersion blender to blend the soup until smooth. If using a countertop blender, scrape the onion and herb mixture into the jar, then add the stock and garlic and blend until smooth. Return the blended soup to the pot.

6. Turn the heat back up to medium and, once at a simmer, add the kale and tortellini. Cover and simmer, stirring occasionally, for 10 minutes, or until the pasta is cooked through and the kale is wilted. Turn off the heat and stir in the heavy cream.

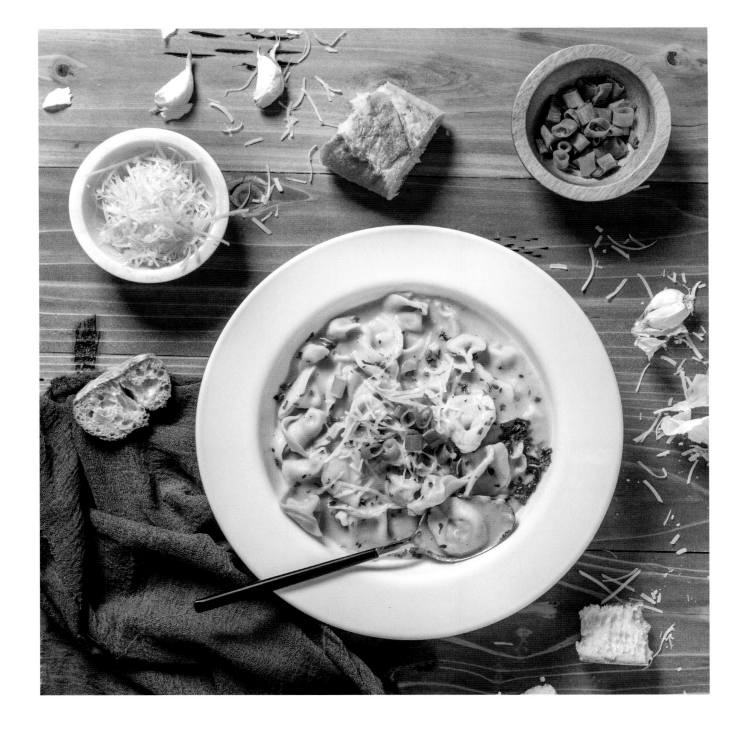

7. Taste and add salt and pepper if needed, then serve immediately in bowls. Top with sliced scallions, fresh or dried parsley, and Parmesan cheese, if desired.

Tip: The cooking time for this recipe is a bit longer than most of the soups in this chapter, but the majority is spent roasting the garlic, which can easily be done a day ahead to save yourself time when making the soup.

Cheesy Cauliflower
& WHITE BEAN SOUP

SERVES
4

PREP TIME
15 minutes

COOK TIME
45 minutes

If you love a rich, creamy, cheesy soup, then this recipe is for you! It makes a slightly thick soup, but you can easily thicken the consistency (if preferred) by reducing the amount of stock by about 1 cup. Using coconut cream instead of milk also helps to create a thicker soup. To give the soup an even bolder cheese flavor, I love to top each serving with extra shredded or shaved cheddar cheese. While cheesy soups like this are a favorite indulgence, I don't consistently consume dairy in large amounts; when I'm looking for nondairy "cheese" options, I enjoy using nutritional yeast as my vegan stand-in for an amazing cheesy flavor without the dairy. So, if you want to make this soup vegan, omit the cheese and add 3 to 4 tablespoons of nutritional yeast instead.

1 tablespoon extra-virgin olive oil

1 medium onion, chopped

1 teaspoon finely ground sea salt

1 teaspoon ground black pepper

1 teaspoon ground cumin

1 teaspoon red pepper flakes

1 teaspoon smoked paprika

½ teaspoon turmeric powder

1 teaspoon dried parsley, plus more for topping if desired

1 large head cauliflower, cut into florets

3 cups low-sodium vegetable stock

3 cups water

1 (15-ounce) can cannellini beans, drained and rinsed

1 cup canned coconut cream or full-fat coconut milk

2 cups shredded white cheddar cheese, plus more for topping if desired

1. Heat the olive oil in a 4-quart soup pot or a Dutch oven over medium-high heat, then add the onion and sauté for 2 to 3 minutes, or until translucent. Reduce the heat to medium-low and add the salt, spices, and parsley. Sauté the mixture for another 30 seconds to 1 minute to bloom the seasonings.

2. Add the cauliflower, stock, and water to the pot. Cover and bring to a boil, then reduce the heat to low and simmer for 15 minutes, or until the cauliflower is tender. Turn off the heat. If you have an immersion blender, use it to blend the soup until smooth. If using a countertop blender, transfer the contents of the pot to the blender and blend until smooth, then return to the pot. You may have to work in batches, depending on the size of your blender.

3. Return the heat to medium-high and stir in the cannellini beans. Cook until the soup is just heated through, then turn off the heat. Stir in the coconut cream until the soup is creamy. Fold in the cheese until it is distributed throughout the soup and has melted.

4. Season to taste with salt and pepper and serve immediately in bowls. Top with dried parsley and extra cheese, if desired.

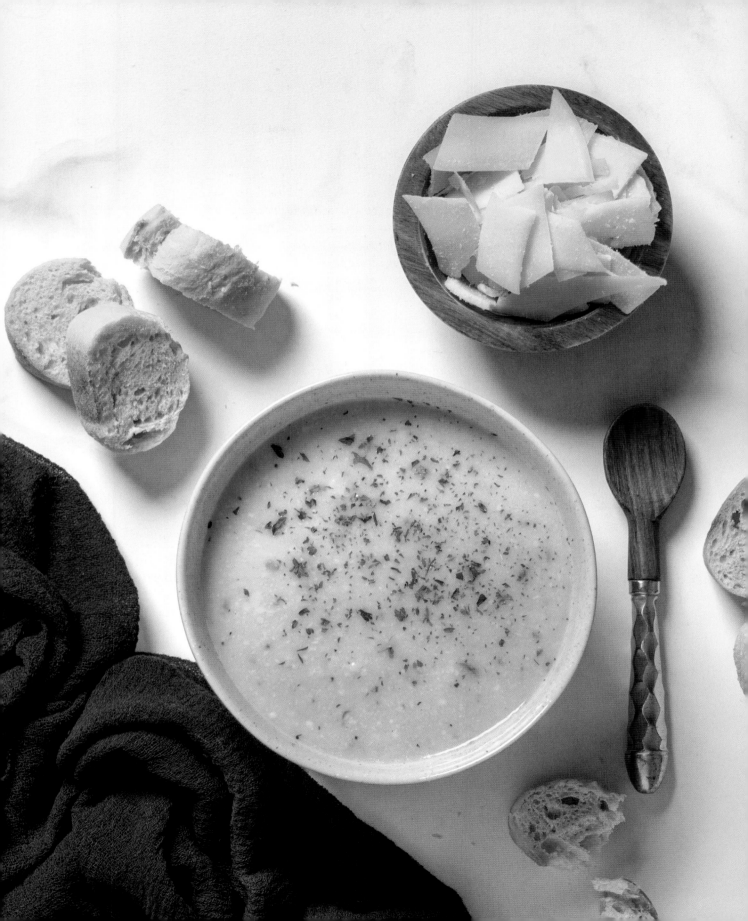

Creamy Cajun
ROASTED CORN, TOMATO & ARUGULA PASTA SALAD

SERVES
6

PREP TIME
15 minutes

COOK TIME
15 minutes

If I'm honest, eating salad wasn't something I was taught to do growing up. I often saw it as a side that might make its way onto your plate if you weren't already full from the rest of your meal. On my personal health journey, I've realized just how important plant foods are, so salad has naturally become an important part of how I eat. But just because salad is good for you doesn't mean it can't be delicious! The creamy Cajun sauce, which is entirely dairy-free and made from my go-to "cream cheese" sauce, makes this salad irresistible. The pasta bulks it up for a nice hearty feel, the roasted veggies add a "meaty" depth of flavor, and the arugula brings a bright burst of flavor, altogether putting this salad on par with comfort food. Of course, you can always load it with more veggies and even add a few pieces of shredded chicken if you're feeling the need for meat.

3 cups cherry tomatoes, halved

2 ears of corn, cut into 2-inch pieces

1 tablespoon extra-virgin olive oil

1 teaspoon finely ground sea salt

1 teaspoon ground black pepper

1 pound bow tie pasta

2 cups Vegan Cream Cheese Sauce (page 48)

2 tablespoons Cajun seasoning, homemade (page 43) or store-bought

6 cups arugula

1 cup crumbled feta cheese, for topping

1. Preheat the oven to 350°F.

2. Toss the halved tomatoes and pieces of corn in the olive oil and season with the salt and pepper. Spread the tomatoes and corn pieces on a sheet pan and roast for 10 to 15 minutes, until the tomatoes have begun to wilt and the corn to char. Set aside to cool.

3. While the tomatoes and corn are roasting, cook the pasta: Bring a large pot of salted water to a boil, then add the pasta and cook according to the package directions. Once done, drain the pasta and pour it into a large mixing bowl. Add the cream cheese sauce and Cajun seasoning and toss until evenly coated, then lightly mix in the arugula.

4. Spread the salad on a serving platter. Cut the kernels off of half of the charred pieces of corn, then add them to the salad along with the remaining pieces of corn and roasted tomatoes. Top with the feta and serve.

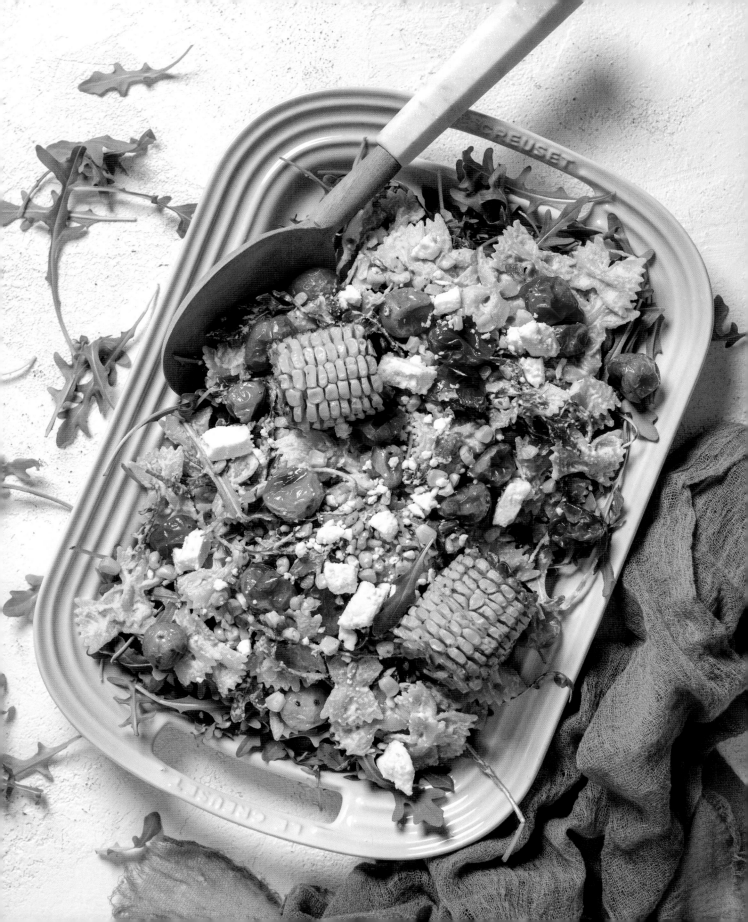

Roasted Jerk
BUTTERNUT SQUASH & VEGGIE SALAD

SERVES
6

PREP TIME
15 minutes

COOK TIME
40 minutes

When it comes to veggie salads, I'm such a huge fan these days! But I'm even more in love with veggie salads that highlight the flavors of Jamaican cooking. This recipe does just that via the jerk-seasoned and roasted butternut squash. The tomatoes, bell peppers, and red onion are roasted as well, which brings out their natural sugars, countering the heat of the jerk seasoning. This easy salad pays homage to the traditional jerk chicken salad through the same use of bold flavors and simple ingredients, but without the need for chicken. (Of course, you can always add some shredded jerk chicken if you like; see my recipe on page 60.) With this salad, you can choose a creamy dressing or something lighter, like a simple seasoned olive oil and vinegar dressing. Either way, you're sure to enjoy every bite.

4 cups peeled, seeded, and chopped butternut squash

2 tablespoons jerk seasoning, homemade (page 42) or store-bought

2 cups cherry tomatoes

1 red bell pepper, chopped

1 yellow bell pepper, chopped

1 medium red onion, chopped

1 tablespoon extra-virgin olive oil

1 teaspoon finely ground sea salt

1 teaspoon ground black pepper

6 cups spinach

2 cups crumbled feta cheese, for topping (optional)

Dressing of choice, for serving

1. Preheat the oven to 400°F.

2. In a medium-size mixing bowl, toss the butternut squash with the jerk seasoning, then transfer to a sheet pan. Add the tomatoes, bell peppers, and onion. Drizzle the olive oil over the vegetables and season with the salt and pepper. Roast the vegetables for 35 to 40 minutes, or until tender. Set aside to cool.

3. Once the roasted vegetables have cooled, transfer them to a large mixing bowl along with the spinach. Toss to combine and top with the feta, if desired. Serve immediately with the dressing of your choice.

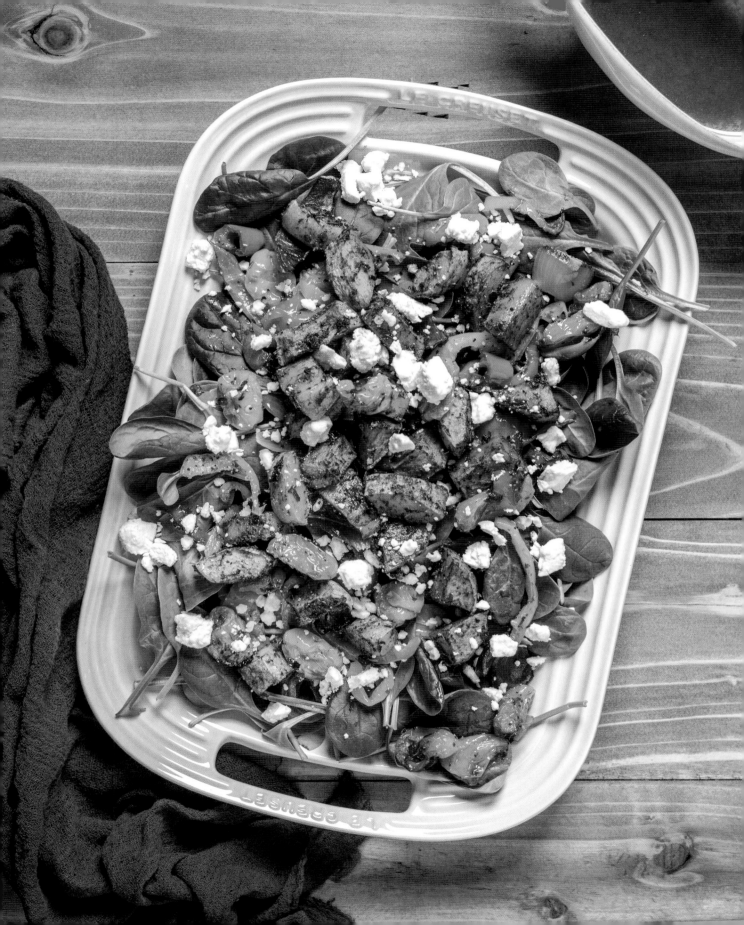

Roasted Vegetable
GREEN GODDESS SALAD

SERVES
6

PREP TIME
20 minutes

COOK TIME
40 minutes

My favorite thing about this salad has to be the green goddess dressing. I'm a huge fan of creamy salad dressings. Growing up, I was completely obsessed with Hidden Valley Ranch. I think it's safe to say that my all-time favorite dressing was ranch before I began reducing dairy. From time to time, I still enjoy a good creamy dressing, especially when the dressing is as bold in flavor as this one. Since I like just about everything spicy, I've added some chili pepper to my green goddess dressing, but feel free to omit it for a more traditional rendition. This roasted vegetable salad is the perfect choice for fall and winter, and the kale gives it a beautiful crunch.

2 medium-size russet potatoes, peeled and diced

2 cups grape tomatoes

1 red onion, chopped

4 carrots, peeled and cut in half lengthwise

1 teaspoon finely ground sea salt

1 teaspoon ground black pepper

1 teaspoon garlic powder

1 teaspoon smoked paprika

2 tablespoons extra-virgin olive oil

6 cups destemmed chopped kale

GREEN GODDESS DRESSING:

½ bunch fresh cilantro

½ bunch fresh parsley

1 cup plain full-fat Greek yogurt

2 scallions, roughly chopped

2 cloves garlic, smashed with the side of a knife

Juice of 1 lime

1 jalapeño pepper, seeded and roughly chopped

¼ cup extra-virgin olive oil

1 tablespoon white wine vinegar

Finely ground sea salt and ground black pepper

TOPPINGS:

Crumbled feta cheese

Pomegranate arils (optional)

ROAST THE VEGGIES:

1. Preheat the oven to 400°F.

2. Place the potatoes, tomatoes, onion, and carrots on a sheet pan. Season with the salt and spices, then drizzle with the olive oil. Toss the vegetables until evenly coated, then spread out on the pan. Roast for 35 to 40 minutes, or until tender. Remove from the oven and set aside to cool.

MAKE THE DRESSING:

3. Place all the ingredients in a blender or food processor and process until smooth. Chill until ready to serve.

ASSEMBLE THE SALAD:

4. To serve, spread out the kale evenly on a platter, then top with the cooled vegetables, dressing, feta, and, if desired, pomegranate arils.

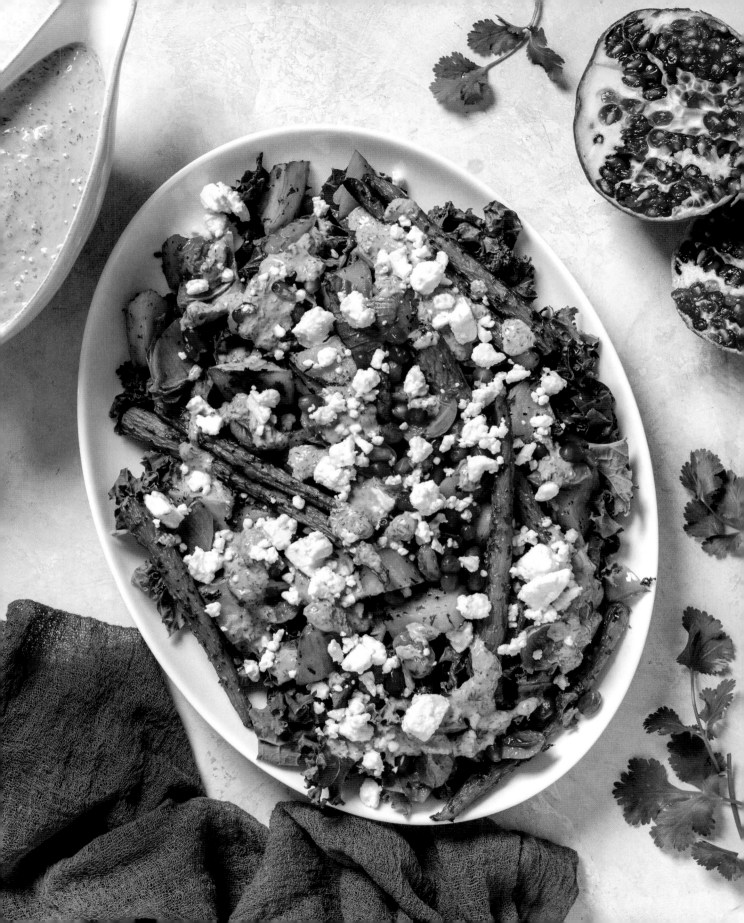

Jerk Shrimp
ASPARAGUS SALAD

SERVES
4

PREP TIME
10 minutes

COOK TIME
25 minutes

If you're looking for a light, flavorful salad, look no further. This recipe marries the bold, fresh flavors of tomato, feta, and asparagus with the spicy flavor of jerk shrimp. It's a match made in heaven, and once you've tried it, it's sure to become one of your staple salads. I enjoy making this salad as an appetizer for special gatherings or as a lunch salad served with toasted rustic bread. Plus, you can always replace the shrimp with chickpeas, chicken, or salmon for a twist!

1 bundle asparagus, tough ends removed

4 medium tomatoes, halved

2 tablespoons extra-virgin olive oil, divided

Finely ground sea salt and ground black pepper

2 tablespoons balsamic vinegar

1 teaspoon dried basil

½ teaspoon dried oregano leaves

8 ounces extra-large shrimp, peeled and deveined

2 tablespoons jerk seasoning, homemade (page 42) or store-bought

1 cup crumbled feta cheese

Fresh thyme sprigs, for topping (optional)

ROAST THE ASPARAGUS AND TOMATOES:

1. Preheat the oven to 425°F.

2. Toss the asparagus and halved tomatoes with 1 tablespoon of the olive oil along with 1 teaspoon each of salt and pepper, then spread out on a sheet pan. Roast for 9 to 12 minutes, or until the asparagus is tender. Remove from the oven and set aside to cool; reduce the oven temperature to 350°F.

MARINATE THE ROASTED TOMATOES:

3. In a small bowl, whisk together the vinegar, basil, and oregano, then season with salt and pepper to taste. Place the roasted tomatoes in a medium-size bowl and pour the vinegar mixture over the top. Gently toss to coat and set aside.

BAKE THE SHRIMP:

4. Put the shrimp, jerk seasoning, and remaining tablespoon of olive oil in a medium-size bowl and toss to coat. Spread the seasoned shrimp on a sheet pan and bake for 15 minutes, or until just cooked through—they will have become opaque and will be turning pink.

ASSEMBLE THE SALAD:

5. Arrange the roasted asparagus on four salad plates, then top with the marinated tomatoes, baked shrimp, and feta. Serve immediately with a sprig of fresh thyme, if desired.

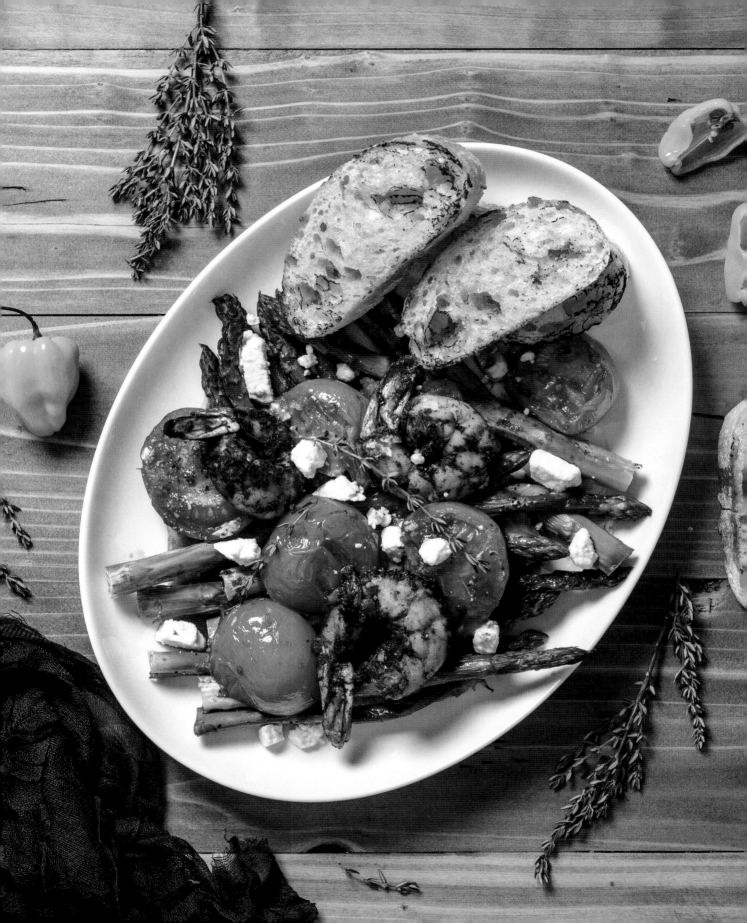

Buffalo Chickpea
KALE SALAD

SERVES
4

PREP TIME
10 minutes

COOK TIME
25 minutes

When it comes to anything spicy, I am completely locked in! My love for spicy food comes from my grandfather; I often watched him eat his Popeye's fried chicken with an entire Scotch bonnet pepper that he carried around in a plastic bag in case he needed it. While I have nowhere near his tolerance for chile heat, I do like to doctor most things—soup, meat, rice, tacos, and so on— with a dash (or two!) of hot sauce. That's why this salad is perfect for me. It has a great amount of spiciness from the Buffalo sauce that works amazingly well with fresh kale, and a creamy dressing helps offset the heat factor. It's simple and healthy yet flavorful—my entire motto, especially with plant-forward eating!

1 (15-ounce) can chickpeas, drained and rinsed

2 tablespoons extra-virgin olive oil, divided

1 cup cherry tomatoes, halved

1 teaspoon dried parsley

1 teaspoon red pepper flakes

1 teaspoon turmeric powder

½ teaspoon ground cumin

½ teaspoon garlic powder

Finely ground sea salt and ground black pepper

2 cups Buffalo sauce, homemade (page 54) or store-bought

1 bunch kale

TOPPINGS:

Creamy salad dressing of choice

Nuts of choice (optional)

1. Preheat the oven to 425°F and line a sheet pan with parchment paper.

2. Put the chickpeas in a medium-size bowl along with 1 tablespoon of the olive oil and toss until fully coated. In a separate bowl, toss the halved tomatoes with the remaining tablespoon of olive oil until fully coated. Place the coated chickpeas and tomatoes on the sheet pan, on opposite sides, and sprinkle the chickpeas with the parsley, red pepper flakes, turmeric, cumin, garlic powder, and 1 teaspoon each of salt and black pepper. Season the tomatoes with a pinch or two of salt and black pepper.

3. Bake the chickpeas and tomatoes for 10 minutes. Give the pan a good shake, then spoon the Buffalo sauce over the chickpeas and tomatoes until they're fully coated. Continue to bake until the sauce is fully baked onto the chickpeas, the chickpeas are crisp, and the tomatoes are slightly blistered around the edges and wilted, another 10 to 15 minutes.

4. Meanwhile, prep the kale: Remove the leaves from the stems, then rinse the leaves and chop them into bite-size pieces. Dress the kale with your favorite creamy dressing and toss until evenly coated.

5. Spread out the coated kale on a platter and top with the Buffalo chickpeas and tomatoes. Garnish with your favorite nuts, if desired. Serve immediately.

Tip: To make this salad dairy-free and vegan, use a vegan Buffalo sauce and salad dressing.

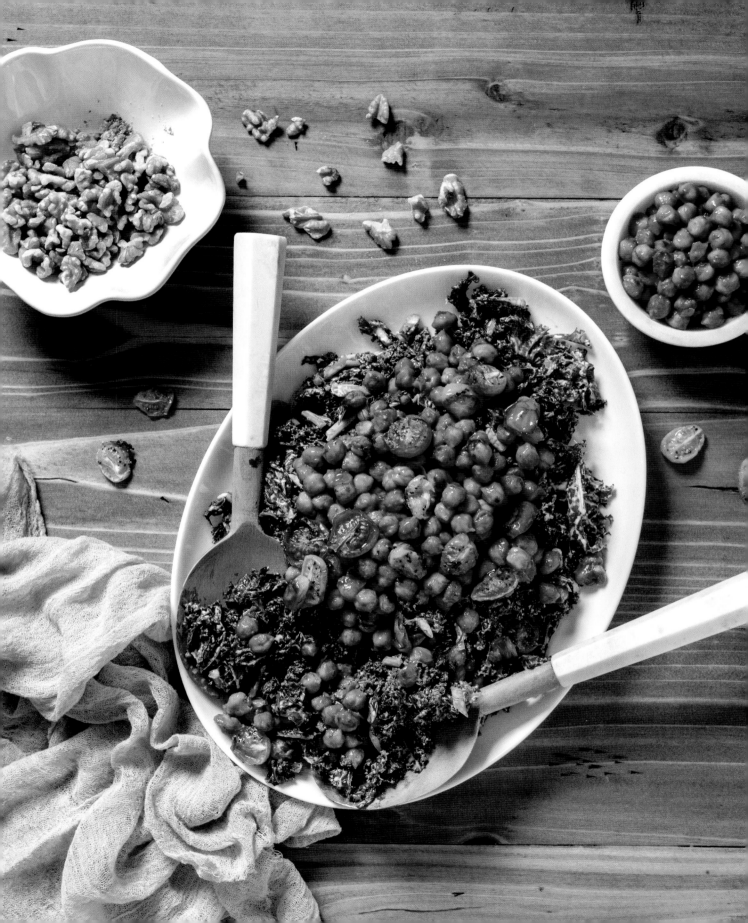

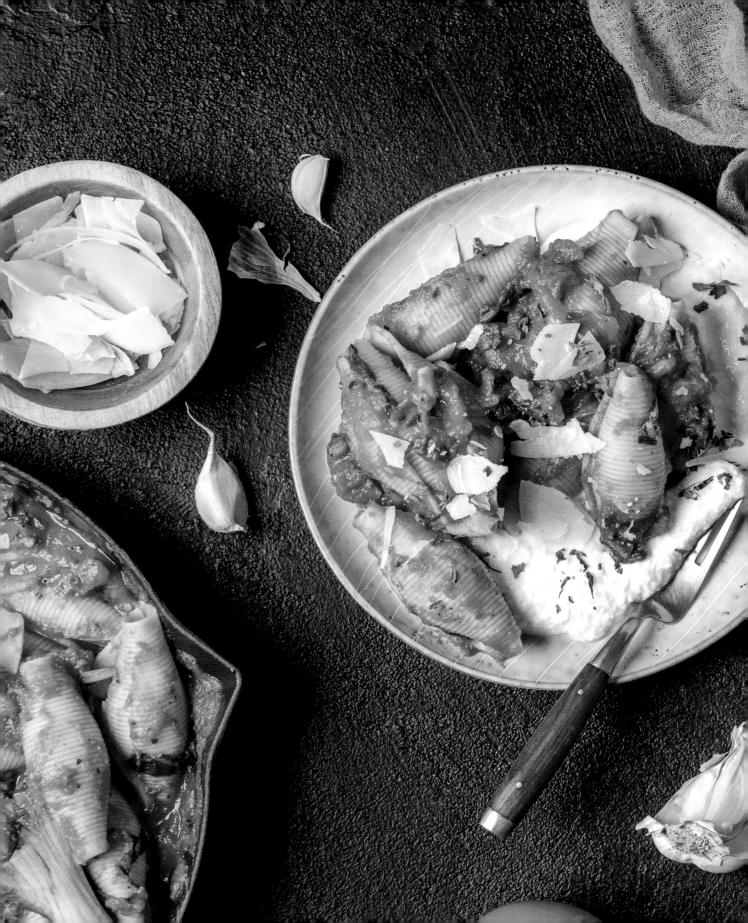

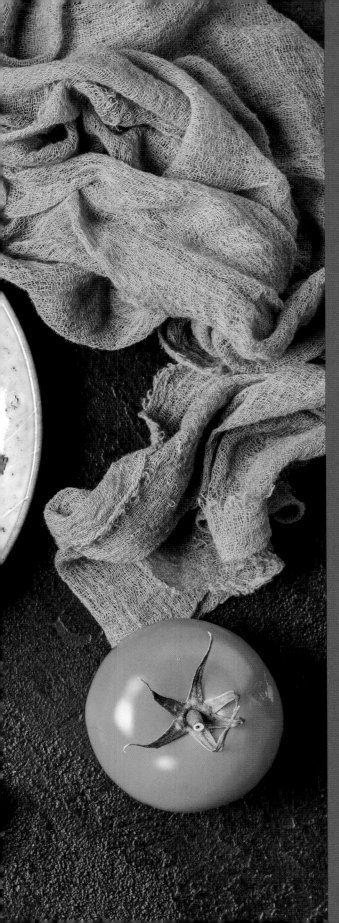

Chapter 9:

DELICIOUS DINNERS

Roasted Bean, Quinoa & SWEET POTATO TACOS

SERVES
3

PREP TIME
15 minutes

COOK TIME
30 minutes

Tacos are my favorite pastime. Taco Tuesdays are great, but it's tacos for me every day. After I began including more plant-based ingredients in my diet, I fell in love with bean and veggie tacos. I enjoy being able to mix and match ingredients, and with tacos, it's so easy to do. This recipe is a great option for enjoying a meatless night with your family, on Tuesdays or otherwise. The toppings can include diced tomatoes, sliced jalapeños, chopped fresh cilantro or parsley, Tabasco, a creamy dressing like ranch—you name it! I chose to use red beans in these tacos, but you can use anything you like here; my runners-up are chickpeas and black beans.

ROASTED RED BEANS:

1 (15-ounce) can small red beans, drained and rinsed

1 teaspoon finely ground sea salt

2 teaspoons garlic powder

2 teaspoons smoked paprika

1 teaspoon ground black pepper

½ teaspoon cayenne pepper

½ teaspoon ground cumin

1 teaspoon dried thyme leaves

1 teaspoon dried parsley

TACOS:

2 cups Simple Sweet Potato Mash (page 56)

1 teaspoon finely ground sea salt

1 teaspoon ground black pepper

2 cups cooked red or tri-color quinoa (see page 58)

2 cups guacamole, homemade (page 62) or store-bought

6 (5-inch) flour tortillas, charred or toasted (see note, page 91)

Lime wedges, for serving

Condiment or sauce of choice, for serving (optional)

1. Preheat the oven to 400°F. Line a sheet pan with parchment paper.

2. In a medium-size bowl, stir together the red beans and seasonings until well coated. Spread out the seasoned beans on the prepared sheet pan and roast for 15 to 20 minutes, tossing them midway through roasting, until browned and crisp.

3. While the beans are roasting, season the sweet potato mash with the salt and pepper and prepare the rest of the taco ingredients.

4. To assemble the tacos, place a spoonful of quinoa, seasoned sweet potato mash, roasted red beans, and guacamole in the center of a tortilla. Serve with lime wedges and the condiments of your choice, if desired.

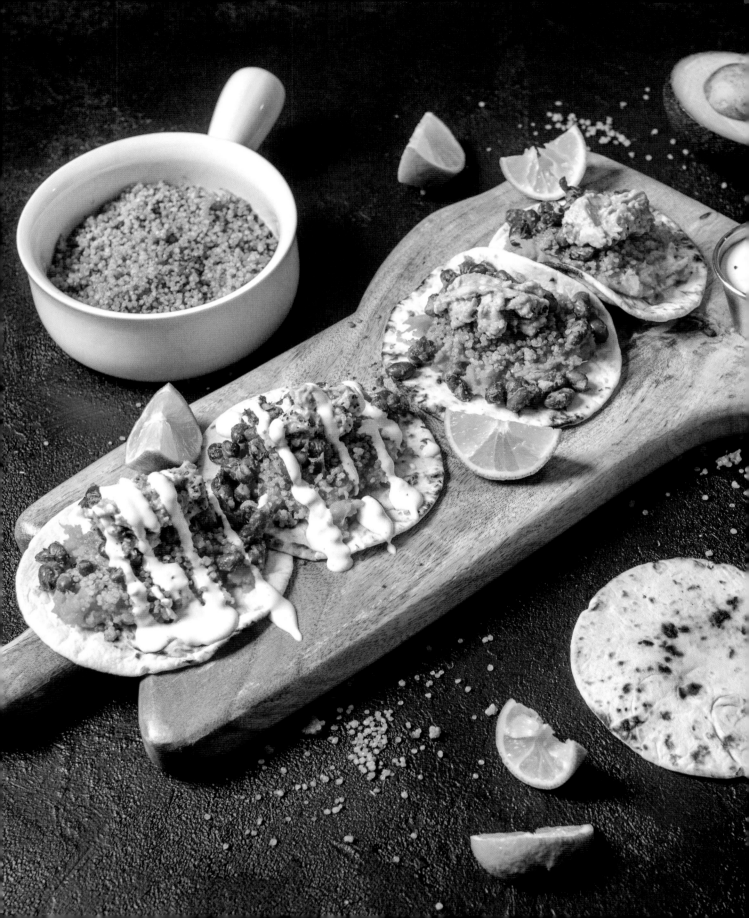

Buffalo Cauliflower Tacos

SERVES
3

PREP TIME
15 minutes

COOK TIME
20 minutes

Cauliflower bites are a staple in my house. They're incredibly versatile! I enjoy adding them to salads, using them to top pizza, waffles, or pancakes, and the list goes on. For this recipe, I wanted to create a taco that didn't include the typical ingredients like beans or rice, but had different elements of crunchiness, softness, and depths of flavor. I chose to add chopped red cabbage to add a nice crunch and freshness, which does a great job of offsetting the heat factor, as does the creamy guacamole, which is used as the base versus being an optional topping. To cool things down even further, opt for a creamy condiment like ranch dressing. Trust me, these tacos are so simple to make, but they are so amazing to eat!

BUFFALO CAULIFLOWER:

1 head cauliflower, chopped into medium florets

1 cup water

1 cup plus 2 tablespoons Buffalo sauce, homemade (page 54) or store-bought

¼ cup raw honey

3 tablespoons BBQ sauce, homemade (page 50) or store-bought

1 tablespoon Sriracha sauce

¾ cup all-purpose flour

1 tablespoon red pepper flakes

1 teaspoon garlic powder

1 teaspoon ground black pepper

1 teaspoon smoked paprika

1 teaspoon dried parsley, plus more for topping if desired

½ teaspoon finely ground sea salt

2 to 3 cups plain breadcrumbs

TACOS:

2 cups guacamole, homemade (page 62) or store-bought

2 cups shredded red cabbage

6 (5-inch) flour tortillas, charred or toasted (see note, page 91)

TOPPINGS (OPTIONAL):

Sliced scallions

Condiment or sauce of choice

MAKE THE BUFFALO CAULIFLOWER:

1. Preheat the oven to 450°F and line a sheet pan with parchment paper.

2. In a medium-size bowl, whisk together the water, 2 tablespoons of the Buffalo sauce, the honey, BBQ sauce, Sriracha, flour, red pepper flakes, garlic powder, black pepper, smoked paprika, parsley, and salt until fully combined. Put the breadcrumbs in a separate medium-size bowl.

3. Dip each cauliflower piece into the batter (shaking off any excess), then toss in the breadcrumbs until fully coated. Lay the cauliflower pieces side by side on the sheet pan about 1 inch apart.

4. Bake for 30 to 35 minutes, or until golden brown and "crunchy" looking. If not crispy enough, turn the oven to broil and broil for 5 to 10 minutes.

ASSEMBLE THE TACOS:

5. Place the guacamole and shredded cabbage in the center of the tortillas, then top with the crispy Buffalo bites. Top with scallions, parsley, and condiments or sauces of your choice, if desired. Serve immediately and enjoy!

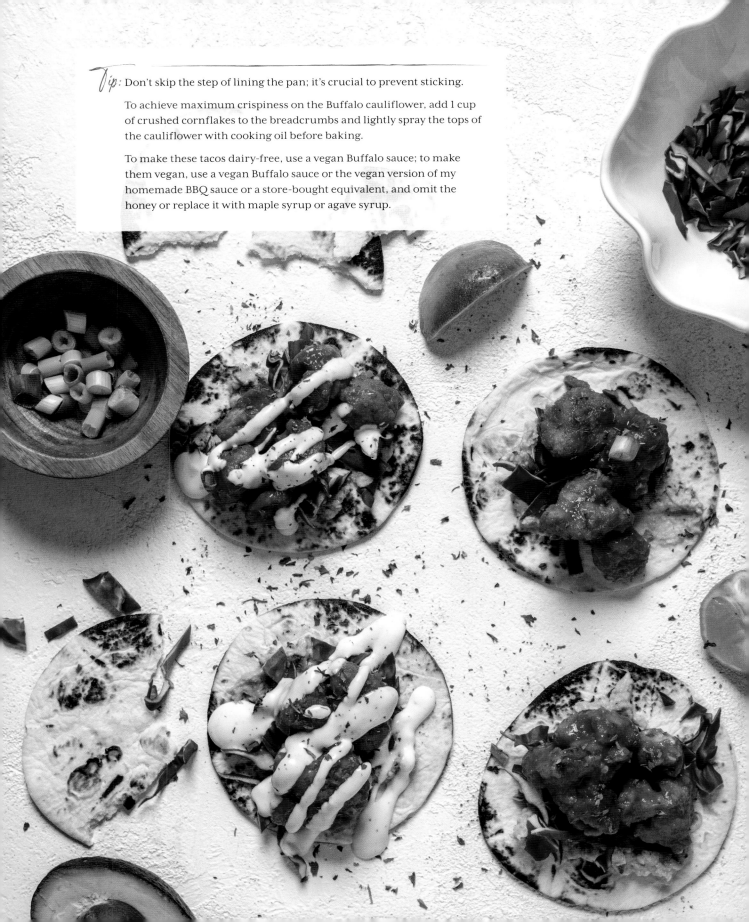

Tip: Don't skip the step of lining the pan; it's crucial to prevent sticking.

To achieve maximum crispiness on the Buffalo cauliflower, add 1 cup of crushed cornflakes to the breadcrumbs and lightly spray the tops of the cauliflower with cooking oil before baking.

To make these tacos dairy-free, use a vegan Buffalo sauce; to make them vegan, use a vegan Buffalo sauce or the vegan version of my homemade BBQ sauce or a store-bought equivalent, and omit the honey or replace it with maple syrup or agave syrup.

Jerk BBQ CHICKEN & VEGGIE PIZZA

SERVES
6

PREP TIME
15 minutes

COOK TIME
25 minutes

This pizza is one of the best examples of taking a traditional staple—in this case Jamaican jerk chicken—and using it to create something entirely new and phenomenal. To keep with the jerk theme, I've chosen to use a spicy-sweet jerk BBQ sauce instead of a traditional pizza sauce, which is then topped with mozzarella cheese, bell peppers, onions, broccolini, and shredded jerk chicken. It's bursting with spicy, sweet, and savory flavors, and it's just too delicious not to try. To make this pizza super quick and easy to whip together on the day you eat it, I recommend making the dough, jerk BBQ sauce, and jerk chicken the day before. You can even sauté the broccolini a day ahead if you like.

2 tablespoons extra-virgin olive oil, divided, plus more for the crust

2 cups chopped broccolini

½ teaspoon finely ground sea salt

½ teaspoon ground black pepper

1 recipe Easy Pizza Dough (page 44), or 1 (12-ounce) package pizza dough

1 cup jerk BBQ sauce, homemade (page 52) or store-bought, plus more for topping if desired

2 cups shredded low-moisture mozzarella cheese

2 medium bell peppers (any color), sliced

½ medium onion, sliced

2 cups Shredded Jerk Chicken (page 60)

TOPPINGS (OPTIONAL):

Sliced scallions

Dried parsley

1. Prepare the broccolini: Heat 1 tablespoon of the olive oil in a medium-size skillet over medium-high heat, then add the broccolini and sauté until tender and slightly charred, 4 to 5 minutes. Season with the salt and black pepper, then remove the broccolini from the pan and set aside.

2. If the pizza dough has been refrigerated, place it on the counter and let it come to room temperature for at least 1 hour.

3. Once the dough is ready to roll out, place an oven rack in the middle of the oven and preheat the oven to 475°F. Grease a pizza pan or baking sheet (preferably one with air holes) with the remaining tablespoon of olive oil.

4. Lightly flour a work surface and place the dough on it. Using a rolling pin, gently roll out the dough into a circle about ½ inch thick. Using your hands, work the dough into a larger circle about 11 inches in diameter. Transfer the dough to the prepared pan. Using your hands, begin lightly working the dough, evenly pressing it and flattening it out to about 12 inches in diameter, then pinch the edges together to form the crust.

5. Spoon a generous amount of the jerk BBQ sauce into the center of the crust and spread it out thinly, leaving a 1-inch border. Sprinkle on the cheese, then top with the remaining ingredients, except for the scallions and parsley, ensuring that the chicken is on top. Lightly brush the edge of the crust with olive oil to ensure that it turns a nice golden brown.

6. Bake for 15 to 20 minutes, until the cheese is melted and bubbly and the crust is golden brown. Remove from the oven and let cool for 5 minutes before slicing with a pizza cutter. Top with scallions, parsley, and/or a drizzle of jerk BBQ sauce, if desired.

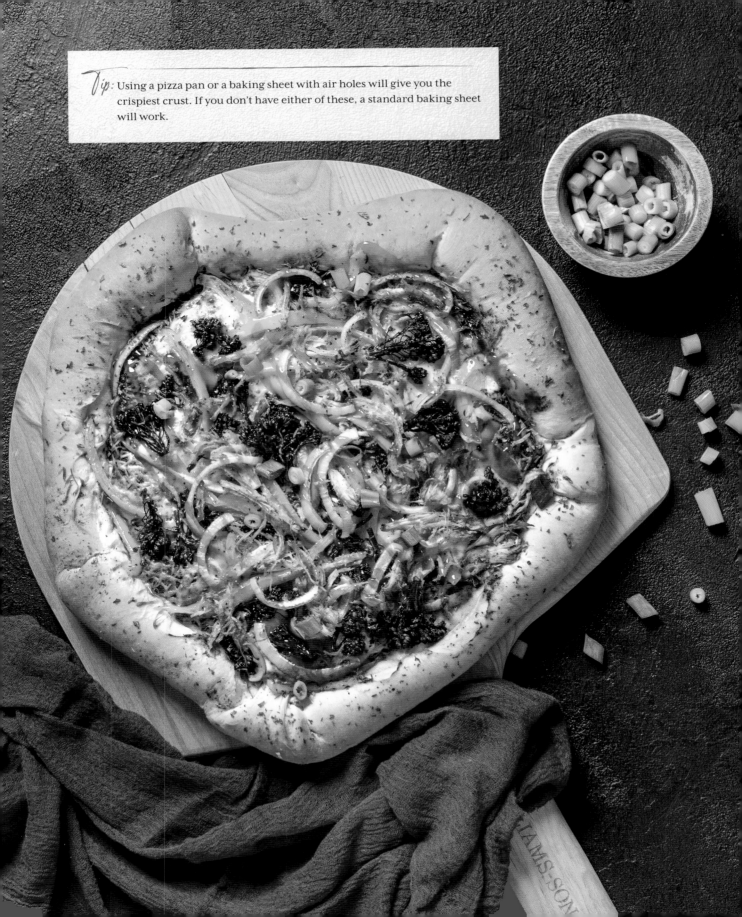

Tip: Using a pizza pan or a baking sheet with air holes will give you the crispiest crust. If you don't have either of these, a standard baking sheet will work.

Dairy-Free
GARLIC ALFREDO SPINACH PASTA

SERVES
4

PREP TIME
10 minutes
(not including
time to soak
cashews)

COOK TIME
30 minutes

Pasta, especially creamy pasta, is just one of those dishes you can't get enough of. When I first began reducing my dairy and gluten intake, I felt so saddened by the idea of no longer being able to enjoy pasta. For years, pasta was the dish I would choose over any other when given the option, so you can imagine the fear I felt. Thankfully, there are so many gluten-free pasta options today, which, in combination with the great dairy substitutes I've found, make it easy to enjoy creamy pasta dishes. This recipe is the epitome of being able to do just that—enjoying all the creamy goodness without the dairy. If you want to add a bit of meat, such as chicken or bacon, or change up the greens by substituting kale or sautéed broccolini for the spinach, feel free! With small tweaks, you can completely recreate this dish.

ALFREDO SAUCE:

1¼ cups raw cashews, soaked, drained, and rinsed (see note, page 48)

1 cup unsweetened, unflavored almond milk

⅓ cup nutritional yeast

4 cloves garlic, peeled

1 tablespoon freshly squeezed lemon juice

1 teaspoon garlic powder

1 teaspoon onion powder

1 teaspoon dried oregano leaves

1 teaspoon finely ground sea salt

¼ teaspoon ground black pepper

1 pound pappardelle pasta

2 cups spinach

TOPPINGS (OPTIONAL):

Chopped walnuts

Dried parsley

Fresh thyme sprigs

1. Make the sauce: Using a blender or food processor, blend the soaked cashews, almond milk, nutritional yeast, garlic cloves, lemon juice, garlic powder, onion powder, oregano, salt, and pepper until a smooth sauce has formed.

2. Bring a large pot of salted water to a boil. Add the pasta and cook according to the package directions. While the pasta cooks, combine the sauce and spinach in a large skillet and cook over medium heat until the spinach has begun to wilt and the sauce is just heated through. Drain the pasta.

3. Pour the sauce over the cooked pasta and toss to coat evenly. Immediately portion the pasta into bowls and top with chopped walnuts, dried parsley, and/or fresh thyme sprigs, if desired.

Tip: For a stronger lemon flavor, wait to mix the lemon juice into the sauce until just before tossing it with the pasta.

To make this dish gluten-free, use 1 pound of your favorite brand of dried gluten-free pasta.

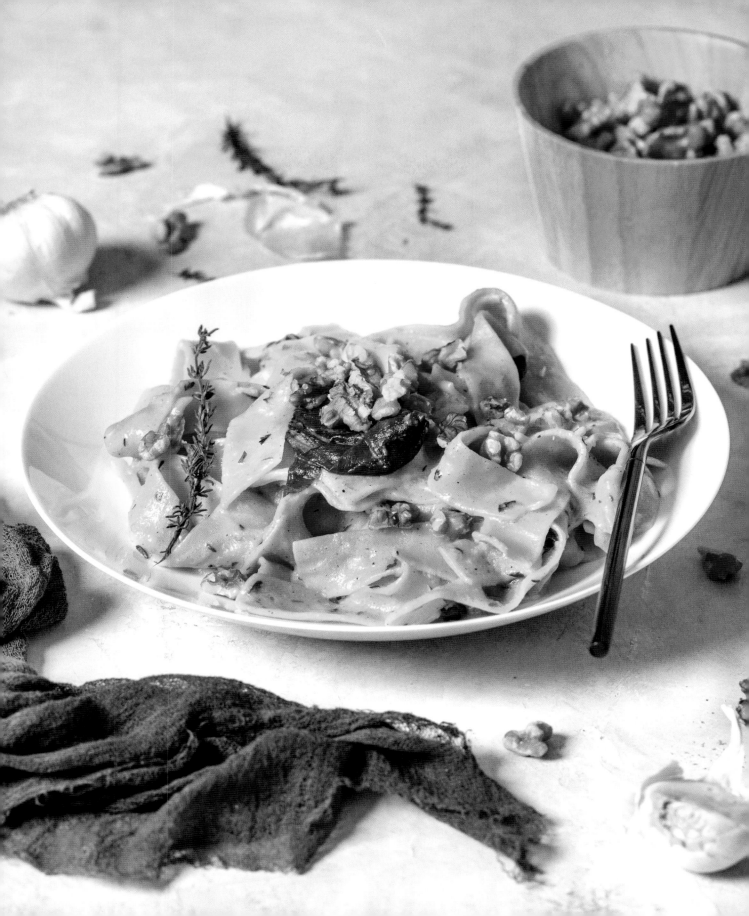

Fire-Roasted Tomato
DECONSTRUCTED STUFFED SHELLS

SERVES
4

PREP TIME
10 minutes

COOK TIME
20 minutes

These deconstructed stuffed shells are heavily inspired by my mother-in-law, who makes traditional shells stuffed with ground turkey, cheese, ricotta, and a well-seasoned sauce. While I still enjoy the traditional version from time to time, I adore this meatless option. Since this recipe isn't loaded with cheese, you are able to enjoy the fire-roasted flavor as well as the lightness of the lemon-ricotta mixture. This recipe makes for such an easy weeknight meal that everyone is guaranteed to enjoy. Oh, and don't worry—you can always change things up by adding ground turkey or beef to the sauce for an even heartier dish.

1 pound jumbo pasta shells

¼ cup plus 2 tablespoons extra-virgin olive oil, divided

3 cloves garlic, minced

1 tablespoon dried parsley, plus more for topping if desired

1 tablespoon fresh oregano leaves, or 2 teaspoons dried

½ teaspoon garlic powder

Pinch of red pepper flakes

1 (6-ounce) can tomato paste

1 (14-ounce) can diced fire-roasted tomatoes

½ cup chopped fresh basil leaves, plus more for topping if desired

Finely ground sea salt and ground black pepper

1 cup skim-milk ricotta cheese, whisked until whipped

Grated zest and juice of 1 lemon (about 3 tablespoons juice)

Shaved Parmesan cheese, for topping (optional)

1. Bring a large pot of salted water to a boil. Add the pasta and cook according to the package directions. Drain, reserving 1¼ cups of the pasta water, and set the cooked shells aside.

2. Heat 2 tablespoons of the olive oil in a sauté pan over medium-high heat. Add the garlic, parsley, oregano, garlic powder, and red pepper flakes. Sauté for 30 seconds to 1 minute, or until the garlic begins to become fragrant. Add the tomato paste and cook, stirring, for 2 minutes.

3. Reduce the heat to medium and add the fire-roasted tomatoes, juices and all, as well as 1 cup of the reserved pasta water. Add the chopped basil and season with 1 teaspoon each of salt and pepper. Stir and allow to simmer until the sauce begins to thicken, about 10 minutes, scraping the sides and bottom of the pan every few moments with a wooden spoon.

4. Add the pasta shells and mix until the shells are evenly coated. Turn off the heat.

5. In a small bowl, whisk together the remaining ¼ cup of reserved pasta water, the ricotta, lemon zest and juice, and a sprinkle of salt.

6. Spread the whipped ricotta mixture on the bottoms of four shallow bowls and spoon the pasta on top. Top with dried parsley, shaved Parmesan, and/or chopped fresh basil leaves, if desired.

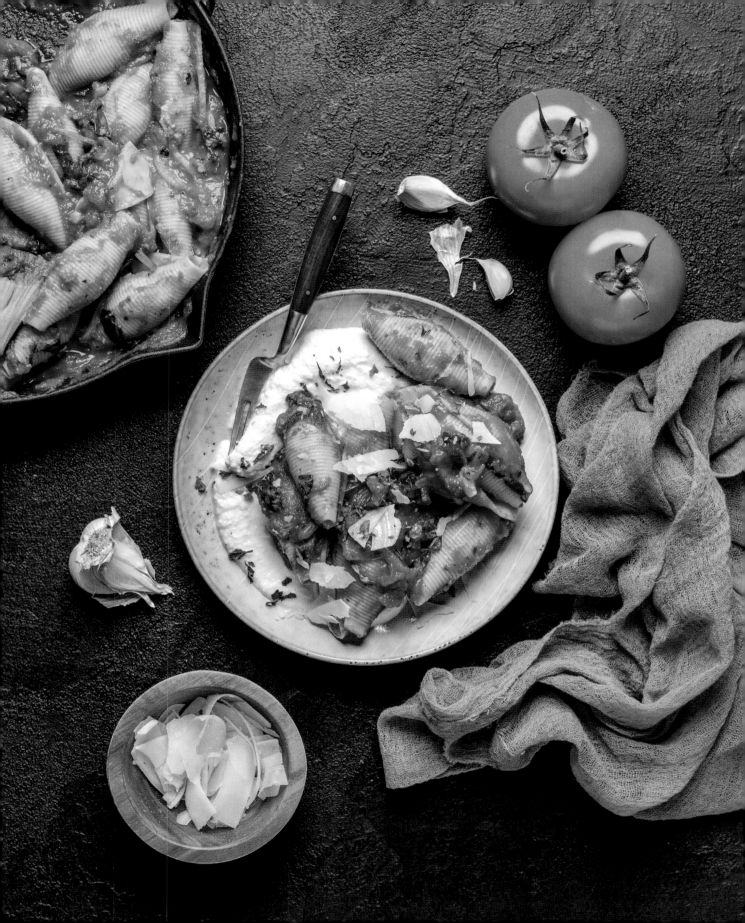

Cajun Sweet Potato
RIGATONI WITH KALE

SERVES
4

PREP TIME
10 minutes

COOK TIME
20 minutes

This sweet potato pasta is the perfect way to enjoy a plate of creamy pasta, but without the dairy and cheese. This recipe is loaded with sweet potato flavor, which marries deliciously with Cajun seasonings and of course the amazing chunkiness of rigatoni. Inspired by my Southern and Jamaican roots, this pasta adds real comfort to dinnertime meals. Whip it together in 20 short minutes and make the sauce ahead for an easier cooking experience.

1 pound rigatoni pasta

1 tablespoon extra-virgin olive oil

3 cloves garlic, minced

Pinch of ground cinnamon

¼ cup all-purpose flour

1 cup low-sodium vegetable stock

1 (13-ounce) can coconut cream or full-fat coconut milk

1 to 2 tablespoons Cajun seasoning, homemade (page 43) or store-bought, plus more for topping if desired

1½ cups Simple Sweet Potato Puree (page 56)

¼ cup nutritional yeast

Pinch of finely ground sea salt

Pinch of ground black pepper

1 tablespoon dry white wine

2 cups destemmed and chopped kale

1. Bring a large pot of salted water to a boil. Add the pasta and cook according to the package directions. While the pasta is cooking, begin preparing the sauce.

2. Heat the olive oil in a large skillet over medium-high heat, then add the garlic and cinnamon and sauté for 30 seconds to 1 minute, until the garlic begins to become fragrant. Reduce the heat to medium and add the flour to the skillet, whisking until well combined and a paste forms.

3. Slowly whisk in the vegetable stock, stirring constantly until a thick sauce begins to form. Repeat this step with the coconut cream, then stir in the Cajun seasoning, sweet potato puree, nutritional yeast, salt, pepper, and wine. Add the kale and simmer for another 3 to 4 minutes, stirring occasionally, until the kale is tender.

4. Drain the pasta, then add it to the sauce. Stir to fully coat the pasta. Remove from the heat and serve immediately in bowls topped with additional Cajun seasoning, if desired.

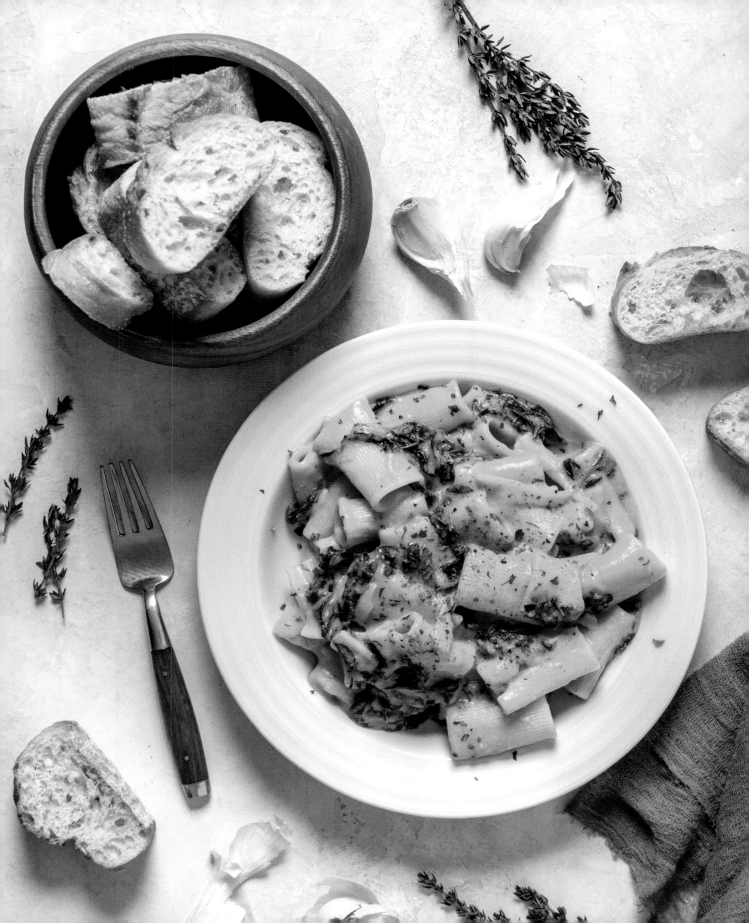

Creamy Lemon-Kale Orzo
WITH ROASTED TOMATOES & VEGETABLES

SERVES
4

PREP TIME
10 minutes

COOK TIME
30 minutes

This is one of my staple weeknight recipes! I was late to the orzo craze; however, after making this dish a few times, I'm a believer. I love how easy it is to pair this small ricelike pasta with any number of favorite ingredients. I felt compelled to make this orzo dish super creamy and bursting with lemony and savory flavors because it works so perfectly. When it comes to sautéed greens, I love using kale or spinach; however, you can use your own favorite here. The roasted veggies lend a hearty "meatiness" to the dish, making it a satisfying meal despite being completely meatless. From time to time, whenever I'm in the mood for a bit of crunchiness, I'll sprinkle chopped nuts on top.

ROASTED VEGETABLES:

10 asparagus spears, tough ends removed

2 cups broccoli florets

2 medium heirloom tomatoes, quartered

4 cloves garlic, minced

1 teaspoon finely ground sea salt

1 teaspoon ground black pepper

1 teaspoon dried parsley

1 teaspoon smoked paprika

½ teaspoon garlic powder

1 tablespoon extra-virgin olive oil

CREAMY ORZO:

1 cup orzo

1 cup low-sodium chicken stock

1 cup heavy cream

2 cups destemmed and finely chopped kale

1 cup shredded low-moisture mozzarella cheese

1 tablespoon freshly squeezed lemon juice

Pine nuts, for topping (optional)

Lemon wedges, for serving

1. Preheat the oven to 350°F.

2. Prepare the roasted vegetables: Put the asparagus, broccoli, tomatoes, and garlic in a medium-size bowl. Season with the salt, pepper, parsley, smoked paprika, and garlic powder. Pour the olive oil over the top and toss until evenly coated. Spread the vegetables out on a sheet pan. Bake for 30 minutes, or until the asparagus and broccoli are tender and the tomatoes are blackened and give off a sweet roast-y smell.

3. When the vegetables are about halfway done, make the orzo: Bring the orzo, chicken stock, and heavy cream to a boil in a 2- to 4-quart saucepan over high heat. Once boiling, reduce the heat and simmer for 10 minutes, stirring occasionally. Remove from the heat. Add the kale and mozzarella and stir until well combined, then place a lid on the pot and let sit for 4 to 5 minutes, until the kale is wilted. The orzo will absorb liquid as it sits, so allow it to sit longer if you find it too soupy.

4. Once the vegetables are roasted, remove them from the oven and set aside. Add the lemon juice to the orzo and mix well. Spoon the pasta into bowls and top with the roasted vegetables and, if desired, pine nuts. Serve immediately with lemon wedges.

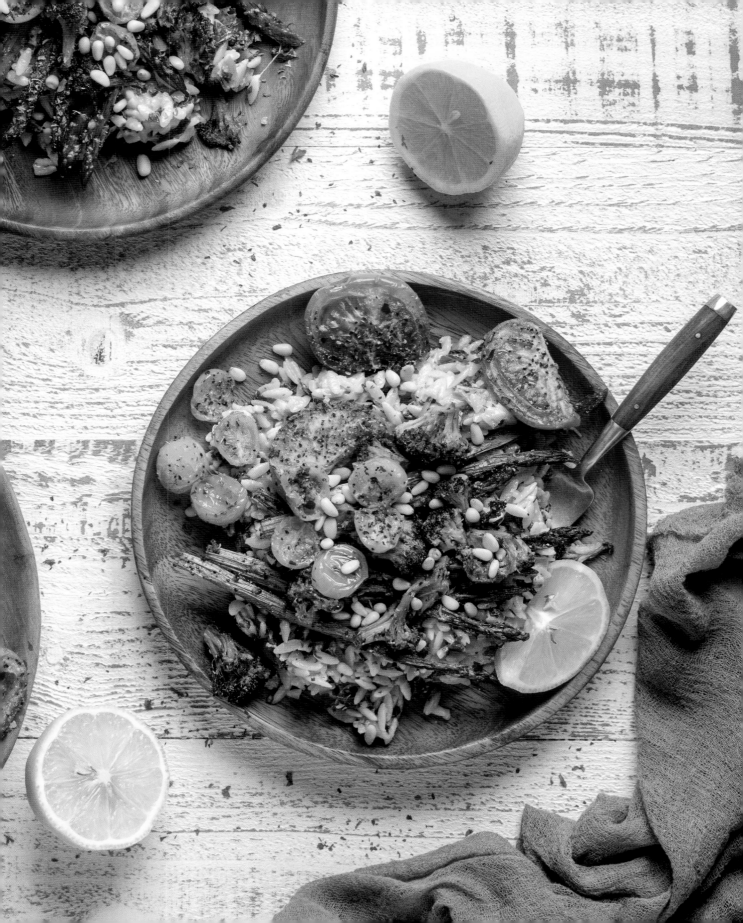

Cajun Quinoa & Brown Rice
STUFFED PEPPERS

SERVES
8

PREP TIME
20 minutes

COOK TIME
30 minutes

These stuffed peppers are a vegetarian twist on a family favorite recipe. Since no one can resist stuffing, not even children, this dish is a great way to keep kids interested in eating colorful vegetables. While these stuffed peppers have a nice kick of heat from the Cajun seasoning, you can omit the seasoning or use a lesser amount if you aren't a fan of spicy flavors.

4 medium bell peppers, any color

2 tablespoons extra-virgin olive oil, divided, plus more for the pan

1 medium onion, chopped

2 cloves garlic, minced

½ cup mini bell peppers, finely diced

1 Scotch bonnet or habanero pepper, minced

2 tablespoons Cajun seasoning, homemade (page 43) or store-bought

2 tablespoons dried basil

1 tablespoon dried oregano leaves

1 tablespoon dried parsley

½ teaspoon red pepper flakes

Finely ground sea salt and ground black pepper

2 cups grape tomatoes, halved

1 cup cooked red or tri-color quinoa (see page 58)

½ cup brown basmati rice, cooked

1 cup shredded low-moisture mozzarella cheese

Fresh thyme sprigs, for topping (optional)

1. Preheat the oven to 425°F and lightly grease a 9 by 13-inch casserole dish with olive oil.

2. Cut the bell peppers in half lengthwise, from the top downward, through their stalks. Scoop out the seeds and white membranes, then rinse and pat dry.

3. Place the peppers cut side up in the prepared casserole dish and drizzle with 1 tablespoon of the olive oil. If the peppers won't stay put, slice off a small amount from their undersides to create an even base. Bake for 15 to 20 minutes, until the peppers are just tender and beginning to brown on the edges.

4. Meanwhile, heat the remaining tablespoon of olive oil in a large skillet over medium-high heat. Add the onion and garlic and sauté for 3 to 4 minutes, until the onion is translucent and the garlic is fragrant. Add the mini bell peppers and Scotch bonnet and sauté for another 1 to 2 minutes.

5. Reduce the heat to medium-low, then add the Cajun seasoning, basil, oregano, parsley, red pepper flakes, and a pinch each of salt and black pepper. Continue to sauté for 30 seconds to 1 minute, then add the tomatoes and cook for another 2 minutes, tossing occasionally. Add the cooked quinoa and rice and stir until fully combined.

6. Once the bell peppers have just cooked through, remove them from the oven and let cool for 2 to 3 minutes.

7. Carefully spoon the quinoa-vegetable mixture into the bell pepper halves, then top with the cheese. Return to the oven for 5 to 10 minutes to melt the cheese.

8. Remove from the oven and serve warm, topped with thyme sprigs, if desired. BAM!

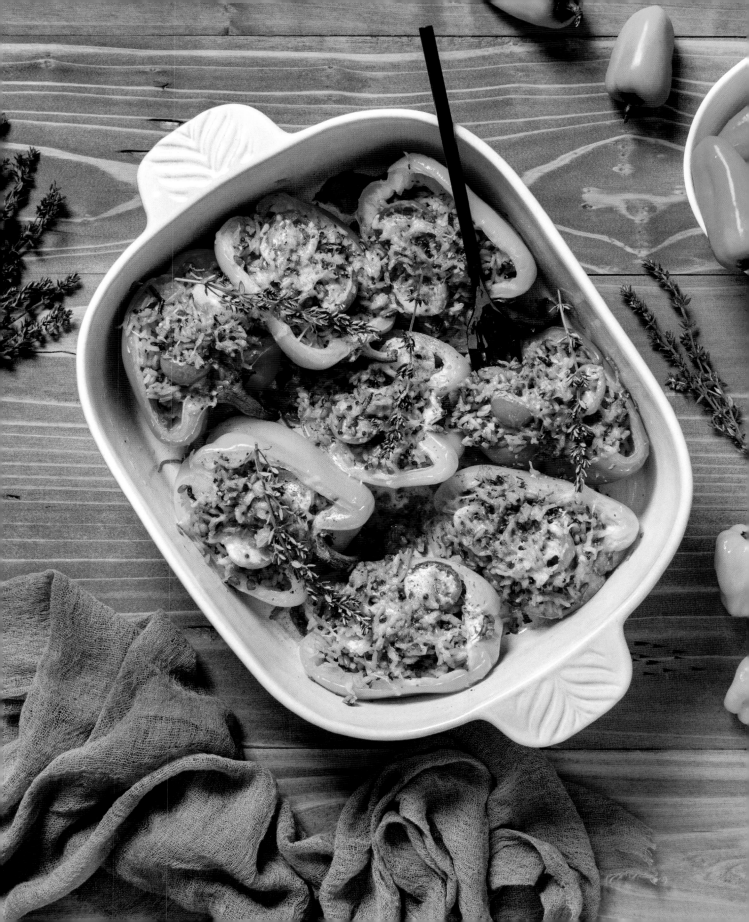

Jerk BBQ Pineapple
BLACK BEAN BURGERS

SERVES
6

PREP TIME
20 minutes

COOK TIME
20 minutes

These jerk BBQ pineapple burgers are some of the best veggie burgers I've had! I love using black beans for burger patties because they hold together so well; however, I occasionally use chickpeas or quinoa as well. Regardless, the flavors in these burgers are insane. The sweetness from the pineapple and the heat and tang from the jerk BBQ sauce will remind you of an island experience. You can keep things simple and enjoy them as is (they're plenty delicious with just the BBQ sauce and pineapple), or top them with a dollop of guacamole, your favorite greens, or coleslaw—whatever your taste buds desire!

BURGERS:

1 (15-ounce) can black beans, drained and rinsed

2 cups grated carrots

2 cloves garlic, peeled

1 Scotch bonnet or habanero pepper, roughly chopped

2 cups plain breadcrumbs, plus more if needed

2 large eggs

1 teaspoon finely ground sea salt

1 teaspoon ground black pepper

1 teaspoon smoked paprika

1 teaspoon garlic powder

1 teaspoon dried thyme leaves

1 teaspoon ground cumin

1 teaspoon dried parsley

1 tablespoon extra-virgin olive oil, for cooking (optional)

FOR SERVING:

12 pineapple rings

6 burger buns, split and toasted

2 cups jerk BBQ sauce, homemade (page 52) or store-bought

Guacamole, homemade (page 62) or store-bought (optional)

1. Preheat the oven to 425°F and line a sheet pan with parchment paper.

2. Put all the burger ingredients in a food processor or blender and pulse until broken down and well combined. If the mixture is too sticky, add more breadcrumbs until it's "paste-y" enough to form into a ball without difficulty.

3. Using your hands, form the mixture into 6 medium-size patties about ¾ inch thick.

4. If you like your veggie burgers with a well-browned crust, pan-fry the patties a bit first. Heat 1 tablespoon of olive oil in a large skillet over medium-high heat. Once hot, add half of the patties and cook until browned on both sides, cooking 2 to 3 minutes per side. Repeat with the remaining patties.

5. Carefully place the patties on the sheet pan and bake for 15 to 20 minutes, or until crispy.

6. Meanwhile, grill the pineapple rings: Preheat a nonstick grill pan over medium-high heat, then place the pineapple rings on the pan and lightly char on each side, 3 to 4 minutes total. Set aside.

7. When the burgers are done, remove them from the oven and serve immediately on toasted buns. Top with jerk BBQ sauce and 2 pineapple rings and, if desired, add a dollop of guacamole.

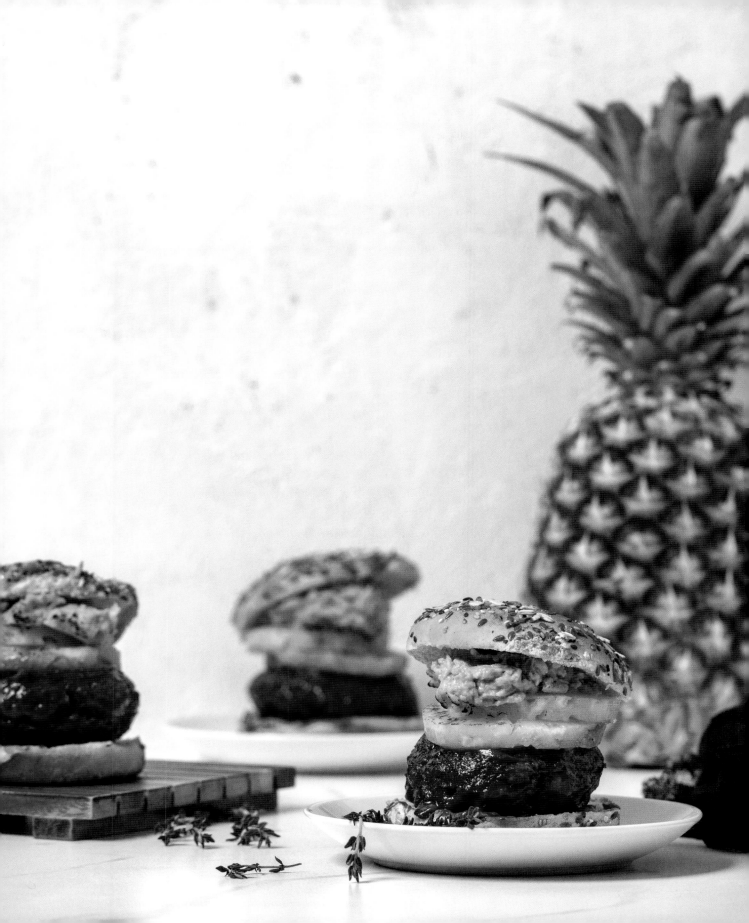

Spicy Sesame Plant-Based Meatballs
WITH CAULIFLOWER RICE

SERVES
4

PREP TIME
20 minutes

COOK TIME
30 minutes

This recipe was inspired by one of my favorite Chinese dishes, sesame chicken and rice. In my teens, I used to get Chinese food from my local restaurant in Brooklyn almost every day after school, and I almost always ordered the same two things—chicken wings and french fries or sesame chicken and rice. Here, I've sought to recreate that eating experience but with plant-forward ingredients. The vegan meatballs are made from chickpeas and quinoa, and of course, the rice isn't actual rice but rather riced cauliflower. Overall, this dish has bold flavors with a slight hint of heat, but a nice amount of sweetness to offset it. All eaters will appreciate this one!

PLANT-BASED MEATBALLS:

1 (15-ounce) can chickpeas, drained and rinsed

1 cup cooked red or tri-color quinoa (see page 58)

½ cup plain breadcrumbs

1 Flaxseed Egg (page 38)

3 cloves garlic, roughly chopped

1 tablespoon nutritional yeast

1 tablespoon dried parsley

1 tablespoon smoked paprika

½ teaspoon finely ground sea salt

½ teaspoon ground black pepper

1 tablespoon extra-virgin olive oil, for cooking

SESAME GLAZE:

1 tablespoon extra-virgin olive oil

3 cloves garlic, minced

1 teaspoon grated fresh ginger

⅓ cup low-sodium soy sauce

¼ cup raw honey

1 tablespoon toasted sesame oil

1 teaspoon unseasoned rice vinegar

1 teaspoon Sriracha sauce

SPICY CAULIFLOWER RICE:

1 medium head cauliflower

1 tablespoon extra-virgin olive oil

4 cloves garlic, minced

¼ cup low-sodium vegetable stock

1 tablespoon freshly squeezed lemon juice

1 tablespoon Tabasco

1 teaspoon finely ground sea salt

1 teaspoon ground black pepper

TOPPINGS:

Sesame seeds

Sliced scallions (optional)

1. Form the meatballs: In a high-powered blender or food processor, pulse all the meatball ingredients, except for the olive oil, until they are well combined and hold together when pinched between your fingers.

2. Scoop up about 2½ tablespoons of the meatball mixture and roll it between your hands to form a ball about 2 inches in diameter. Set aside on a piece of parchment paper. Repeat with the rest of the meatball mixture.

3. Make the glaze: Heat the olive oil in a medium-size saucepan over medium-high heat. Add the garlic and sauté for 2 to 3 minutes, or until lightly golden brown.

4. Reduce the heat to low, then add the ginger, soy sauce, honey, sesame oil, rice vinegar, and Sriracha. Whisk to combine and simmer until thickened, 2 to 3 minutes, whisking occasionally to prevent clumps from forming. Once slightly thickened, remove the pan from the heat and set aside to cool and thicken further.

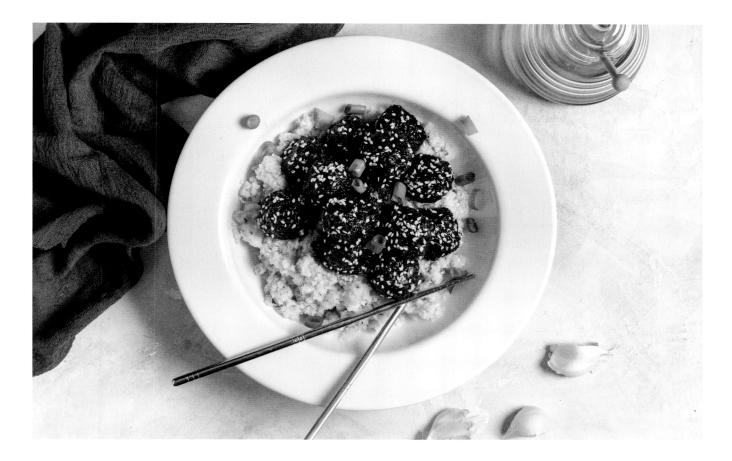

5. Make the cauliflower rice: Remove the florets from the head of cauliflower; discard the core and place the florets in a food processor. Pulse the florets until they are broken down into very small pieces about the size of rice.

6. Heat the olive oil in a large skillet over medium-high heat. Once hot, add the garlic and sauté for 30 seconds to 1 minute. Reduce the heat to medium-low and add the vegetable stock, lemon juice, Tabasco, and cauliflower rice. Season with the salt and pepper and continue to cook until the cauliflower rice is tender and the liquid is mostly absorbed. Turn off the heat and set aside.

7. Cook the meatballs: Heat a tablespoon of olive oil in a large skillet over medium heat. Once hot, add the meatballs one at a time, making sure not to overcrowd the pan, and fry until they are golden brown on all sides, turning them from time to time.

8. Toss the browned meatballs with the sesame glaze and serve immediately in bowls over the cauliflower rice. Top with sesame seeds and, if desired, sliced scallions.

Tip: To make these meatballs vegan, replace the honey with a vegan sweetener such as agave or maple syrup. Also, ensure that the breadcrumbs are vegan-friendly.

Maple Brown Butter Chicken
& WILD RICE SKILLET
WITH BRUSSELS SPROUTS

SERVES
4

PREP TIME
10 minutes

COOK TIME
1 hour

When it comes to chicken, I am the biggest fan. I do love seafood on occasion, but I hardly ever eat red meat, leaving chicken as my main source of meat. During my childhood, chicken was the one thing I'd never refuse to eat, to the point that my nickname was "Chicken Wing." So, of course, you can only imagine how happy I am whenever I get a chance to make a chicken dish for dinner. This recipe pairs chicken thighs with the bold flavors of maple, brown butter, and wild rice. If you are a fan of skillet meals, then this one is for you!

6 tablespoons (¾ stick) unsalted butter, divided

4 boneless, skinless chicken thighs, patted dry

Finely ground sea salt and ground black pepper

1 tablespoon dried parsley, plus more for garnish if desired

½ cup pure maple syrup

4 cloves garlic, minced

7 ounces Brussels sprouts, halved (about 2 cups)

1 onion, diced

½ teaspoon dried thyme leaves

¼ teaspoon onion powder

2 cups low-sodium chicken stock

1 cup dry white wine

1½ cups wild rice blend

1. Preheat the oven to 400°F.

2. Heat 1 tablespoon of the butter in a large skillet over medium heat. Lightly season both sides of the chicken thighs with salt and pepper, then sprinkle with the parsley. When the butter is hot, add the chicken to the skillet and brown on one side, about 5 minutes. Flip the chicken and brown on other side, about 5 more minutes. Remove the chicken and set aside.

3. Drain most of the excess fat from the pan, leaving about 2 tablespoons of drippings for flavor. Add 4 more tablespoons of the butter and allow it to melt, scraping any browned bits from the bottom of the skillet. Continue to lightly stir the butter until the foam dissipates and the butter begins to brown, 3 to 5 minutes. Gently stir in the maple syrup until it dissolves into the butter, then add the garlic and simmer for 30 seconds to 1 minute.

4. Return the chicken to the pan and cook for 20 to 25 minutes, or until it is cooked through (it will no longer be pink in the middle when pierced with a knife). After about 5 minutes, turn the thighs over so they cook evenly. In the final 10 minutes of cooking, add the Brussels sprouts and cook them until fork-tender.

5. While the chicken finishes cooking, make the rice: Melt the remaining tablespoon of butter in a separate large skillet over medium-high heat, then add the onion, thyme, and onion powder and sauté for 3 minutes, or until the onion is translucent. Add the chicken stock and wine and stir in the wild rice. Cover and bring to a boil, then reduce the heat to low and simmer until all the liquid is absorbed, 40 to 45 minutes.

6. Spoon the rice onto plates, then top with the chicken and Brussels sprouts. Garnish with parsley, if desired.

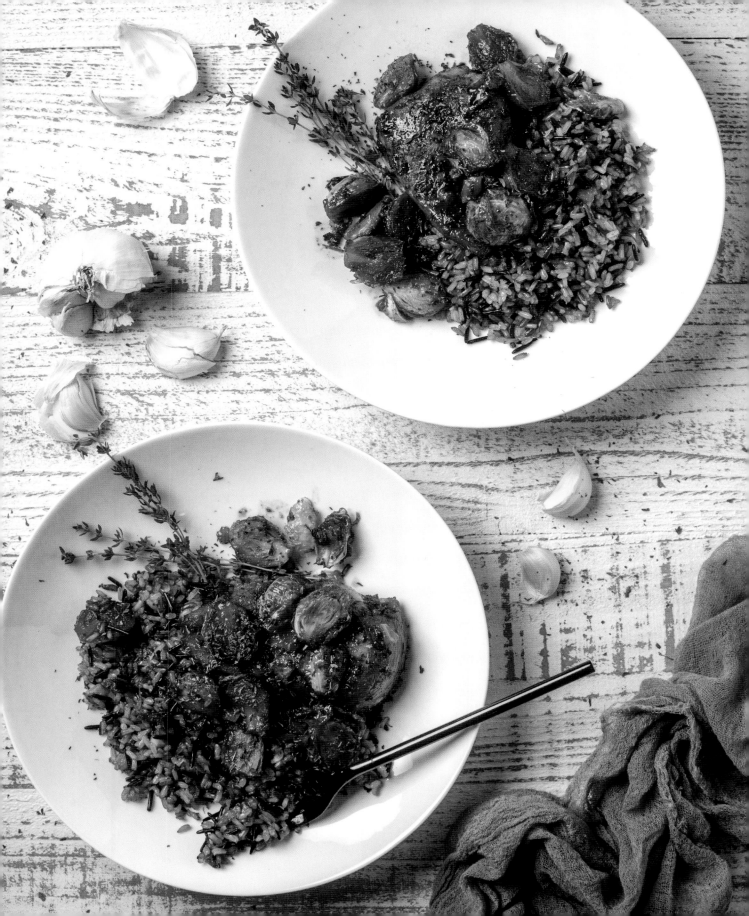

Savory Vegetarian
JERK POT PIES

SERVES
6

PREP TIME
15 minutes

COOK TIME
45 minutes

As a kid, I remember eating single-serving pot pies that came frozen in aluminum pie plates. The white sauce filling was jam-packed with frozen veggies and chicken and was enveloped top and bottom with a semi-flaky crust. Back then, I used to pick around the filling and ate mostly the crust, avoiding the liquid-y sauce as best I could (I was super sensitive to textures as a young and very picky eater). Now that I make my own version of pot pie, I can make the creamy filling just how I like it. With this recipe, I chose to create something new and interesting that draws from both my backgrounds—Southern and Jamaican—going with a jerk theme for the filling and biscuits in lieu of the usual pie pastry crust for the topping. The filling has the perfect amount of heat, which is offset by the cheese, and the savory cheddar herb biscuit topping makes this the best comfort food ever. This dish is guaranteed to be your newest family favorite!

FILLING:

3 tablespoons unsalted butter

1 medium red onion, finely chopped

1 tablespoon jerk seasoning, homemade (page 42) or store-bought

4 to 5 cups frozen mixed vegetables

1 teaspoon finely ground sea salt

½ teaspoon ground black pepper

¼ cup plus 2 tablespoons all-purpose flour

1 cup low-sodium chicken stock

¾ cup unsweetened, unflavored almond milk

2 tablespoons dry white wine

1 cup shredded mild white cheddar cheese

½ cup grated Parmesan cheese

CHEDDAR HERB BISCUIT TOPPING:

2 cups all-purpose flour

2 teaspoons baking powder

½ teaspoon baking soda

1 teaspoon finely ground sea salt

2 tablespoons dried parsley

1 teaspoon dried thyme leaves

½ teaspoon dried oregano leaves

1 teaspoon garlic powder

1 cup shredded mild white cheddar cheese

½ cup (1 stick) cold unsalted butter, cubed

1 cup Vegan Buttermilk (page 46), made with lemon juice

1 large egg

Splash of unsweetened, unflavored almond milk

(Recipe continues on page 229)

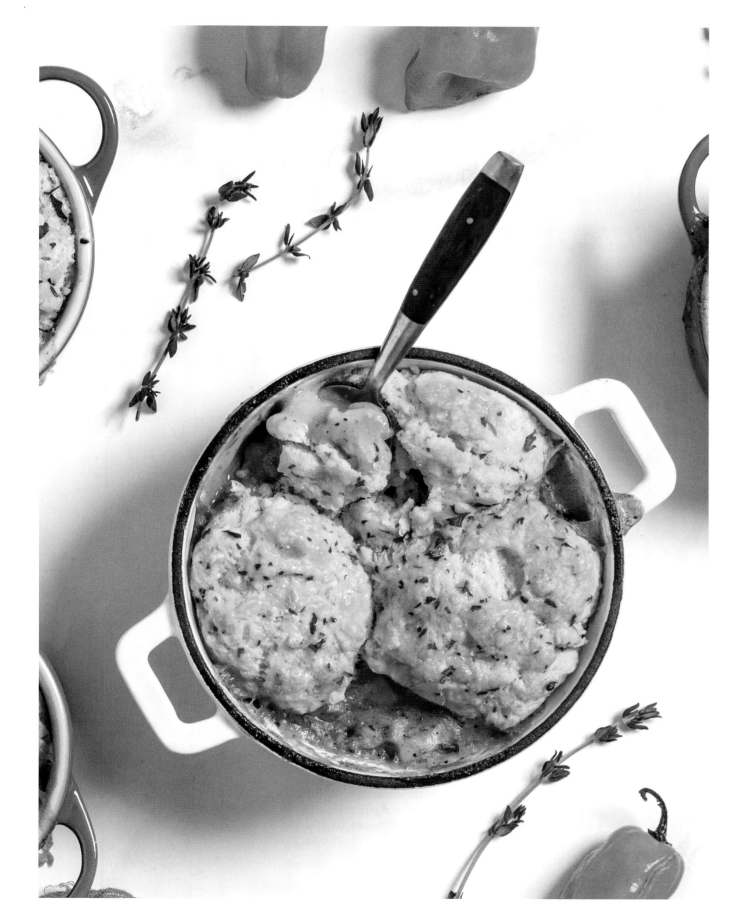

Plant-Based
JERK BBQ MEATBALL PO' BOYS

SERVES
4

PREP TIME
20 minutes

COOK TIME
45 minutes

In recent years, I've grown to love sandwiches of any kind. Growing up in Florida, my favorite sandwich was a classic grilled cheese or hot dog; after moving to New York, I began loving other types, like heroes, meatball subs, and BLTs. This Jamaican twist on the po' boy features bold jerk BBQ flavors while paying homage to the classic Southern sandwich, which hails from New Orleans. Traditional po' boys include some sort of roast or fried seafood (such as oysters, shrimp, crab meat, crawfish, or fish), but this plant-based meatball version creates a nice "meatiness" without using actual meat. Of course, to make the entire recipe vegan, you can substitute the buns and butter with vegan-friendly options.

PLANT-BASED MEATBALLS:

1 (15-ounce) can chickpeas, drained and rinsed

1 cup cooked red or tri-color quinoa (see page 58)

½ cup vegan plain breadcrumbs

1 Flaxseed Egg (page 38)

3 cloves garlic, roughly chopped

1 tablespoon nutritional yeast

1 tablespoon dried parsley

1 tablespoon smoked paprika

½ teaspoon finely ground sea salt

½ teaspoon ground black pepper

1 tablespoon extra-virgin olive oil, for cooking

PO' BOYS:

4 hotdog buns

2 tablespoons unsalted butter, for the buns

1 cup shredded red cabbage

2 cups jerk BBQ sauce, homemade (page 52) or store-bought

Dried parsley, for garnish

1. Preheat the oven to 400°F. Line a sheet pan with parchment paper.

2. In a high-powered blender or food processor, pulse all the meatball ingredients, except for the olive oil, until they are well combined and hold together when pinched between your fingers.

3. Working with about 1½ tablespoons of the meatball mixture at a time, use your hands to roll it into balls about 2 inches in diameter. Set aside on the prepared pan. Drizzle the olive oil over the meatballs and bake for 15 minutes, or until browned.

4. Meanwhile, toast the buns: Heat a large skillet over medium heat. Butter the insides of the buns, then place them buttered side down in the skillet, flattening them slightly to ensure the surface toasts evenly. Remove the toasted buns from the pan and set aside.

5. To assemble the po' boys, place several meatballs in each toasted bun and top evenly with the shredded cabbage and jerk BBQ sauce. Garnish with parsley and serve immediately.

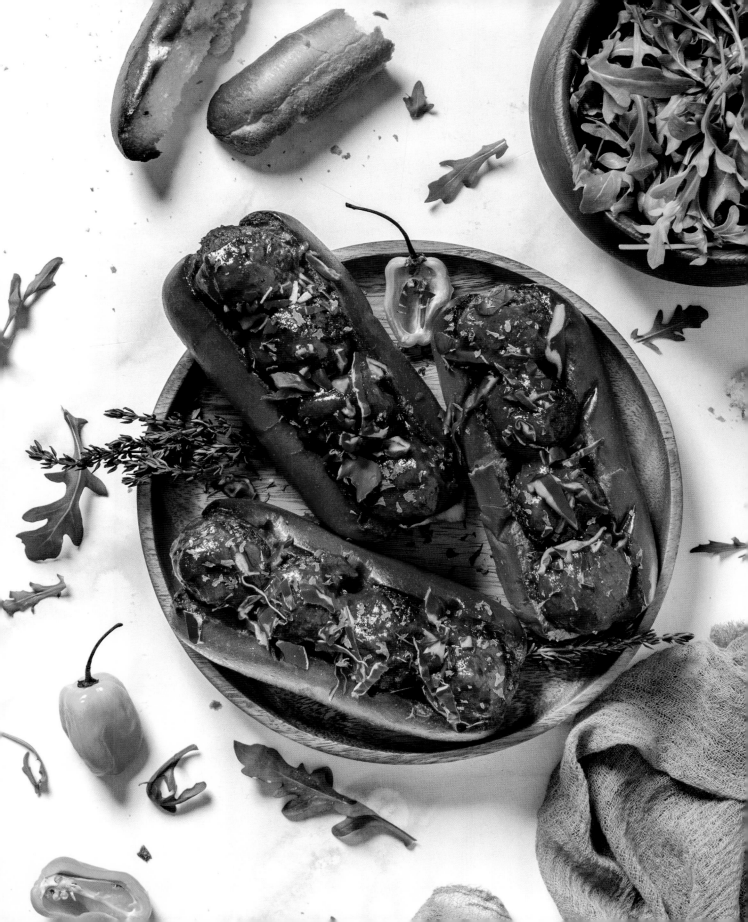

Curry Shrimp
WITH CAULIFLOWER RICE

SERVES
4

PREP TIME
10 minutes, plus
20 minutes to
marinate

COOK TIME
20 minutes

Curry shrimp and rice was something my parents always cooked at home. Though rather simple, it's so delicious and often comes with a great amount of gravy to pour over the rice. This dish is very hot, but it can be as spicy as you want it to be; to make it less spicy, use just one Scotch bonnet pepper, and for even less heat, remove the seeds and membranes. You can also omit the hot sauce from the rice if you prefer. If you're looking for something quick and easy, then this dish is a perfect fit; as a bonus, it includes a few veggies to create a well-rounded meal. For a healthier twist, I chose cauliflower rice instead of conventional rice and often use wild-caught shrimp to ensure that all the ingredients are sustainable.

CURRY SHRIMP:

8 ounces extra-large shrimp, peeled and deveined

2 tablespoons extra-virgin olive oil, divided

2 teaspoons finely ground sea salt

1½ tablespoons curry powder

2 teaspoons garlic powder

2 teaspoons ginger powder

1 teaspoon ground allspice

1 teaspoon ground black pepper

1 teaspoon paprika

3 bay leaves

5 baby red potatoes

2 carrots

2 Scotch bonnet or habanero peppers

3 cloves garlic

SPICY CAULIFLOWER RICE:

1 head cauliflower

1 tablespoon extra-virgin olive oil

4 cloves garlic, minced

¼ cup low-sodium vegetable stock

1 tablespoon Tabasco

1 teaspoon finely ground sea salt

1 teaspoon ground black pepper

1 tablespoon freshly squeezed lemon juice

TOPPINGS (OPTIONAL):

Sliced scallions

Dried parsley

1. In a large bowl, combine the shrimp, 1 tablespoon of the olive oil, the salt, and spices. Cover and marinate for at least 20 minutes or up to overnight.

2. While the shrimp marinates, scrub the potatoes and carrots, then peel them if desired. Chop the potatoes and carrots into bite-size chunks. Finely chop the Scotch bonnet pepper (deseeded first if you prefer less heat), then mince the garlic.

3. Heat the remaining tablespoon of olive oil in a 4-quart soup pot or Dutch oven over medium-high heat. Once hot, add the garlic and sauté for 30 seconds to 1 minute, until it becomes fragrant. Add the vegetables and Scotch bonnet with just enough water to cover them. Bring to a boil, then lower the heat and simmer until the vegetables are tender, about 20 minutes.

4. While the vegetables cook, make the cauliflower rice: Remove the florets from the head of cauliflower; discard the core and place the florets in a food processor. Pulse the florets until they are broken down into very small pieces about the size of rice.

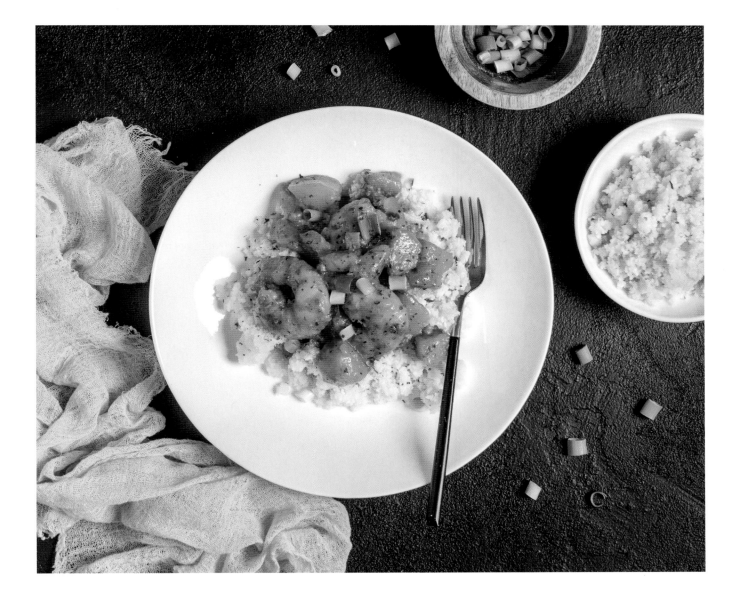

5. Heat the olive oil in a large skillet over medium-high heat. Once hot, add the garlic and sauté for 30 seconds to 1 minute, until it becomes fragrant. Reduce the heat to medium-low and add the vegetable stock, Tabasco, and cauliflower rice. Season with the salt and pepper and simmer until the cauliflower is tender and the liquid is mostly absorbed. Turn off the heat, toss with the lemon juice, and set aside.

6. Once the vegetables are tender, add the shrimp and remaining marinade to the pot. Simmer for another 4 to 5 minutes, until the shrimp are just cooked through. Remove the pot from the heat.

7. Portion the cauliflower rice into shallow bowls and ladle the curry shrimp over the top. Top with sliced scallions and dried parsley, if desired, and serve immediately.

Creamy Southern Grits
WITH SAUTÉED COLLARDS, CANDIED BACON & ROASTED CORN

SERVES
4

PREP TIME
10 minutes, plus
20 minutes to
marinate

COOK TIME
35 minutes

I've gotten my husband to love Southern grits, and I'm very proud of it. Born and raised in Brooklyn, he wasn't accustomed to grits. For me, though, grits were a part of everyday life; you couldn't have breakfast without grits, eggs, bacon, sausage, and the whole works! While this dish is perfect for dinner, if you're like me and you love to enjoy an occasional savory dish for breakfast, it is perfect for that too. I add my favorite type of bacon—candied—for a bit of sweetness with all the savory, but you can skip the candying step or replace the bacon with thin slices of cooked chicken or even shrimp. The number of elements in this dish may look intimidating, but they come together quicker than you might think: the bacon and corn are cooked in the oven at the same time, and when they're underway, you can get the grits going. Likewise, the collards can be prepared as the grits cook.

CANDIED BACON:

1 pound thick-cut bacon

½ cup pure maple syrup

½ cup firmly packed brown sugar

ROASTED CORN:

2 ears of fresh corn, husked and rinsed

1 tablespoon extra-virgin olive oil

1 teaspoon finely ground sea salt

1 teaspoon ground black pepper

½ teaspoon smoked paprika

½ teaspoon garlic powder

GRITS:

3 cups water

3 cups low-sodium chicken stock

1 cup grits or polenta (coarse cornmeal)

1 tablespoon unsalted butter

1 cup shredded smoked Gouda cheese

Pinch of finely ground sea salt

Dried parsley, for topping

COLLARD GREENS:

1 tablespoon extra-virgin olive oil

4 cloves garlic, minced

1 bunch collard greens, chopped

¼ teaspoon finely ground sea salt

¼ teaspoon smoked paprika

¼ teaspoon ground black pepper

⅛ teaspoon red pepper flakes

MAKE THE CANDIED BACON AND ROASTED CORN:

1. Place one oven rack in the bottom position and a second rack in the middle position. Preheat the oven to 400°F and line two sheet pans with parchment paper.

2. Lay the bacon on one of the prepared pans. Brush the tops with half of the maple syrup and sprinkle on half of the brown sugar. Coat the ears of corn with the olive oil, then place them on the second prepared pan. Sprinkle the ears all over with the seasonings.

3. Put the pans of bacon and corn in the oven at the same time, placing the bacon on the middle rack and the corn on the bottom rack. Cook as follows:

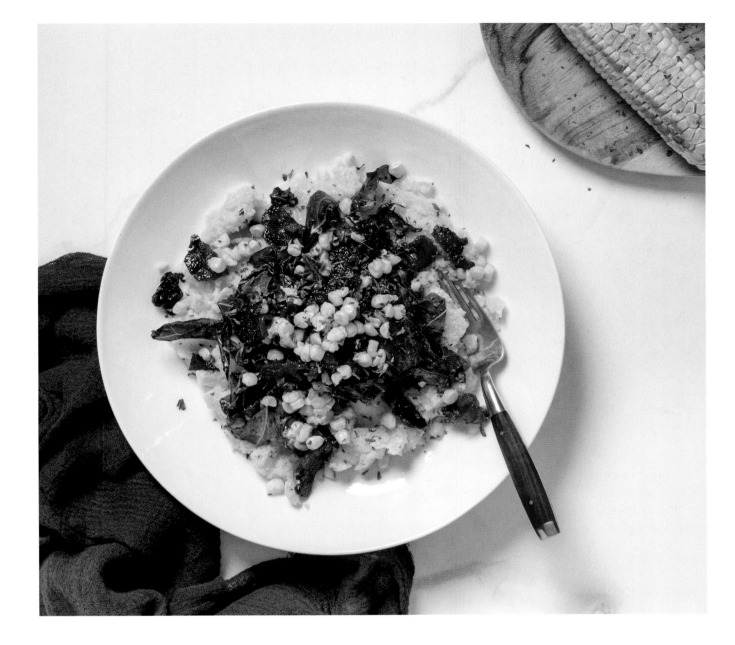

For the bacon, bake for 10 to 15 minutes, then flip and brush the opposite sides with the remaining maple syrup and sprinkle with the remaining brown sugar. Bake for another 10 to 15 minutes, or until the bacon is completely caramelized and crispy. Remove from the oven and allow to cool slightly, then roughly chop and set aside.

For the corn, roast for 20 to 25 minutes, or until the kernels are charred and tender. Remove from the oven and let cool completely, then cut the kernels off the cobs. Set aside.

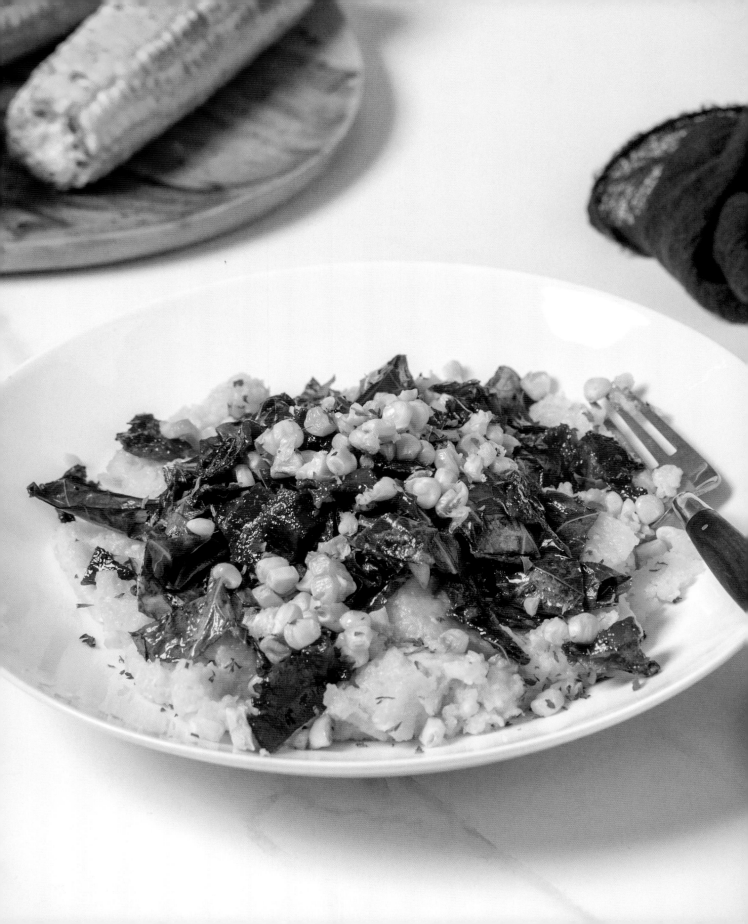

MAKE THE GRITS:

4. Bring the water and chicken stock to a low boil in a heavy 3- to 4-quart pot (such as a Dutch oven) or saucepan. Whisk in the grits and cook for 15 to 20 minutes, until most of the water has been absorbed and the grits are tender but not mushy. Stir in the butter and cheese until melted. Season with the salt, then garnish with dried parsley and cover with a lid to keep warm.

MAKE THE COLLARDS:

5. Heat the olive oil in a large skillet over medium-high heat. Once hot, add the garlic and sauté for 30 seconds to 1 minute, until the garlic begins to become fragrant. Reduce the heat to medium and add the collards, salt, paprika, black pepper, and red pepper flakes. Continue to sauté, stirring frequently, for 3 to 5 minutes, or until the collards are wilted.

6. To serve, spread the cooked grits in the bottoms of four serving bowls and top with the collards. Sprinkle the candied bacon and corn kernels over the top and serve immediately.

Cajun Shrimp
WITH GARLIC BUTTER ZUCCHINI NOODLES & TOMATOES

SERVES
2

PREP TIME
25 minutes

COOK TIME
15 minutes

This dish tops my list of easy meals to make during the week. Flavor is a must for me, regardless of the type of dish, and this recipe brings major flavor! Cajun shrimp is near and dear to my heart because of my Southern roots, and while it can easily be added to your favorite gumbo, rice dish, po' boy, or anything else, the pairing with garlic butter zucchini noodles will have you obsessed. Rich and creamy sauces have their place, but I've always felt that the best pasta dishes come lightly sauced. Growing up, I loved my spaghetti and meatballs with more chunks of meat than sauce, and this dish is a nod in that direction, with just enough sauce and more shrimp and noodle in every bite. Dig those forks in!

CAJUN SHRIMP:

8 ounces extra-large shrimp, peeled and deveined

2 tablespoons garlic powder

2 tablespoons Italian seasoning

2 tablespoons smoked paprika

1 tablespoon onion powder

1 tablespoon dried parsley

1 tablespoon ground dried thyme

1 teaspoon cayenne pepper

1 teaspoon finely ground sea salt

1 teaspoon ground black pepper

NOODLES:

2 medium zucchinis

4 tablespoons unsalted butter, divided

4 cloves garlic, minced

1 tablespoon freshly squeezed lemon juice

1 tablespoon Sriracha sauce

Finely ground sea salt and ground black pepper

1 cup cherry or grape tomatoes, halved

TOPPINGS:

Thyme sprigs, fresh or dried

Fresh or dried parsley

Lemon wedges

SPECIAL EQUIPMENT:

Spiral slicer

MAKE THE SHRIMP:

1. Put the shrimp in a medium-size bowl. Add the garlic powder, Italian seasoning, smoked paprika, onion powder, dried parsley, dried thyme, cayenne, salt, and black pepper and stir until the shrimp are well coated. Cover the bowl and place in the refrigerator for 10 minutes to marinate the shrimp.

2. Meanwhile, cut the ends off the zucchinis, then use a spiral slicer to slice them into thin noodles. Place the zucchini noodles in a large bowl and gently pat dry using a paper towel to remove the excess water. Set aside.

3. Remove the marinated shrimp from the refrigerator and let sit at room temperature for 5 minutes.

4. Melt 2 tablespoons of the butter in a large skillet over medium-high heat. Add the shrimp and cook until the tails and bodies begin to turn pink, 3 to 4 minutes, then turn them over and cook for another 3 to 4 minutes, or until bright pink. Remove the shrimp from the pan and place them on a plate.

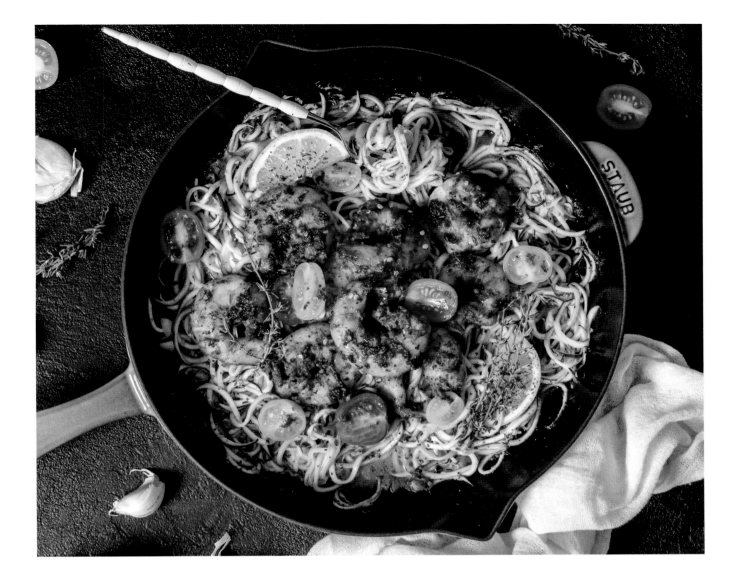

5. In the same skillet, melt the remaining 2 tablespoons of butter. Add the garlic and sauté until fragrant and golden brown, 2 to 3 minutes. Add the zucchini noodles, lemon juice, and Sriracha, season lightly with salt and pepper, and toss the noodles until fully coated with the garlic butter.

6. Add the halved tomatoes and cooked shrimp and toss everything together before removing the pan from the heat.

7. To serve, divide between two bowls or plates and top with thyme and parsley, tucking lemon wedges in on the sides.

Tip: Instead of Sriracha, you can use another medium-hot hot sauce of your choice.

If you don't have smoked paprika, you can substitute the same amount of chili powder.

Vegan Loaded Quinoa Nachos

SERVES
6

PREP TIME
15 minutes
(not including
time to soak
cashews)

COOK TIME
20 minutes

When it comes to nachos, I'm always first in line. Growing up, I enjoyed chips and queso or traditional nachos at the movie theater; however, this vegan version has become my go-to since I've reduced my intake of dairy and gluten. The best part? These nachos can easily be customized by adding beans along with the quinoa or other toppings such as jalapeños, corn, arugula, or fresh cilantro. Regardless of which toppings you choose to add, this dish is the best weeknight meal or weekend comfort food for the entire family.

NACHOS:

1 (12-ounce) bag unsalted tortilla chips

1 cup cooked red or tri-color quinoa (see page 58)

3 tablespoons chili powder

1 teaspoon finely ground sea salt

1 teaspoon ground black pepper

1 teaspoon garlic powder

1 teaspoon onion powder

1 teaspoon ground dried oregano

1 teaspoon smoked paprika

1 teaspoon dried parsley

½ teaspoon ground cumin

1 (10-ounce) can red or green enchilada sauce

1 onion, chopped

2 cups chopped red cabbage

VEGAN WHITE QUESO SAUCE:

1 cup raw cashews, soaked, drained, and rinsed (see note, page 48)

2 cloves garlic, peeled

1 jalapeño pepper, seeded and roughly chopped

¼ cup plus 1 tablespoon nutritional yeast

1 tablespoon freshly squeezed lemon juice

1 teaspoon finely ground sea salt

1 teaspoon ground black pepper

½ teaspoon chili powder

Pinch of ground cumin

TOPPINGS (OPTIONAL):

Halved grape tomatoes or diced tomatoes

Freshly squeezed lime juice

Guacamole, homemade (page 62) or store-bought

Finely chopped fresh cilantro

1. Preheat the oven to 400°F and line a large skillet with parchment paper cut into a circle to fit neatly in the bottom.

2. Lay the tortilla chips in the prepared skillet, spreading them evenly until the bottom of the skillet is covered.

3. Put the quinoa and seasonings in a large bowl and stir until well combined.

4. Spoon the enchilada sauce evenly over the tortilla chips, then sprinkle on the chopped onion and cabbage. Spoon the seasoned quinoa evenly over the top until everything is mostly covered.

5. Bake the nachos for 15 to 20 minutes, or until the vegetables are soft and tender.

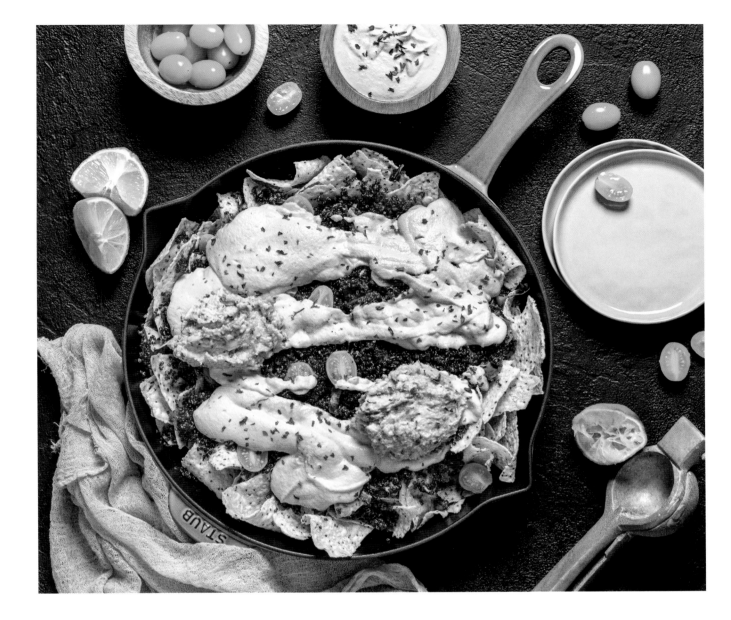

6. Meanwhile, make the queso sauce: Put all the ingredients in a high-powered blender and blend until completely smooth and creamy, 2 to 3 minutes. Season to taste with additional salt, if needed.

7. Once done, remove the nachos from the oven and top with the queso sauce and, if desired, tomatoes, lime juice, guacamole, and/or cilantro. Serve immediately.

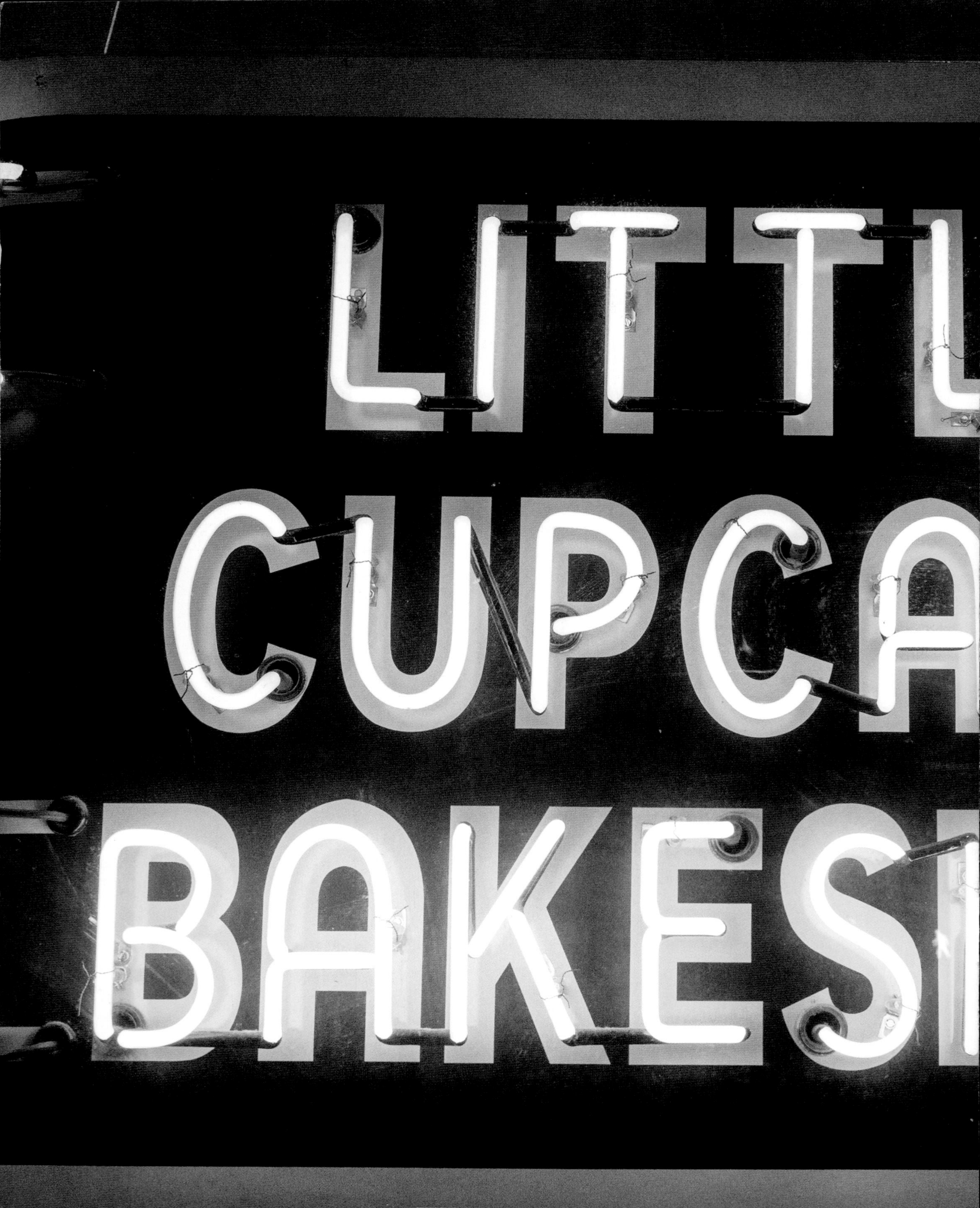
LITTL
CUPCA
BAKESI

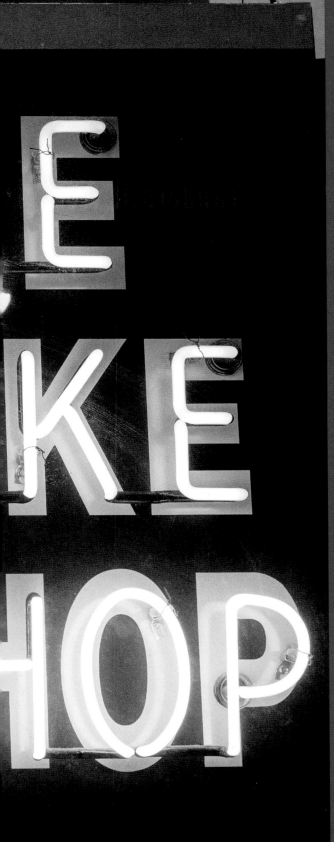

Easy Fudgy
VEGAN AVOCADO BROWNIES

MAKES
8 brownies

PREP TIME
15 minutes

COOK TIME
40 minutes

I don't bake brownies often, but when I do, I'm always hooked. These timeless sweet treats are just so good—am I right? Give me a glass of plant-based milk and two or three of these homemade brownies and I'm one happy camper. If you want to make the brownies gluten-free, don't worry—they won't lose their fudginess or richness. Plus, I love the idea of changing things up whenever my taste buds are ready for something new. So it's totally OK to experiment by leaving out the avocado or subbing one small zucchini, peeled and grated, or natural peanut butter or replacing the chocolate chips with caramel baking chips or something else along those lines. If you'd like to dress up these brownies, try serving them with your favorite nondairy ice cream or fresh fruit or sprinkling them with powdered sugar.

½ cup vegan butter, melted, plus more for the pan

1 cup cane sugar

4 Flaxseed Eggs (page 38) or Chia Eggs (page 39)

½ cup unsweetened almond milk

½ Hass avocado, peeled, pitted, and mashed

1 tablespoon vanilla extract

1 cup all-purpose flour

¾ cup cacao powder

1 teaspoon baking powder

½ teaspoon finely ground sea salt

1 cup vegan semi-sweet chocolate chips, divided

1. Preheat the oven to 350°F. Grease an 8-inch square baking pan with vegan butter, then line it with parchment paper, leaving some paper overhanging the sides.

2. In a large bowl, whisk the melted butter and sugar until the mixture looks like wet sand. Add the flaxseed eggs, almond milk, mashed avocado, and vanilla extract and whisk to combine.

3. In a medium-size bowl, whisk together the flour, cacao powder, baking powder, and salt.

4. Add the dry ingredients to the bowl with the wet ingredients and mix using a rubber spatula or wooden spoon just until fully combined. The batter will be quite thick—almost as stiff as cookie dough.

5. Gently fold in half of the chocolate chips.

6. Scrape the batter into the prepared baking pan and spread it out evenly. Sprinkle the remaining chocolate chips on top and gently press them into the batter.

7. Bake for 35 to 40 minutes, or until a toothpick inserted in the center comes out mostly clean. Remove from the oven and let cool for 20 minutes, then lift the brownie out of the pan and transfer to a cooling rack to finish cooling.

8. Once completely cool, slice into 8 squares and serve. Store leftover brownies in a tightly sealed container for up to 3 days at room temperature or refrigerate for up to 5 days. To freeze, wrap the brownies tightly in plastic wrap followed by foil and freeze for up to 3 months. Shortly before serving, thaw at room temperature.

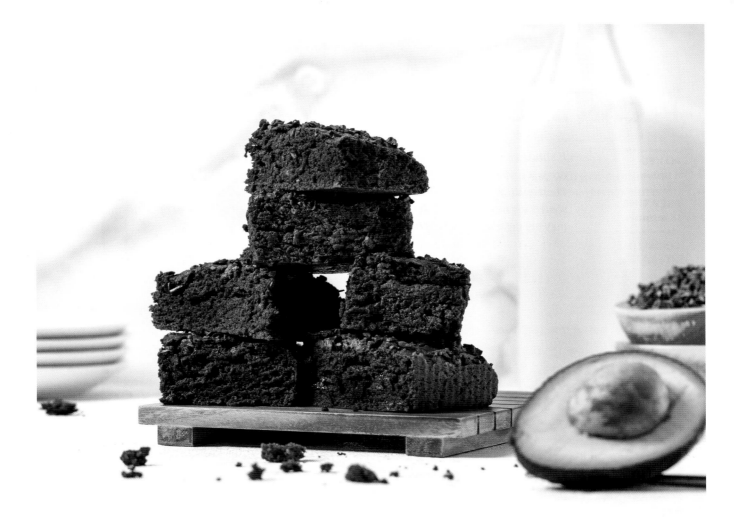

VARIATION: Gluten-Free Fudgy Avocado Brownies.

Substitute gluten-free 1-to-1 baking flour for the all-purpose flour. Also reduce the almond milk to ⅓ cup and the vegan butter to ⅓ cup.

 Tip: **FOR MAKING THE BEST BROWNIES:**

#1: Don't overmix the batter.

#2: Use an appropriate egg substitute. This recipe uses flaxseed eggs or chia eggs as the binder, but those are not the only choices. See page 23 for other options.

#3: Use the right baking pan. Metal pans are the best ones to use because the brownies bake faster; glass baking dishes make them take longer. If using a 9-inch pan instead of an 8-inch pan, the batter will spread out thinner, causing it to bake more quickly.

#4: Use parchment paper! This helps the brownies come out easily, beautifully formed with nice clean edges.

#5: Always wait for the brownies to *fully* cool before cutting them. Brownies have the best texture and structure when entirely cool.

Chocolate Cheesecake Bites
WITH MIXED BERRIES

MAKES
12 cheesecake bites

PREP TIME
15 minutes, plus 1 hour to chill

COOK TIME
30 minutes

Cheesecake bites are one of the few desserts that my son and I make together. He loves using our handheld mixer, and as I organize the remaining ingredients, I let him beat the cream cheese. It feels like a full-circle moment because cheesecake was the first dessert that I learned to make and perfect. I was right out of high school and looking for a way to impress my now-husband, who was my sweetheart at the time. I baked him a New York–style cheesecake with a strawberry topping as a way to impress him. Well, it worked. Back then, I used mostly premade ingredients, but today, I enjoy making my cheesecake from scratch and showing my son how to do the same.

GRAHAM CRACKER CRUST:

1½ cups roughly chopped graham crackers (10 to 12 full sheets)

2 tablespoons lightly packed brown sugar

¼ teaspoon ground cinnamon

3 tablespoons unsalted butter, melted

CHOCOLATE CHEESECAKE FILLING:

12 ounces cream cheese, room temperature

½ cup cane sugar

3 tablespoons all-purpose flour

2 tablespoons cacao powder

3 tablespoons plain Greek yogurt (full-fat)

2 teaspoons vanilla extract

2 large eggs, room temperature

4 ounces semi-sweet chocolate, melted

TOPPINGS:

Sliced fresh strawberries

Fresh blueberries

Fresh blackberries

MAKE THE GRAHAM CRACKER CRUST:

1. Place one oven rack in the lowest position and a second rack in the middle. Preheat the oven to 325°F. Line a 12-cavity muffin pan with cupcake liners.

2. Using a food processor, crush the graham crackers until they're mostly finely ground. (It's OK to leave a few medium-size pieces if you're a lover of a little crunch!) Alternatively, you can put the crackers in a zip-top bag and crush them with a rolling pin. Combine the crushed graham crackers, brown sugar, cinnamon, and melted butter in a small bowl and mix with a rubber spatula until well incorporated.

3. Divide the mixture evenly among the cupcake liners, using about 2 tablespoons per cup, and press down on the crust with your fingers to ensure that it's perfectly covering the bottoms.

4. Bake the crusts for 5 minutes, then remove the pan from the oven and set aside to cool.

MAKE THE CHEESECAKE BITES:

5. Using a large mixing bowl and hand mixer or a stand mixer fitted with the paddle attachment, beat the cream cheese, sugar, flour, and cacao powder on high speed until well combined. Scrape down the sides of the bowl as needed.

6. Add the yogurt and vanilla extract and beat on low speed. Scrape the sides of the bowl again. Then add the eggs one at a time, all the while mixing on low speed until combined.

7. Gently fold in the melted chocolate until no streaks remain, scraping the sides and bottom of the bowl to eliminate any lumps.

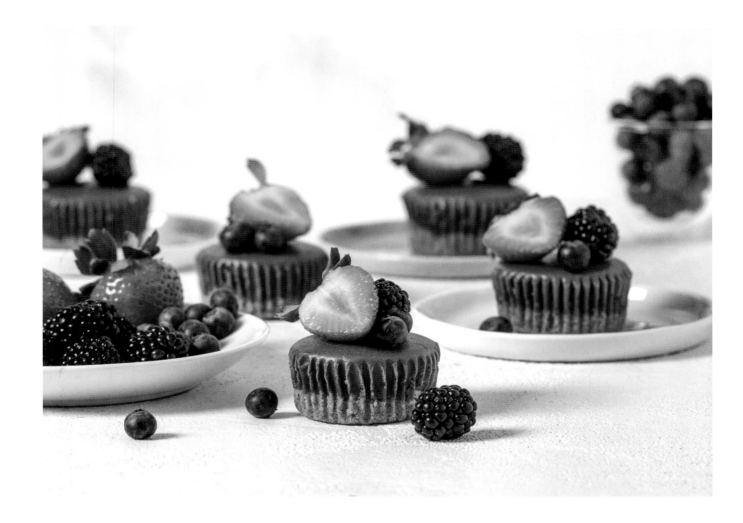

8. Divide the cheesecake filling evenly among the cupcake liners, using about 2 tablespoons per cup. Fill a baking pan with at least 2-inch sides about halfway with warm water and carefully place it on the bottom rack in the oven; this ensures the cheesecakes remain moist as they bake. Place the muffin pan with the cheesecakes on the middle rack, above the pan of water.

9. Bake the cheesecakes for 20 to 25 minutes, then turn off the oven and allow them to sit in the oven with the door halfway open for another 5 minutes to keep the cheesecakes from deflating.

10. Remove the cheesecakes from the oven and allow them to cool completely, then put them in the refrigerator to chill for at least 1 hour before serving.

11. Once cool, top with fresh berries and enjoy. Leftovers can be stored tightly wrapped in the refrigerator for up to 5 days. To freeze, wrap the cheesecakes tightly in plastic wrap followed by foil and freeze for up to 1 month. For best results, keep them in the freezer until the night before you're ready to serve them; place the frozen cakes in the refrigerator to defrost overnight.

Vegan Strawberry Funfetti
BIRTHDAY CAKE

MAKES
one three-layer
8-inch cake, or
one two-layer
9-inch cake
(16 servings)

PREP TIME
25 minutes

COOK TIME
35 minutes

The first time I perfected a vegan cake was for my thirtieth birthday. To celebrate the occasion, I decided to make myself a funfetti cake. It came out perfect! I remember feeling so accomplished because until then I'd struggled with vegan cakes. This recipe is that very same cake but with the addition of a delicious strawberry buttercream that makes it even more special. If you're looking to bake something festive for a loved one's birthday or to celebrate a "just because" moment, then this cake is the one. Plus, you can transform it into cupcakes for the perfect bite if you'd like (see the variation on page 253).

CAKE:

Vegan butter, for the pans

1½ cups all-purpose flour

¾ cup cane sugar

1½ teaspoons baking powder

½ teaspoon baking soda

½ teaspoon finely ground sea salt

1 cup Vegan Buttermilk (page 46)

¼ cup vegetable oil

1 teaspoon vanilla extract

½ cup vegan rainbow sprinkles

STRAWBERRY BUTTERCREAM:

(makes enough for a two-layer 9-inch cake)

½ cup vegan butter, room temperature

4 cups powdered sugar, sifted, divided, plus more if needed

2 tablespoons strawberry preserves or jam

1 tablespoon unsweetened almond milk, plus more if needed

1 teaspoon vanilla extract

Pinch of finely ground sea salt

TOPPINGS:

1 cup vegan rainbow sprinkles

Sliced or halved strawberries

MAKE THE CAKE:

1. Preheat the oven to 350°F. Lightly grease either three 8-inch round cake pans or two 9-inch round cake pans with vegan butter, then line the greased pans with parchment paper.

2. In a large bowl, whisk together the flour, sugar, baking powder, baking soda, and salt. Set aside.

3. In a stand mixer fitted with the whisk attachment, beat the buttermilk with the vegetable oil and vanilla extract until the ingredients are combined and the mixture becomes slightly foamy. Turn off the mixer and change the attachment to the paddle.

4. With the mixer running on low speed, add the dry ingredients and continue to mix until well incorporated and the batter is smooth, 3 to 4 minutes. Fold in the sprinkles.

5. Pour the batter evenly into the prepared pans, then spread it out evenly. (See the tip on page 252 regarding the use of cake strips.)

6. Place the cake pans on the top rack of the oven and bake for 25 to 30 minutes (if making three 8-inch cakes) or 30 to 35 minutes (if making two 9-inch cakes), or until a toothpick inserted in the center of a cake comes out clean.

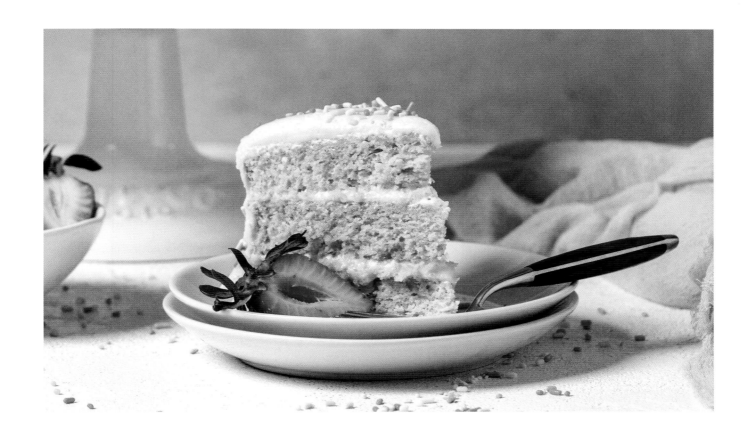

7. Remove the cakes from the oven and let cool for at least 30 minutes. Carefully turn them upside down, allow the cakes to slide out, and place them on a cooling rack to cool completely before frosting. *Note:* To accelerate cooling, you can allow the cakes to cool on the counter until they are barely warm to the touch, about 30 minutes, then place them in the refrigerator for another hour or so to cool completely.

MAKE THE BUTTERCREAM:

8. If making a three-layer cake, you will need to increase the quantity of buttercream slightly; see the tip on page 252 before proceeding with this step. In a stand mixer fitted with the paddle attachment, beat the butter on high speed until smooth and creamy, about 2 minutes. Turn the mixer to low and add half of the powdered sugar, the strawberry preserves, almond milk, and vanilla extract; continue mixing until well combined. Add the remaining powdered sugar and pinch of salt and mix again for 1 minute before increasing the speed to medium-high and mixing until smooth. If the frosting is too thick, add more almond milk 1 tablespoon at a time; if the frosting is too thin, add more powdered sugar 1 tablespoon at a time.

Vegan Red Velvet Sheet Cake
WITH BOURBON BUTTERCREAM

MAKES
one 8-inch
square cake
(12 servings)

PREP TIME
20 minutes

COOK TIME
20 minutes

When it comes to red velvet anything, you will probably agree that it's something special, especially during the holiday season. There's nothing like a delicious slice of red velvet cake, which often comes paired with a beautiful cream cheese topping—am I right? Believe it or not, the awesome thing about this recipe is that it doesn't use a traditional cream cheese topping, but the bourbon buttercream doesn't miss a beat. You can always omit the bourbon and reduce the powdered sugar by ½ cup to create a traditional vanilla buttercream for the kids to enjoy along with you, if needed! It'll still taste just as decadent.

CAKE:

Vegan butter, for the pan
(optional)

3 cups all-purpose flour

1½ cups cane sugar

½ cup cacao powder

1 tablespoon baking powder

½ teaspoon baking soda

½ teaspoon finely ground sea salt

Pinch of ground cinnamon

1 cup Vegan Buttermilk (page 46)

¼ cup vegetable oil

2 teaspoons vanilla extract

2 to 3 tablespoons natural red
food coloring (see Tip)

BOURBON BUTTERCREAM:

½ cup vegan butter, room
temperature

5 cups powdered sugar, sifted,
divided, plus more if needed

3 tablespoons bourbon

1 tablespoon unsweetened
almond milk, plus more if
needed

1 teaspoon vanilla extract

Pinch of finely ground sea salt

Sliced or halved strawberries,
for topping (optional)

MAKE THE CAKE:

1. Preheat the oven to 350°F. Lightly grease an 8-inch square cake pan with vegan butter or line it with parchment paper.

2. In a large mixing bowl, whisk together the flour, sugar, cacao powder, baking powder, baking soda, salt, and cinnamon.

3. Add the buttermilk, vegetable oil, vanilla extract, and food coloring to the dry ingredients. Using a rubber spatula, mix just until well combined and smooth; make sure no lumps are visible, but be careful not to overmix.

4. Pour the batter into the prepared pan, then use a rubber spatula to spread it out as evenly as possible. Bake for 15 to 20 minutes, or until a toothpick inserted in the center comes out clean.

5. Remove from the oven and let cool completely.

Tip: For a cake with a lighter red color, use just 2 tablespoons of food coloring; if you'd like a deep red cake, as shown in the photo, use 3 tablespoons.

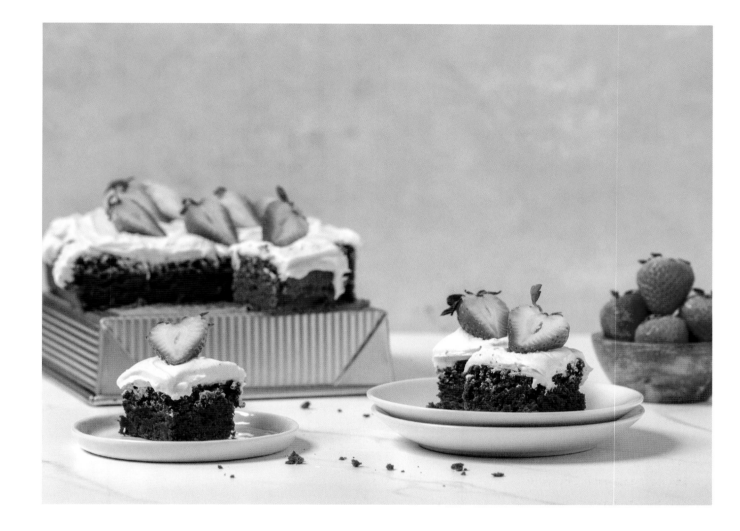

MAKE THE BUTTERCREAM:

6. In a stand mixer fitted with the paddle attachment, beat the butter on high speed until smooth and creamy, about 2 minutes. Turn the mixer to low and add half of the powdered sugar, the bourbon, almond milk, and vanilla extract; continue mixing until well combined. Add the remaining powdered sugar and pinch of salt, increase the mixer speed to medium-high, and continue mixing until well combined. If the frosting is too thick, add more almond milk 1 tablespoon at a time; if it is too thin, add more powdered sugar 1 tablespoon at a time.

7. Once the cake is completely cool, use a metal frosting spatula to top the cake with the bourbon buttercream, gently spreading it out until the cake is fully covered and the frosting is even. Slice into squares, top with sliced strawberries, and enjoy! Store leftovers tightly wrapped in an airtight container in the refrigerator for up to 4 days. You can also freeze leftover cake tightly wrapped in plastic wrap followed by foil for up to 3 months. Before serving, defrost the cake on the counter.

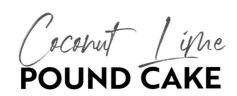

Coconut Lime POUND CAKE

MAKES
1 Bundt or
loaf cake
(16 servings)

PREP TIME
15 minutes

COOK TIME
1 hour
15 minutes

While most of the pound cakes I make are inspired by my Southern roots, this recipe was inspired by my Jamaican background. Coconut and lime is one of the most island-y combinations to exist, and you can really appreciate both flavors in this cake. The batter for this dense, fluffy, spongy cake is whipped together in just 15 minutes and then baked to perfection. To up the island theme, you can add a bit of rum (see the tip below). For a nice crunch, I like to add coconut flakes to the batter; however, you can use them just on the top of the cake if you prefer. Either way, you're going to love this recipe!

CAKE:

2 cups all-purpose flour, plus more for the pan

1 cup unsweetened coconut flakes

1 teaspoon baking powder

1 teaspoon finely ground sea salt

1 cup (2 sticks) unsalted butter, room temperature, plus more for the pan

1½ cups cane sugar

4 large eggs

¾ cup plain Greek yogurt (full-fat)

1 teaspoon coconut extract

1 tablespoon grated lime zest

1 teaspoon freshly squeezed lime juice

GLAZE:

1½ cups powdered sugar

2 to 3 tablespoons heavy cream

1 teaspoon freshly squeezed lime juice

TOPPINGS:

1 tablespoon grated lime zest

½ cup unsweetened coconut flakes

MAKE THE CAKE:

1. Preheat the oven to 325°F. Generously grease and flour a 12-cup Bundt pan.

2. In a medium-size bowl, whisk together the flour, coconut flakes, baking powder, and salt. Set aside.

3. In a separate medium-size bowl, cream the butter and sugar with a hand mixer on medium speed until well combined and the mixture becomes pale yellow. Turn the mixer to high, add the eggs one at a time, and mix until light and fluffy. Add the yogurt, coconut extract, and lime zest and juice and mix until combined.

4. Turn the mixer to low speed and slowly add half of the flour mixture to the wet mixture; mix until well combined. Then mix in the remaining flour mixture. Once it's mostly incorporated, increase the speed to medium-high and mix just until thick and smooth, being careful not to overmix. Allow the batter to rest for 5 minutes.

5. Pour the batter into the prepared pan and smooth the top. Bake for 60 to 75 minutes, or until a toothpick inserted in the center comes out clean. Remove the cake from the oven, place on a cooling rack, and allow to cool completely before removing from the pan.

MAKE THE GLAZE:

6. In a small bowl, mix together all the glaze ingredients, using 2 tablespoons of heavy cream, until well combined. If the glaze is too thick to run off a spoon, add up to 1 tablespoon more cream to thin it.

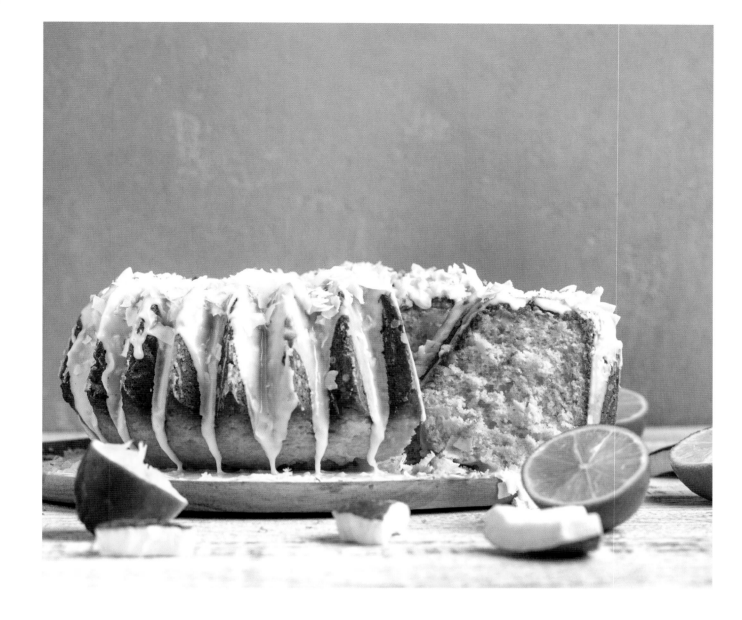

7. Once the cake is cool, run a butter knife around the edge of the pan to loosen the cake, then turn the pan over onto a cake plate. The cake should slide out of the pan onto the plate. Drizzle the glaze over the top and sides of the cake. Top with the lime zest and coconut flakes. Slice and serve. Store any leftovers in an airtight container in the refrigerator for up to 5 days. To freeze, tightly wrap leftover cake in plastic wrap followed by foil and store in the freezer for up to 3 months.

Tip: To give this cake a touch of rum flavor, you can add ¼ cup to ⅓ cup of white rum to the batter and omit the almond milk. Besides adding flavor, the rum will give the cake a more tender crumb.

Vegan Oat Cupcakes
WITH STRAWBERRY BUTTERCREAM

MAKES
12 cupcakes

PREP TIME
10 minutes

COOK TIME
18 minutes

This recipe was inspired by a cake that I made for Valentine's Day and published on my blog. It was a hit, so I decided to reinvent it for you here, in cupcake form. The best part is that while these cupcakes are entirely plant-based, you don't need any fancy ingredients to whip them together. However, if I'm honest, the true highlight is the strawberry buttercream. Usually, I make my own strawberry compote before adding it to the buttercream, but for this recipe, I kept things simple and used natural strawberry preserves, which adds bits of strawberries throughout the frosting's velvety base.

OATMEAL CUPCAKES:

1 cup all-purpose flour

1 cup rolled oats (gluten-free)

¾ cup cane sugar

1½ teaspoons baking powder

½ teaspoon baking soda

½ teaspoon finely ground sea salt

½ teaspoon ground cinnamon

1 cup Vegan Buttermilk (page 46)

⅓ cup vegan butter, melted

2 Flaxseed Eggs (page 38) or Chia Eggs (page 39)

Unsweetened almond milk, if needed to thin batter

STRAWBERRY BUTTERCREAM:

½ cup vegan butter, room temperature

4 cups powdered sugar, sifted, divided, plus more if needed

2 tablespoons strawberry preserves or jam

1 tablespoon unsweetened almond milk, plus more if needed

1 teaspoon vanilla extract

Pinch of finely ground sea salt

12 strawberry halves or slices, for topping

MAKE THE CUPCAKES:

1. Preheat the oven to 350°F. Line a 12-cavity muffin pan with cupcake liners.

2. In a large bowl, whisk together the flour, oats, sugar, baking powder, baking soda, salt, and cinnamon until combined. Add the buttermilk, melted butter, and flaxseed eggs and mix with a hand mixer on high speed until just combined. Do not overmix. If the batter is extremely thick, add almond milk 1 tablespoon at a time until the batter is pourable but not thin or runny.

3. Pour the batter into the cupcake liners until they are about two-thirds of the way full, using about 2 tablespoons of batter per cupcake. Bake for 15 to 20 minutes, or until a toothpick inserted in the center of a cupcake comes out clean. Remove the cupcakes from the oven and let cool completely in the pan.

MAKE THE BUTTERCREAM:

4. In a stand mixer fitted with the paddle attachment, beat the butter on high speed until smooth and creamy, about 2 minutes. Turn the mixer to low and add half of the powdered sugar, the strawberry preserves, almond milk, and vanilla extract; continue mixing until well combined. Add the remaining powdered sugar and pinch of salt, increase the speed to high, and mix again until well combined. If the frosting is too thick, add more almond milk 1 tablespoon at a time; if it is too thin, add more powdered sugar 1 tablespoon at a time. (*Note:* Any leftover buttercream can be stored in an airtight container in the refrigerator for up to 1 week or frozen for up to 3 months.)

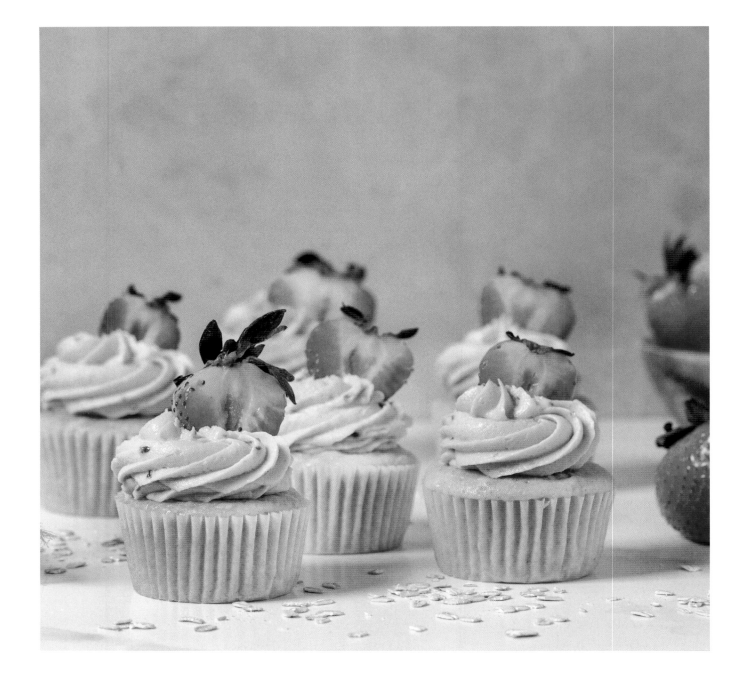

5. Remove the cooled cupcakes from the pan and frost them with the buttercream, using a pastry bag and icing tip for a pretty presentation. Decorate each cupcake with a strawberry half or slice. Enjoy! Leftover cupcakes can be stored in an airtight container in the refrigerator for up to 1 week if unfrosted or up to 4 days if frosted. Unfrosted cupcakes can be frozen for up to 6 months and thawed at room temperature; wrap them in plastic wrap and then foil before freezing them.

Ginger Cupcakes
WITH CHAI CREAM CHEESE FROSTING

MAKES
12 cupcakes

PREP TIME
15 minutes

COOK TIME
18 minutes

Who doesn't love a good cupcake? This version packs incredible flavor into every bite. Inspired by my Jamaican background, these ginger-filled cupcakes pay homage to the heavy use of gingerroot in Jamaican cuisine. Growing up, I remember having ginger everything, including ginger tea, which was used as a healing remedy due to ginger's powerful health benefits. Here the bold flavors of ginger and other spices combine with the coolness and spiciness of a chai-infused cream cheese frosting. You're sure to make these more than once.

CUPCAKES:

1½ cups all-purpose flour

1½ teaspoons baking powder

½ teaspoon baking soda

½ teaspoon finely ground sea salt

2 teaspoons ginger powder

½ teaspoon ground cinnamon

½ cup lightly packed brown sugar

2 tablespoons vegetable oil

2 teaspoons golden syrup

2 teaspoons molasses

1 large egg, room temperature

¾ cup unsweetened almond milk

CHAI CREAM CHEESE FROSTING:

4 ounces cream cheese, room temperature

½ cup (1 stick) unsalted butter, room temperature

1 teaspoon vanilla extract

1 tablespoon chai spice mix, homemade (page 40) or store-bought

4 cups powdered sugar, sifted, divided

2 to 3 tablespoons heavy cream or milk

Ground nutmeg, for sprinkling

MAKE THE CUPCAKES:

1. Preheat the oven to 350°F. Line a 12-cavity muffin pan with cupcake liners.

2. In a medium-size mixing bowl, whisk together the flour, baking powder, baking soda, salt, ginger, and cinnamon. Add the brown sugar, oil, syrup, molasses, egg, and almond milk. Using a hand mixer, mix on medium speed until just combined; do not overmix.

3. Pour the batter into the cupcake liners until they are about two-thirds full, using about 2 tablespoons of batter per cupcake. Bake for 15 to 20 minutes, or until a toothpick inserted in the center of a cupcake comes out clean. Remove the cupcakes from the oven and set aside to cool completely.

MAKE THE FROSTING:

4. In a large mixing bowl, using the hand mixer, cream the cream cheese and butter on medium-high speed until completely combined and all the lumps are gone. Add the vanilla extract and chai spice and mix until just combined. Add half of the powdered sugar and mix until well combined. Add 2 tablespoons of the heavy cream and the remaining powdered sugar and mix until the frosting is fluffy; if it's too thick, add up to 1 tablespoon more cream.

5. Once the cupcakes are completely cool, remove them from the pan and frost them with the cream cheese frosting, using a pastry bag and icing tip for a pretty presentation. Sprinkle the tops with nutmeg and enjoy! Leftover cupcakes can be stored in an airtight container in the refrigerator for up to 1 week if unfrosted or up to 4 days if frosted. Unfrosted cupcakes can also be wrapped in plastic wrap and then foil and frozen for up to 6 months; thaw at room temperature.

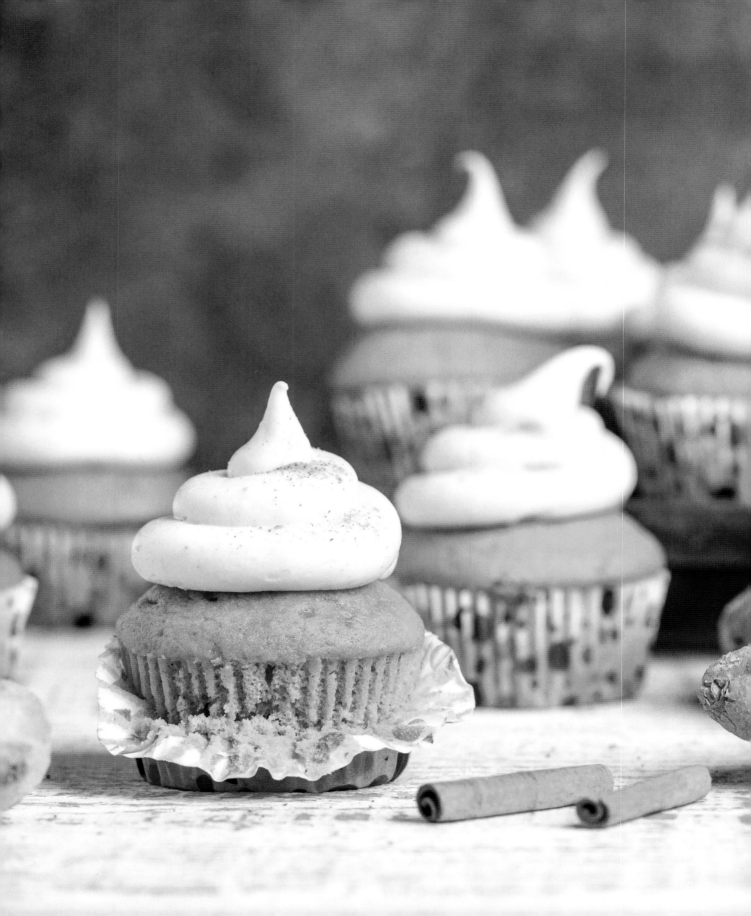

Southern BANANA PUDDING

SERVES
8

PREP TIME
20 minutes,
plus 1 hour to
chill

Banana pudding was one of the desserts that my grandmother used to make for our weekend movie nights during my childhood, right before we binge-watched thrillers and horror films. It was our love language, much like my ice cream adventures with my grandfather. Her version of banana pudding was simple, and she would bake everything together, which gave you a warm experience in every spoonful. Now that I live in NYC and have tried so many different variations of sweets and other foods, I've grown accustomed to creating twists on old favorites, like this one. My version of banana pudding is made with sweetened condensed milk for an extra rich and velvety texture that is lightened with homemade whipped cream and layered with lots of banana slices and vanilla wafers—just how I like it!

WHIPPED CREAM TOPPING:

1½ cups heavy whipping cream

3 tablespoons powdered sugar

1½ teaspoons vanilla extract

PUDDING:

1½ cups ice-cold water

1 (14-ounce) can sweetened condensed milk

1 (3-ounce) box vanilla instant pudding mix

1 tablespoon vanilla extract

Pinch of finely ground sea salt

Pinch of ground cinnamon

1 (12-ounce) box vanilla wafers

4 ripe bananas, sliced

1. Make the whipped cream topping: Pour the heavy whipping cream into a medium-size mixing bowl, preferably chilled (see Tip, opposite), then add the powdered sugar and vanilla extract. Beat on high speed with a hand mixer until soft peaks form, then reduce the speed to medium and continue whipping until stiff peaks form. Store in the refrigerator until ready to use.

2. Make the pudding: In a large bowl, using an electric mixer, mix together the ice-cold water, sweetened condensed milk, and pudding mix on medium-high speed until thick and puddinglike, about 10 minutes. Add the vanilla extract, salt, and cinnamon to the pudding and mix for another minute or so.

3. Gently fold the whipped cream into the pudding using a rubber spatula until well incorporated.

4. In a trifle bowl or other serving dish, create a single layer of vanilla wafers, banana slices, and pudding mixture; repeat the layering until all the ingredients have been used, reserving 10 to 12 wafers for the top.

5. Place about half of the reserved vanilla wafers on top, then crush the remaining wafers and sprinkle them on top, around the whole wafers. Refrigerate for at least an hour before serving; it's best if chilled overnight. Store leftovers in an airtight container or sealed serving bowl in the refrigerator for 3 days.

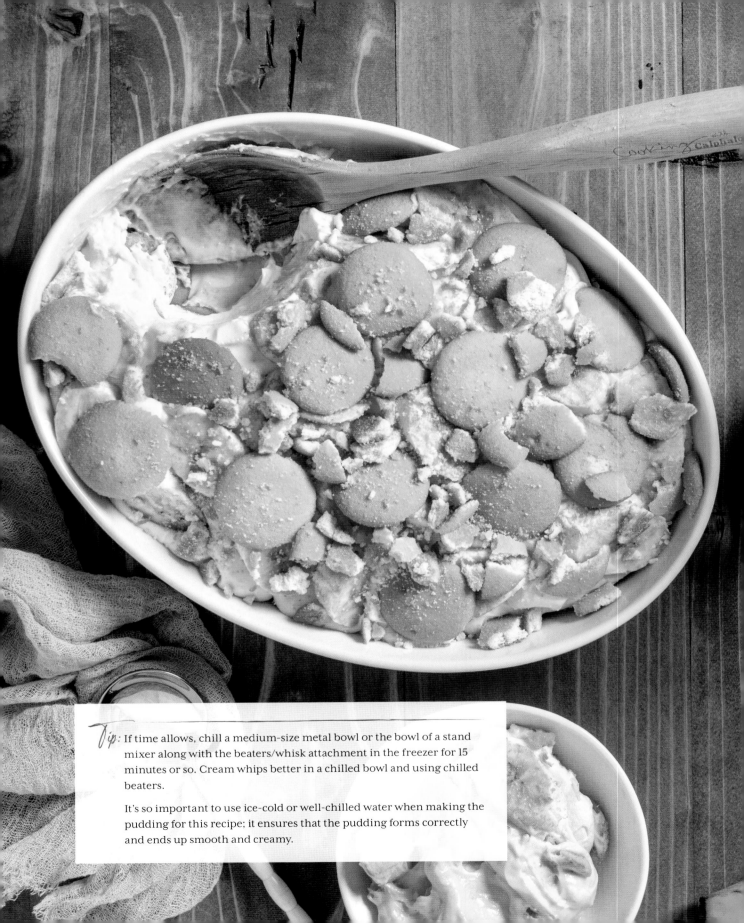

Tip: If time allows, chill a medium-size metal bowl or the bowl of a stand mixer along with the beaters/whisk attachment in the freezer for 15 minutes or so. Cream whips better in a chilled bowl and using chilled beaters.

It's so important to use ice-cold or well-chilled water when making the pudding for this recipe; it ensures that the pudding forms correctly and ends up smooth and creamy.

Vegan Maple
BLACKBERRY CRISPS

SERVES
4

PREP TIME
5 minutes

COOK TIME
35 minutes

These warm crisps are the epitome of everything nice: a tart berry filling flavored with rich, aromatic spices and sweetened with pure maple syrup, covered with a crunchy golden topping. This is one of my favorite summertime desserts to make when blackberries are in season. It's so easy! I love to serve these with a scoop of dairy-free ice cream when they're still warm from the oven so that it melts nicely. So good!

FILLING:

5 cups fresh blackberries

⅓ cup pure maple syrup

¼ cup arrowroot starch

1 tablespoon freshly squeezed lemon juice

1 tablespoon ground cinnamon

1 teaspoon ground nutmeg

½ teaspoon ginger powder

CRUMBLE TOPPING:

1 cup rolled oats (gluten-free)

½ cup all-purpose flour

½ cup firmly packed brown sugar

¼ cup chopped pecans, toasted (see note, page 107)

1 teaspoon ground cinnamon

Pinch of finely ground sea salt

½ cup vegan butter, room temperature, plus more for the pans

TOPPINGS (OPTIONAL):

Fresh mint leaves

Dairy-free ice cream of choice

1. Preheat the oven to 350°F.

2. Put the filling ingredients in a medium-size bowl and toss until the berries are evenly coated. Set aside.

3. In a separate medium-size bowl, whisk together the oats, flour, brown sugar, pecans, cinnamon, and salt. Using a pastry blender or two forks, cut the butter into the flour mixture until it becomes crumbly and the butter is evenly mixed in. Set aside.

4. Lightly grease four mini ceramic tart pans, 4 to 5 inches in diameter, and spread the fruit filling evenly in the pans. Evenly top with the crumble mixture. Place the tart pans on a sheet pan to catch any overflow during baking. Place the sheet pan in the oven and bake for 30 to 35 minutes, or until the fruit mixture is bubbly and the topping is golden.

5. Remove the crisps from the oven and let rest for 5 to 10 minutes. Top with mint leaves and your favorite dairy-free ice cream, if desired. Serve and enjoy.

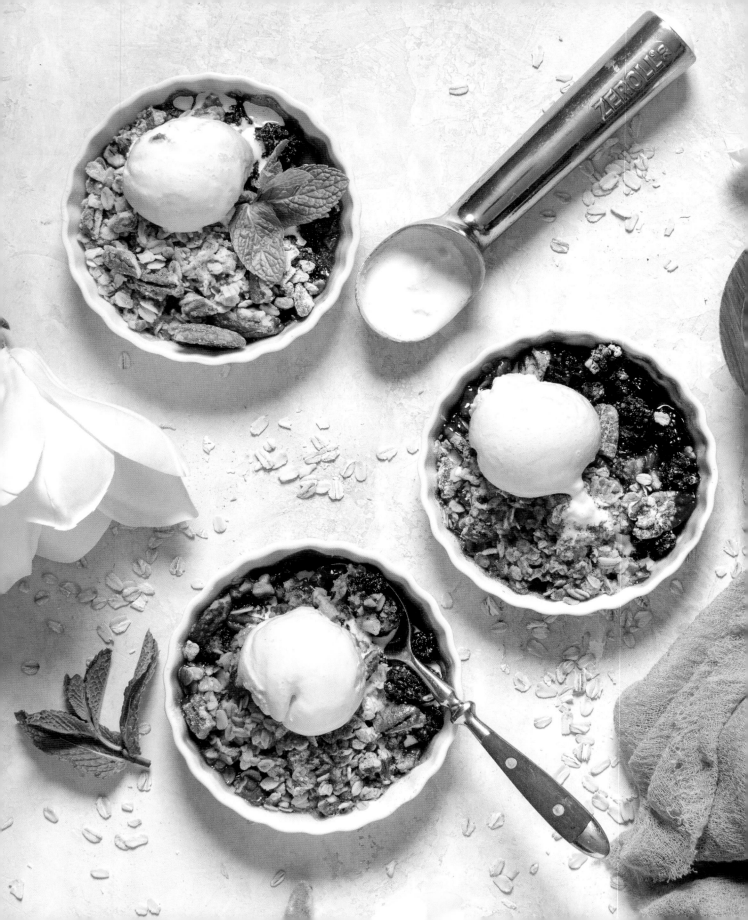

Cheddar TRIPLE APPLE PIE

SERVES
8

PREP TIME
20 minutes

COOK TIME
1 hour

What more is there to say about a cheddar triple apple pie? This incredible savory-sweet pie is by far one of my favorite versions of apple pie that I've made in all my years of baking. As the name suggests, this pie filling uses three types of apples—Gala, Honeycrisp, and Granny Smith—creating a complex burst of apple flavor in every mouthful, and the crust is as flaky and buttery as you could hope for. It does not disappoint! For most cheddar apple pies, the cheese is placed on top of the baked pie as a serving option. Here, the cheese is mixed right into the filling, infusing the pie with a sweet, tart, and savory balance. Going with the savory theme, the pie is garnished with dried herbs. I tend to use parsley, but you can use any herb that complements the flavors of apple and cheddar; rosemary and thyme are good options as well.

Butter, for the pan

FILLING:

3 Granny Smith apples, peeled and sliced

3 Honeycrisp apples, peeled and sliced

2 Gala apples, peeled and sliced

¾ cup cane sugar

¼ cup arrowroot starch

1½ tablespoons ground cinnamon

1 teaspoon ground nutmeg

½ teaspoon ground cloves

½ teaspoon ground allspice

½ cup shredded mild cheddar cheese

1 double recipe Everyday Pie Crust (page 46)

1 large egg

1 tablespoon unsweetened almond milk

1 tablespoon dried herb of choice

Dairy-free ice cream of choice, for serving (optional)

1. Preheat the oven to 400°F. Grease a 9-inch pie pan with butter.

2. In a large bowl, stir the filling ingredients together until well combined. Set aside.

3. On a lightly floured surface, roll out the first disk of pie dough into a circle about ⅛ inch thick. Gently place the dough circle in the prepared pan, then press the dough into the bottom and up the sides. Roll out the second disk of dough to the same size and set aside.

4. Pour the filling into the pie pan.

5. Use a sharp knife or wheeled pastry cutter to cut the dough circle into eight to ten ½-inch-wide strips. To make the strips easier to transfer, gently fold them over, then place them on top of the pie and unfold them, being sure to place the longer strips in the middle and working the shorter ones toward either side of the pie. To create a lattice pattern, place one long strip of dough perpendicular to the parallel strip, then unfold the folded strips over the perpendicular strip. Lay a second perpendicular strip of dough next to the first one with some space between them and unfold the folded parallel strip over the second one. Continue with each strip until a complete weave is made over the top of the pie. (See Tip, opposite, for a simpler option.)

6. Firmly pinch the top and bottom crust together to seal all around the edge of the pie. Cut away the excess dough before tucking or folding the remaining crust.

7. Beat the egg with the almond milk to make a wash, then lightly brush the top of the dough lattice and edges with the wash. Sprinkle the top of the pie with the dried herb of your choice.

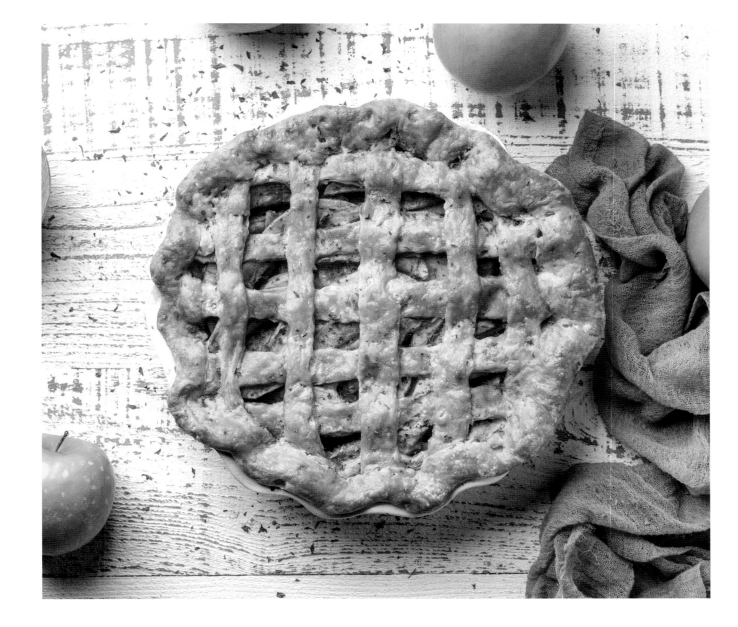

8. Bake for 45 minutes to 1 hour, until the top is golden brown and the apple filling is bubbling. Remove from the oven and let cool completely, about 2 hours.

9. Slice the pie and serve with a few scoops of ice cream, if desired. Store any leftovers tightly wrapped with plastic wrap and foil in the refrigerator for up to 4 days. Reheat each slice when ready to serve.

Tip: For a simpler top crust, simply roll out the second disk of pie dough like the first one, then carefully place it atop the pie filling, cutting off all the excess. Firmly pinch the top and bottom crusts together to seal around the edges of the pie, cut some air vents in the top, and continue with the remaining steps.

Brown Butter Pecan CHOCOLATE CHIP COOKIES

MAKES
1½ dozen cookies

PREP TIME
15 minutes, plus 30 minutes to chill

COOK TIME
15 minutes

I'm an avid chocolate chip cookie lover, especially the really soft and chunky kind. However, this brown butter–pecan version is number one on my chocolate chip cookie list. The flavors in these cookies are insane, and I don't even know if you'll still love classic chocolate chip cookies as much after trying these. To bring out the nuttiness of the pecans, I toast them and let them cool before adding them to the batter. Whether you choose to add a ton of chocolate chips or just a little, these cookies are delicious dunked in a glass of your favorite milk.

1 cup (2 sticks) unsalted butter

1 cup plus 1 tablespoon firmly packed brown sugar

⅓ cup cane sugar

2½ cups all-purpose flour

2 teaspoons cornstarch

1 teaspoon baking soda

1 teaspoon finely ground sea salt

Pinch of ground cinnamon

2 large eggs, room temperature

2 teaspoons vanilla extract

1½ cups chopped pecans, toasted (see note, page 107)

½ cup semi-sweet chocolate chips

1. Preheat the oven to 375°F. Line a baking sheet with parchment paper.

2. Make the brown butter: Melt the butter in a medium-size saucepan over medium-high heat, stirring occasionally. Continue to cook the butter, stirring occasionally, until dark flecks begin to form, the butter becomes fragrant (the aroma will be sweet and slightly nutty), and the color darkens, 3 to 4 minutes. Remove the pan from the heat and allow to cool until no longer hot.

3. In a stand mixer fitted with the paddle attachment, beat the cooled brown butter and the sugars on medium-high speed until well combined and light and fluffy, 2 to 3 minutes.

4. Meanwhile, in a medium-size bowl, whisk together the flour, cornstarch, baking soda, salt, and cinnamon.

5. Continuing to mix on medium-high, add the eggs one at a time to the butter mixture, then add the vanilla extract. Continue beating for 1 minute. Reduce the speed to low and slowly begin adding the dry ingredients to the wet, mixing until well combined. Add the toasted pecans and chocolate chips and mix for just a few seconds more, until they are well distributed in the dough.

6. Using a 1-tablespoon cookie scoop, scoop up portions of the dough and place them on the prepared baking sheet at least 1 inch apart.

7. Bake for 3 to 4 minutes, or until the cookies are slightly puffed in the center. Then lift the baking sheet and let it drop down against the oven rack. This allows the edges of the cookies to set and the centers to fall. If needed, repeat once or twice more to make sure

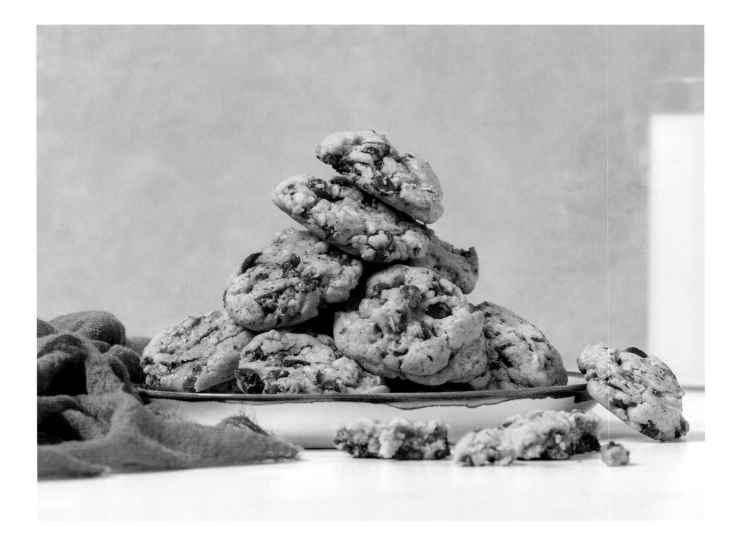

the centers have fallen. Close the oven door and bake for another 3 minutes. Repeat the lifting and dropping process. Bake for another 3 minutes, then lift and drop a third time.

8. Remove the cookies from the oven once they are slightly browned around the edges. The centers may still look soft but will set and harden more as the cookies cool.

9. Allow the cookies to cool on the baking sheet for 5 minutes, then transfer them to a cooling rack to cool completely.

10. Once the cookies are cool, grab a glass of milk and a cookie and enjoy! Leftovers can be stored in an airtight container at room temperature for up to 1 week.

Tip: Unbaked cookie dough balls can be placed in a freezer-safe zip-top bag and stored in the freezer for up to 3 months.

Vegan Chai Latte & Salted Caramel Cashew
ICE CREAM FLOAT

MAKES
two 12-ounce
servings

PREP TIME
10 minutes,
plus 6 minutes
to steep

COOK TIME
7 minutes

Conventionally, floats are made by topping scoops of ice cream with sugary soda; however, I just can't wrap my head around that notion. That's why I chose to create my own version, using my favorite flavor of store-bought vegan ice cream—salted caramel cashew—and topping it with my homemade chai latte. It's so good! I enjoy this decadent dairy-free drink as a sweet treat after dinner or as a midday pick-me-up.

CHAI LATTE:

2 cups unsweetened almond milk

2 black tea bags

1 tablespoon chai spice mix, homemade (page 40) or store-bought, plus more for topping

2 tablespoons agave syrup

1 tablespoon vanilla extract

COCONUT WHIPPED CREAM:

(Makes about 3 cups)

1 (14-ounce) can coconut cream, chilled, or cream from 2 (14-ounce) cans full-fat coconut milk, chilled overnight (see Tip)

3 tablespoons powdered sugar

½ teaspoon vanilla extract

1 pint dairy-free cashew salted caramel ice cream

1. Make the latte: Bring the almond milk to a boil in a medium-size saucepan over medium-high heat, then continue to boil for 1 to 2 minutes. Remove the pan from the heat, add the tea bags, and let steep for 5 to 6 minutes. Once fully steeped, remove the tea bags and whisk in the chai spice mix along with the agave and vanilla extract until well combined. Let the latte cool to room temperature before using.

2. Make the coconut whipped cream: Put the chilled coconut cream in a medium-size mixing bowl, preferably chilled (see Tip, opposite). Add the powdered sugar and vanilla extract and beat on high speed with a hand mixer until soft peaks form, then reduce the speed to medium and continue whipping until stiff peaks form. Store in the refrigerator until ready to use. Leftover whipped cream can be stored in an airtight container in the refrigerator for up to 4 days.

3. To serve, scoop the ice cream into two 12-ounce glasses, until each glass is about three-quarters filled. Pour the chai tea over the ice cream until the glasses are full, then top each float with coconut whipped cream and a pinch of chai spice mix. Grab your favorite straw and enjoy.

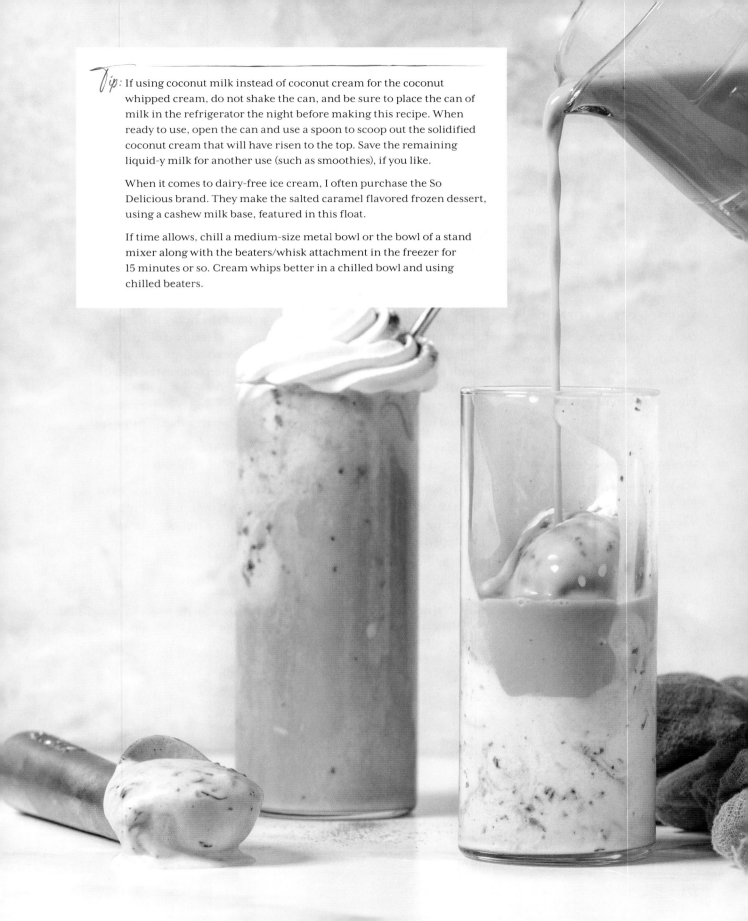

Tip: If using coconut milk instead of coconut cream for the coconut whipped cream, do not shake the can, and be sure to place the can of milk in the refrigerator the night before making this recipe. When ready to use, open the can and use a spoon to scoop out the solidified coconut cream that will have risen to the top. Save the remaining liquid-y milk for another use (such as smoothies), if you like.

When it comes to dairy-free ice cream, I often purchase the So Delicious brand. They make the salted caramel flavored frozen dessert, using a cashew milk base, featured in this float.

If time allows, chill a medium-size metal bowl or the bowl of a stand mixer along with the beaters/whisk attachment in the freezer for 15 minutes or so. Cream whips better in a chilled bowl and using chilled beaters.

White HOT CHOCOLATE

MAKES
two 8-ounce
servings

PREP TIME
5 minutes

COOK TIME
10 minutes

Enjoying a nice cup of hot chocolate is a holiday tradition that my husband introduced to me. While we usually stick to dark chocolate, I enjoyed experimenting with white chocolate for this version. When white chocolate is gently melted into hot milk, the resulting drink has such a nice creaminess, and when you use a premium white chocolate, the flavor is undeniably decadent. The great part about this recipe is that you have the option of keeping it simple or changing it up by adding more vanilla for a bolder flavor or some peppermint to get in the holiday spirit. Either way, I top this white hot chocolate with whipped cream followed by chopped white chocolate and voilà!

4 cups unsweetened almond milk

4 ounces white chocolate, chopped, or ⅔ cup white chocolate chips, plus more for topping if desired

1 teaspoon vanilla extract

Whipped cream, for topping (optional)

Bring the almond milk to a simmer in a medium-size saucepan over medium heat. Reduce the heat to low and add the white chocolate and vanilla extract, stirring until the chocolate is completely melted. Remove from the heat and ladle into two 8-ounce mugs. Top with whipped cream and more white chocolate, if desired.

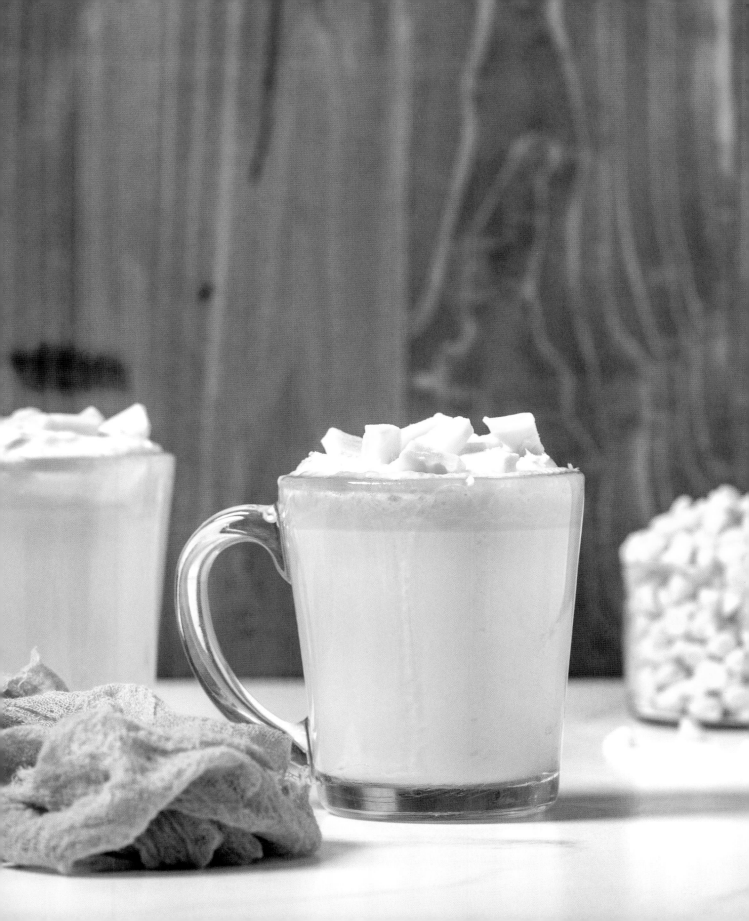

Vegan Spiced
HOT CHOCOLATE

MAKES
two 8-ounce servings

PREP TIME
5 minutes

COOK TIME
10 minutes

In this recipe, I've added a bit of arrowroot starch to create a luxuriously thick hot chocolate, almost thick enough to eat with a spoon. I love this gluten-free option for thickening recipes, but if you don't have arrowroot on hand, you can use cornstarch. I don't know about you, but I can enjoy hot chocolate any time of the year, but I do love having a cup around the Christmas tree with carols playing in the background. Regardless of when you choose to make this recipe, I can guarantee that you'll enjoy every sip!

3½ cups unsweetened almond milk

2 teaspoons arrowroot starch

2 teaspoons cacao powder

12 ounces vegan dark chocolate, chopped (about 2 cups)

2 to 3 tablespoons agave syrup

1 teaspoon vanilla extract

1 teaspoon ground cinnamon

¼ teaspoon ground nutmeg

⅛ teaspoon ground allspice

Pinch of ground cloves

TOPPINGS (OPTIONAL):

Vegan marshmallows

Grated vegan dark chocolate

1. Pour the almond milk into a medium-size saucepan, then add the arrowroot starch and bring to a boil over medium-high heat. Once at a boil, reduce the heat to medium-low and simmer for 1 to 2 minutes, whisking frequently to prevent lumps.

2. Add the cacao powder and continue to whisk until fully incorporated. Turn off the heat and add the chopped chocolate, 2 tablespoons of the agave, the vanilla extract, and spices. Continue to whisk until the mixture is completely smooth and thickened. Taste the hot chocolate and, if you find it isn't sweet enough, add another tablespoon of agave.

3. To serve, pour the hot chocolate into two 8-ounce mugs. Top with marshmallows and a sprinkle of grated chocolate, if desired.

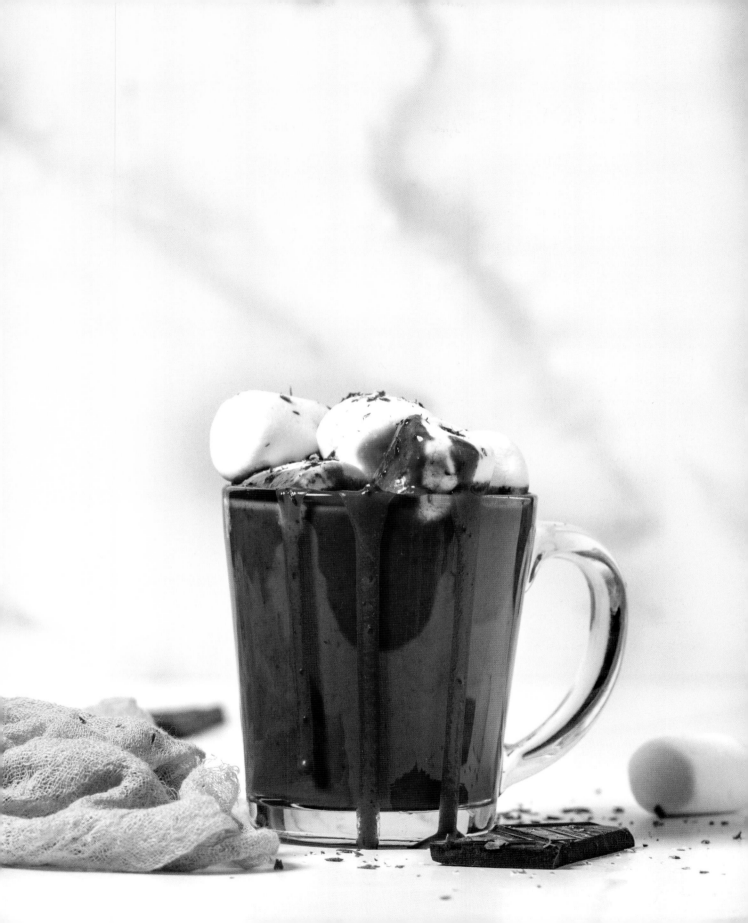

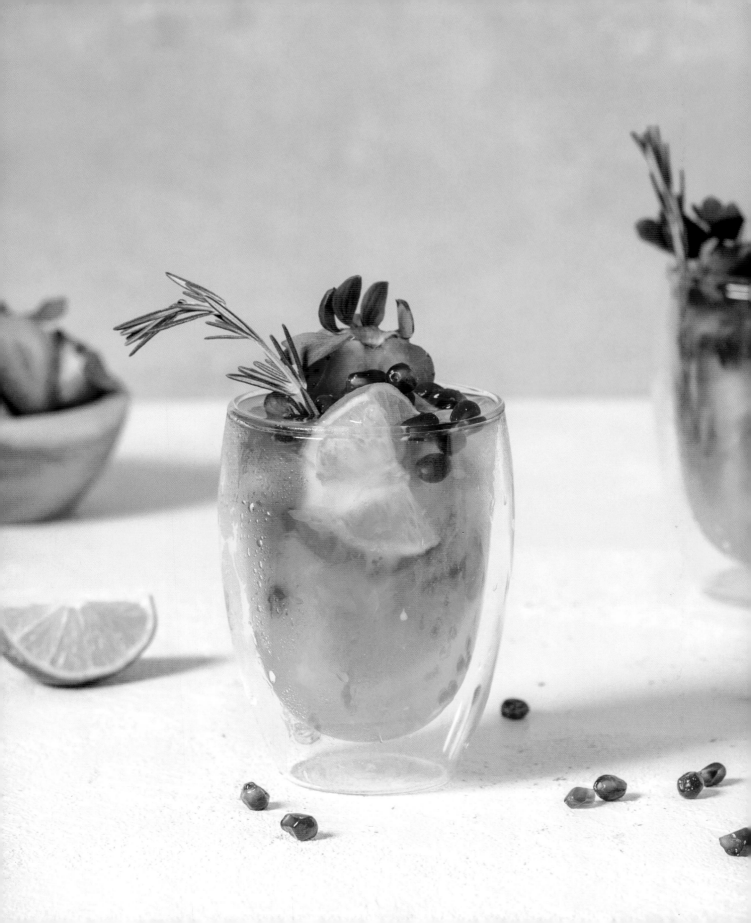

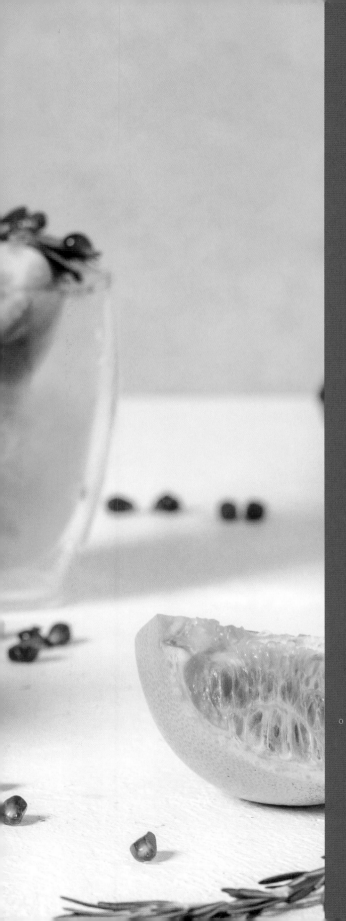

Chapter 11:
HEALTHY JUICES, MOCKTAILS & TEAS

Healthy Cranberry POMEGRANATE JUICE

MAKES
two 8-ounce
servings

PREP TIME
10 minutes

Whether or not you're used to mixing together your own juice concoctions, this recipe is a great place to start. The unbelievably delicious combination of cranberry, lemon, and pomegranate is a guaranteed favorite. I didn't have a clue about making my own juices or mocktails prior to starting my blog; since then, I have learned just how easy they are to make. You simply need the right ingredients, a few tools, and voilà! Drinks have become some of my favorite things to make because I can let my creativity run wild. Cheers to enjoying great drink options!

1 cup unsweetened cranberry juice

Juice of 1 lemon

1 cup pomegranate arils, plus more for garnish

¼ cup agave syrup

2 cups water

Crushed ice, for serving

FOR GARNISH:

Lemon wedges

Fresh cranberries

Fresh rosemary sprigs (optional)

1. Pour the cranberry juice, lemon juice, and pomegranate arils into a pitcher, then lightly crush the arils using the back of a wooden spoon until they are broken down slightly and the mixture becomes a little thick. Add the agave and water and stir to combine. If not using right away, refrigerate until ready to serve.

2. To serve, fill two 8-ounce glasses with crushed ice and pour in the juice mixture, filling the glasses three-quarters full. Garnish with pomegranate arils, lemon slices, cranberries, and rosemary sprigs, if desired.

Tip: One large pomegranate (4 to 5 inches in diameter) should yield the 1 cup of arils needed for this recipe plus a little extra for garnish.

You can also top this drink with a carbonated mixer like sparkling water for a little fizz.

Leftover juice mixture can be stored in a sealed jar in the refrigerator for up to 3 days.

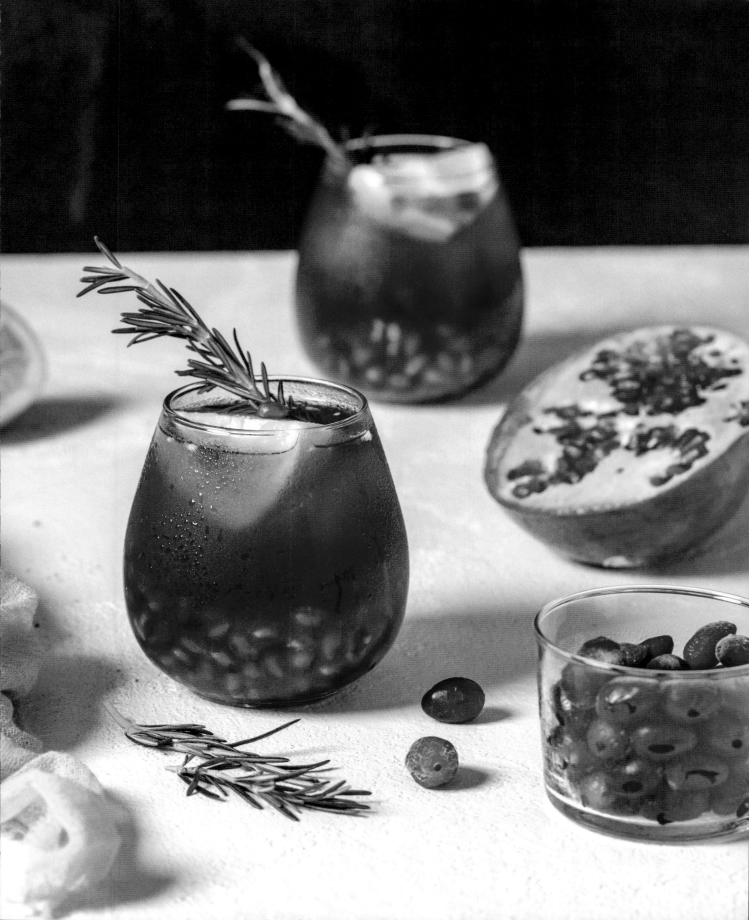

Cucumber Ginger Lemon
DETOX JUICE

MAKES
four 8-ounce
servings

PREP TIME
10 minutes, plus
20 minutes to
infuse

COOK TIME
15 minutes

This juice is an incredible way to boost your immune system. I love this recipe because I often use food as a natural remedy. This juice is a nutrient-dense, easy way to help your body reset and rejuvenate through the use of lemon and ginger together with cucumber, thyme, apples, and more. I consider this easy drink to be a real powerhouse when it comes to the host of health benefits and enjoy drinking it at least once per week.

4 cups water

2 to 3 (2-inch) pieces gingerroot, peeled and roughly chopped

Handful of fresh mint leaves

Leaves from 2 sprigs fresh thyme, plus more sprigs for garnish if desired

2 cucumbers, peeled and chopped

1 Granny Smith apple, sliced

Juice of 1 lemon

½ cup agave syrup

1. Bring the water to a boil in a medium-size saucepan over medium-high heat. Once boiling, add the chopped ginger, mint leaves, and thyme leaves and boil for 5 minutes, then reduce the heat to low and let simmer for another 10 minutes.

2. Remove the pan from the heat, cover, and let the mixture cool and infuse for 15 to 20 minutes.

3. Pour the herb and ginger–infused water into a high-powered blender (including the leaves and chopped ginger). Add the cucumbers, apple, lemon juice, and agave and blend on high speed until smooth and foamy at the top, 2 to 3 minutes.

4. Set a fine-mesh strainer atop a large pitcher, then pour the juice through the strainer into the pitcher, squeezing the pulp against the strainer to ensure that all the juice is extracted. If not using right away, refrigerate until ready to serve.

5. To serve, pour the strained juice into four 8-ounce glasses, filling the glasses all the way to the top. Garnish with thyme sprigs, if desired.

6. Leftover juice can be stored in a tightly sealed pitcher or sealed jar in the refrigerator for up to 2 days. Stir before serving.

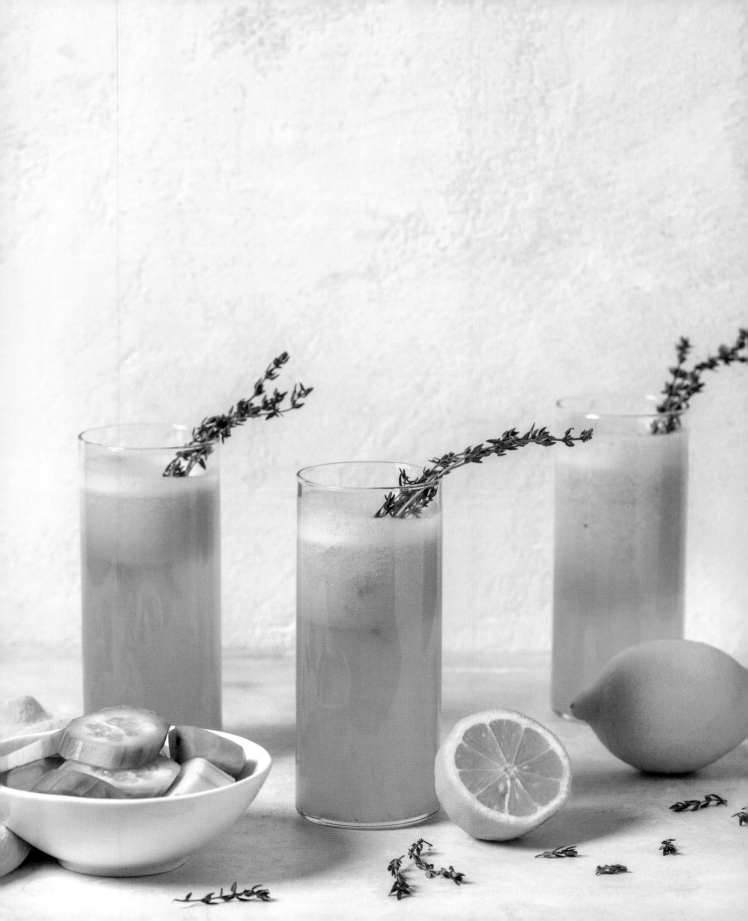

Jamaican Hibiscus Drink

MAKES
six 8-ounce
servings

PREP TIME
10 minutes,
plus 8+ hours
to steep

COOK TIME
20 minutes

Known in Jamaican culture as "sorrel," this drink is the perfect blend of spices and refreshing hibiscus flavors and is often enjoyed on ice. Sorrel also includes the bold flavors of dried sorrel (aka dried hibiscus), pimento seeds (aka allspice berries), cinnamon sticks, orange slices, and sometimes lime. I grew up drinking and loving sorrel in my teen years; however, I fell in love with this drink again as an adult after my mother-in-law made a large bottle of it for Thanksgiving one year. Since then, it has become a tradition for her to make us this drink at Thanksgiving and Christmas. The traditional version also contains rum, which strengthens the flavors even more. My recipe is alcohol-free, but you have the option to add your own for a celebratory moment. The most fascinating thing I've learned from making this drink is that the longer you allow it to ferment—ideally for a year!—the more winelike it becomes, with a deep burgundy color.

8 cups water

2 cups dried hibiscus, thoroughly rinsed

2 (2-inch) pieces gingerroot, peeled and grated

½ navel orange, skin on and sliced (optional)

10 allspice berries

¼ cup whole cloves, plus more for garnish if desired

1½ to 2 cups cane sugar, to taste

½ to 1 cup white rum, to taste (optional)

Crushed ice, for serving

Fresh mint leaves, for garnish (optional)

1. Bring the water, rinsed hibiscus, grated ginger, orange slices (if using), and allspice berries to a boil in a large pot over medium-high heat, then continue to boil for about 5 minutes. Turn off the heat, cover the pot, and let the mixture steep for a minimum of 8 hours; you'll get the best results if you allow it to steep overnight.

2. Once the steeping time is completed, put the cloves in a large pitcher. Set a fine-mesh strainer on top of the pitcher and strain the drink into the pitcher; discard the allspice berries, orange slices, ginger, and hibiscus. Whisk in the sugar, sweetening the drink to your liking, until completely dissolved.

3. Add the rum, if desired. If not using the drink right away, refrigerate until ready to serve.

4. To serve, fill six 8-ounce glasses with ice and pour the drink into the glasses, filling them all the way to the top. Garnish with additional whole cloves and mint leaves, if desired.

5. Leftover juice can be stored in a tightly sealed pitcher or sealed jar in the refrigerator for up to 1 year.

Tip: After completing Step 3, for best flavor, store the drink in the refrigerator for 3 days before serving. This additional resting time allows the flavors to settle in more and become even richer.

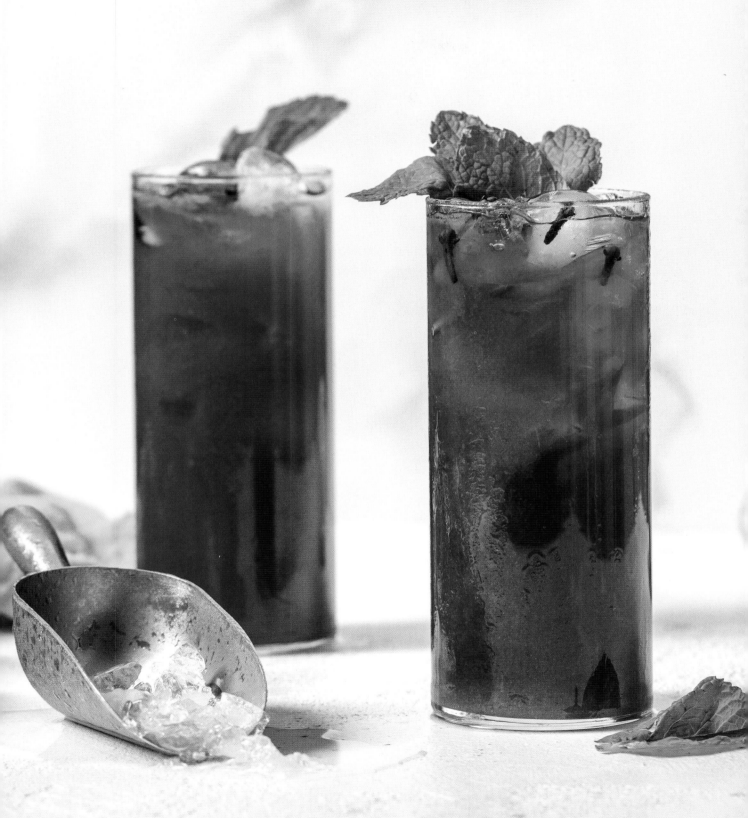

Blueberry Thyme
MOCKTAIL

I love mocktails. They're incredibly fun to make, allowing you to experiment with so many different ingredients, including fresh fruit and herbs. Plus, making your own drinks allows you to control what goes into your libations and customize them to your taste. The ginger beer, a nod to my Jamaican roots, combines with blueberries and thyme to create a fresh flavor that is naturally sweet. Cheers!

½ cup water

1 cup fresh blueberries, plus more for garnish

Juice of ½ lime

4 sprigs fresh thyme, plus more for garnish

Crushed ice, for serving

Ginger beer, for topping

1. In a pitcher, combine the water, blueberries, lime juice, and thyme sprigs, then lightly crush everything using the back of a wooden spoon until the blueberries are broken down and the mixture becomes a little thick and mushy-looking. Remove the thyme springs.

2. To serve, fill two 4-ounce glasses halfway with ice and spoon the blueberry-thyme mixture over the ice. Top the mixture with ginger beer and garnish with more blueberries and thyme sprigs.

Tip: Leftover juice mixture can be stored in a sealed jar in the refrigerator for up to 3 days.

You can top this drink with an alternate carbonated mixer like sparkling water for some fizz with no added sugar.

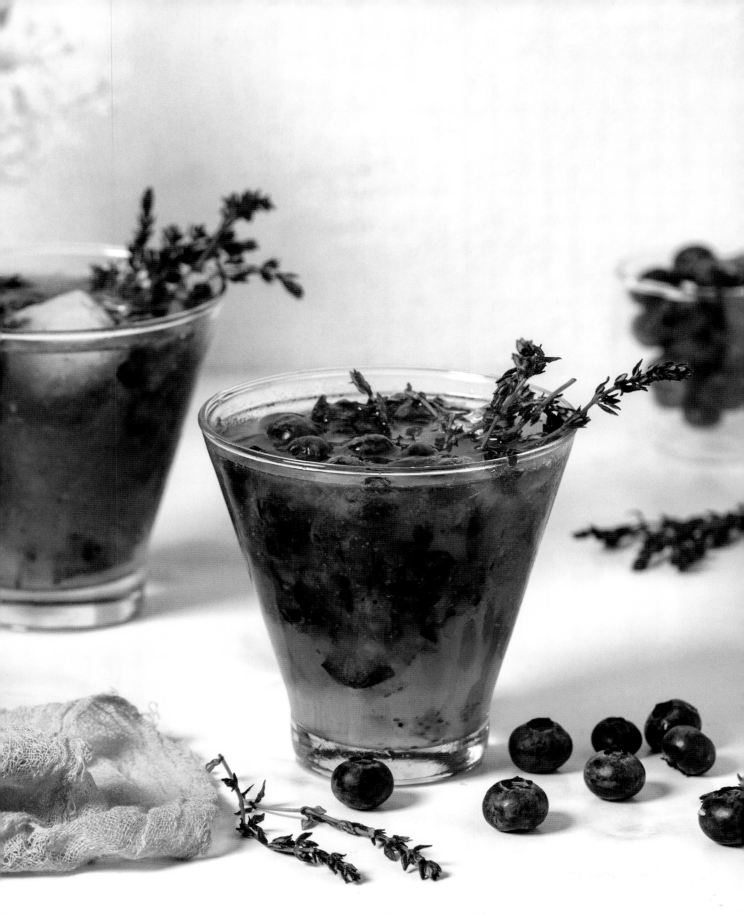

Citrus Cucumber MOCKTAIL

MAKES
four 4-ounce
servings

PREP TIME
10 minutes

Citrus fruits create a naturally refreshing taste, regardless of the ingredients they are paired with. This mocktail pairs orange juice with mandarins and cucumbers, which creates a fruity, fresh blend. I really enjoy making and drinking these mocktails on Fridays to celebrate making it through the week, and I'm sure you will want to add this drink to your end-of-the-week roster as well. This mocktail is naturally sweetened with honey, but you can substitute agave syrup if you prefer a vegan option.

3 mandarin oranges, peeled, divided

1 cucumber, peeled and sliced, divided

1 cup freshly squeezed orange juice

¼ cup raw honey

Crushed ice, for serving

Ginger beer, for topping

Fresh mint leaves, for garnish

1. Separate the oranges into sections and set one-third of the sections aside for garnish. Drop the remaining sections into a pitcher along with half of the cucumber slices, the orange juice, and honey. Using the back of a wooden spoon, lightly crush everything until the orange sections and cucumber slices are mostly broken down and the mixture becomes a little thick and mushy-looking.

2. To serve, fill four 4-ounce glasses halfway with ice and spoon the citrus-cucumber atop the ice. Top the mixture with ginger beer until the glasses are three-quarters filled. Garnish with the remaining orange sections, remaining cucumber slices, and mint leaves.

Tip: You can also top this drink with an alternate carbonated mixer like sparkling water for a little fizz with no added sugar.

Leftover juice mixture can be stored in a sealed jar in the refrigerator for up to 3 days.

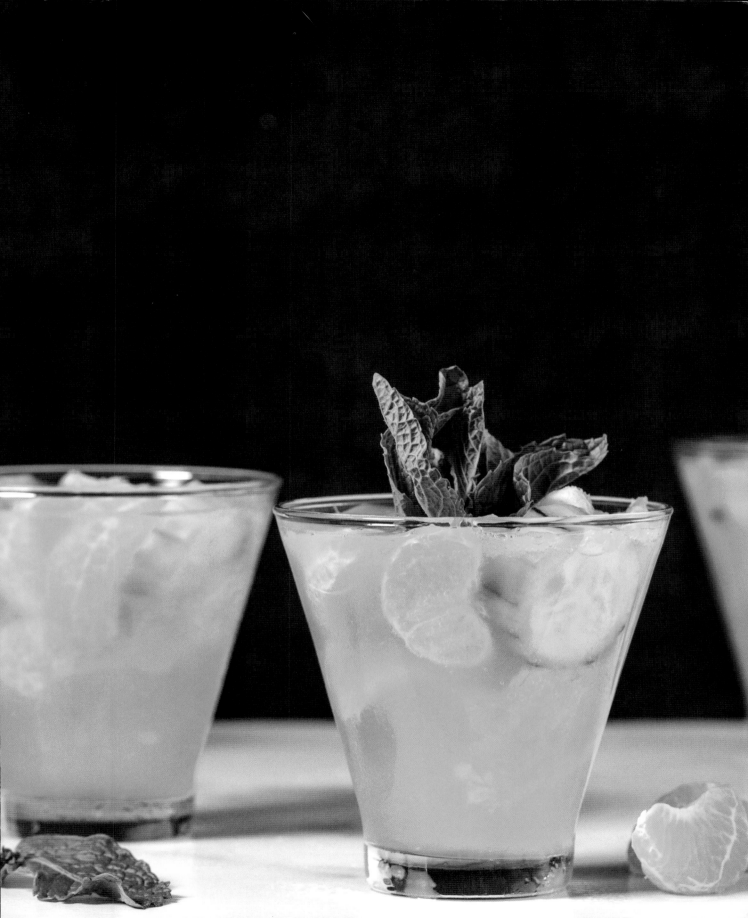

Slim's Grapefruit Rosemary
MOCKTAIL

MAKES
two 8-ounce
servings

PREP TIME
10 minutes

This drink reminds me so much of my grandfather and his love for grapefruit. I remember watching him plant a grapefruit tree in his backyard, which eventually grew into a massive tree that bore many beautiful pink grapefruits. He would pick a few off the tree, slice one, and enjoy it with a few pinches of salt—that was our thing together. In memory of those moments, and in celebration of his life and legacy, I felt compelled to create this mocktail. Filled with not only grapefruit, but also strawberries, lime, pomegranate, and rosemary, and topped with ginger beer, this mocktail is a perfectly refreshing alcohol-free option for any day.

½ cup freshly squeezed grapefruit juice (about 2 grapefruits)

2 cups fresh strawberries, halved, plus more for garnish

2 tablespoons freshly squeezed lime juice (about 1 lime)

Arils from 1 pomegranate

8 fresh rosemary leaves

Crushed ice, for serving

Ginger beer, for topping

FOR GARNISH:
Lime wedges

Fresh rosemary sprigs

1. Pour the grapefruit juice into a pitcher, then add the strawberries. Using the back of a wooden spoon, lightly crush the berries until they are mostly broken down. Transfer the mixture to a pitcher, then add the lime juice, most of the pomegranate arils, setting some aside for garnish, and the rosemary leaves. If not using right away, refrigerate until ready to serve.

2. To serve, fill two 8-ounce glasses with ice and pour in the juice mixture, filling the glasses three-quarters full. Top with ginger beer and garnish with halved strawberries, the reserved pomegranate arils, lime wedges, and rosemary sprigs.

Tip: You can make this drink with other fruit, such as mango, pineapple, or lemon, or an alternate carbonated mixer, like sparkling water.

Leftover juice mixture can be stored in a sealed jar in the refrigerator for up to 3 days.

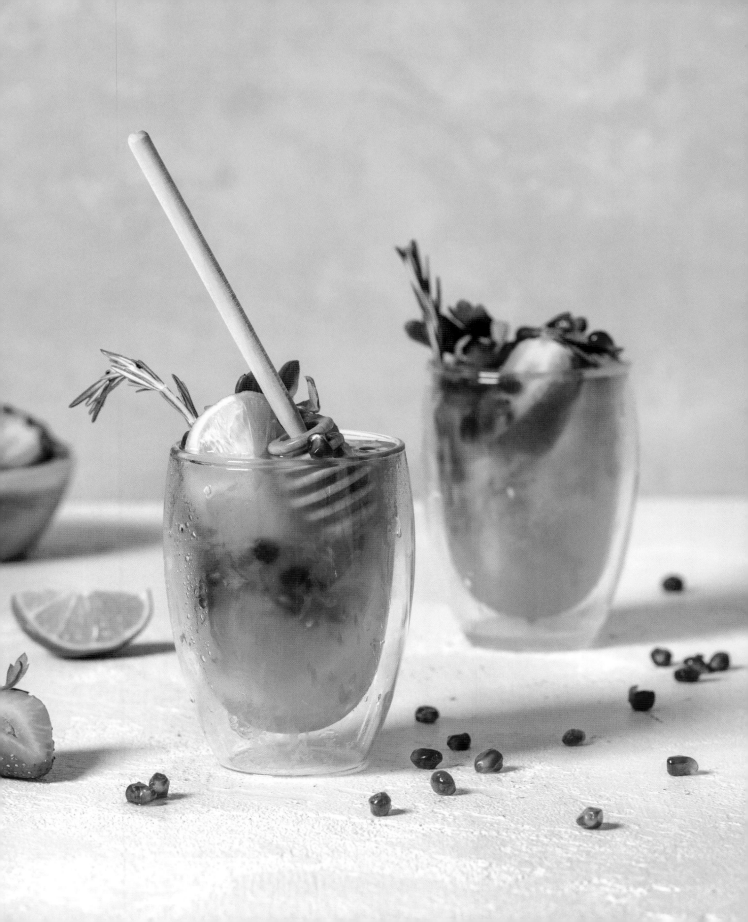

Spicy Kiwi Lime
MOCKTAIL

MAKES
two 4-ounce
servings

PREP TIME
10 minutes

This spicy drink is one you will remember. On my blog, Orchids + Sweet Tea, I created a jalapeño and pineapple mocktail that got so much rave, and I understand why. Sweet and spicy work so well together, and this drink is no different. I've always loved kiwi fruit; therefore, drinking an entire mocktail filled with it is rather enjoyable for me. Don't worry, you can adjust the spiciness if you aren't a huge fan by adding a sweetener such as honey or agave syrup or by halving the number of jalapeños used. Either way, this mocktail is sure to become your newest crave!

4 kiwis, peeled and sliced, plus more for garnish

2 jalapeño peppers, sliced, plus more for garnish

Juice of 1 lime

Crushed ice, for serving

Ginger beer (about 2 ounces), for topping

FOR GARNISH:

Lime wedges

Fresh mint leaves

1. In a pitcher, combine the kiwis, jalapeños, and lime juice, then lightly crush everything using the back of a wooden spoon until the kiwis are mostly broken down, the jalapeños are crushed, and the mixture becomes a little thick and mushy-looking.

2. To serve, fill two 4-ounce glasses halfway with ice and spoon the muddled kiwi-jalapeño mixture over the ice. Top with the ginger beer until the glasses are three-quarters filled. Garnish with kiwi slices, sliced jalapeños, lime wedges, and mint leaves.

Tip: You can top this drink with an alternate carbonated mixer like sparkling water for a little fizz with no added sugar.

Leftover kiwi mixture can be stored in a sealed jar in the refrigerator for up to 3 days.

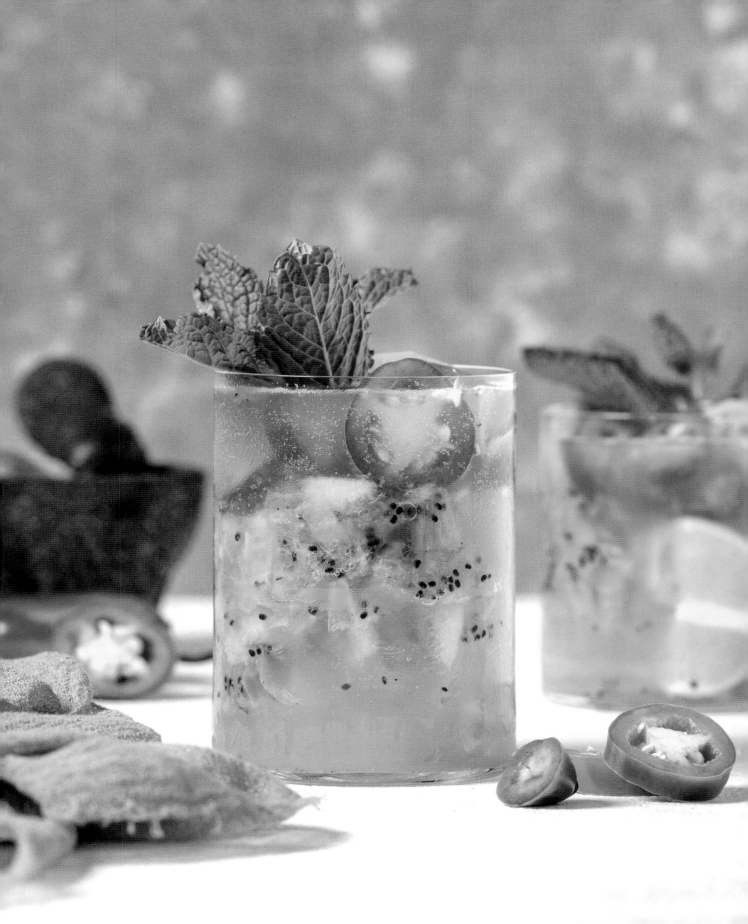

Apple Ginger Peach MOCKTAIL

MAKES
two 8-ounce servings

PREP TIME
10 minutes

After testing this mocktail, I was pleasantly surprised at just how amazing apple, ginger, and peach are together. I'm a fan of quick, easy mocktails, and this version tops my list! In all of ten minutes (or less), you simply muddle the peaches and a few of the apple slices until they are majorly broken down. Then you add lemon juice, mix in a sweetener such as agave, and top these beauties with ginger beer. I love the strong ginger flavor that natural ginger beer adds; therefore, it's my go-to! However, you can change it up by adding a ginger-blood orange beer (yes, that exists) or another fizzy alternative.

3 medium peaches, thinly sliced

1 Granny Smith apple, sliced

½ cup freshly squeezed lemon juice

¼ cup agave syrup

Crushed ice, for serving

Ginger beer, for topping

Fresh rosemary sprigs, for garnish (optional)

1. Place most of the peach and apple slices in a pitcher, reserving the rest for garnish. Add the lemon juice and lightly crush everything using the back of a wooden spoon until the fruits are mostly broken down and the mixture becomes a little thick and mushy-looking. Add the agave and stir until combined.

2. To serve, fill two 8-ounce glasses halfway with ice and spoon the muddled fruit mixture over the ice. Top with ginger beer until the glasses are three-quarters filled. Garnish with the reserved peach and apple slices and, if desired, rosemary sprigs.

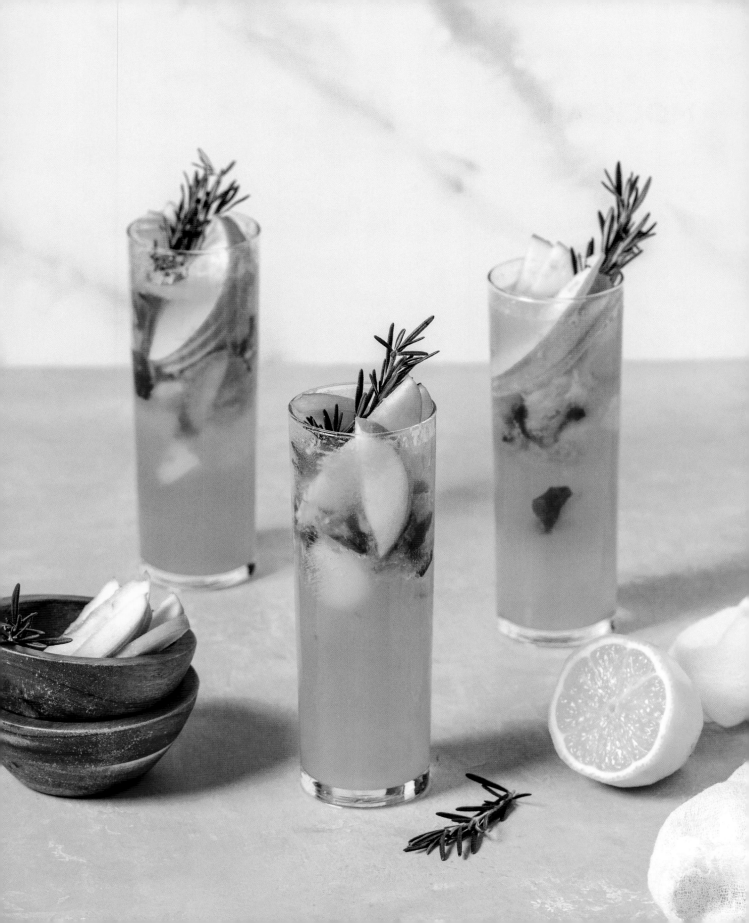

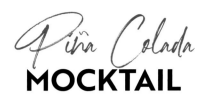
MOCKTAIL

MAKES
two 10-ounce
servings

PREP TIME
5 minutes

I love reinventing classic drinks, and this piña colada mocktail is so good! Though alcohol-free, it's worthy of drinking during a celebratory moment. I enjoy making easy and delicious mocktails with a small number of ingredients and even less effort, and this recipe is no different. You can either grab a bag of frozen pineapple chunks or use fresh. Regardless, you'll need only a high-powered blender, some coconut water and pineapple juice, as well as a sweetener, if desired.

1 cup pure coconut water, plus more if needed

1 cup pineapple juice

1 cup frozen or fresh pineapple chunks (see Tip)

1 to 2 tablespoons agave syrup, to taste (optional)

2 cups ice cubes (if using fresh pineapple chunks)

TOPPINGS (OPTIONAL):

Fresh pineapple chunks

Unsweetened shredded coconut

Fresh mint leaves

1. In a high-powered blender, blend the coconut water, pineapple juice, pineapple chunks, agave (if using), and ice cubes (if using fresh pineapple) on high speed until smooth and thick and no chunks remain, 2 to 3 minutes. If at any point the mixture is too thick to blend easily, add another ¼ cup of coconut water.

2. To serve, pour the drink into two 10-ounce glasses. Garnish with skewered pineapple chunks, shredded coconut, and mint leaves, if desired.

Tip: If you are not using frozen pineapple chunks for this recipe, be sure to add the ice cubes to ensure that the drink has a slushy consistency.

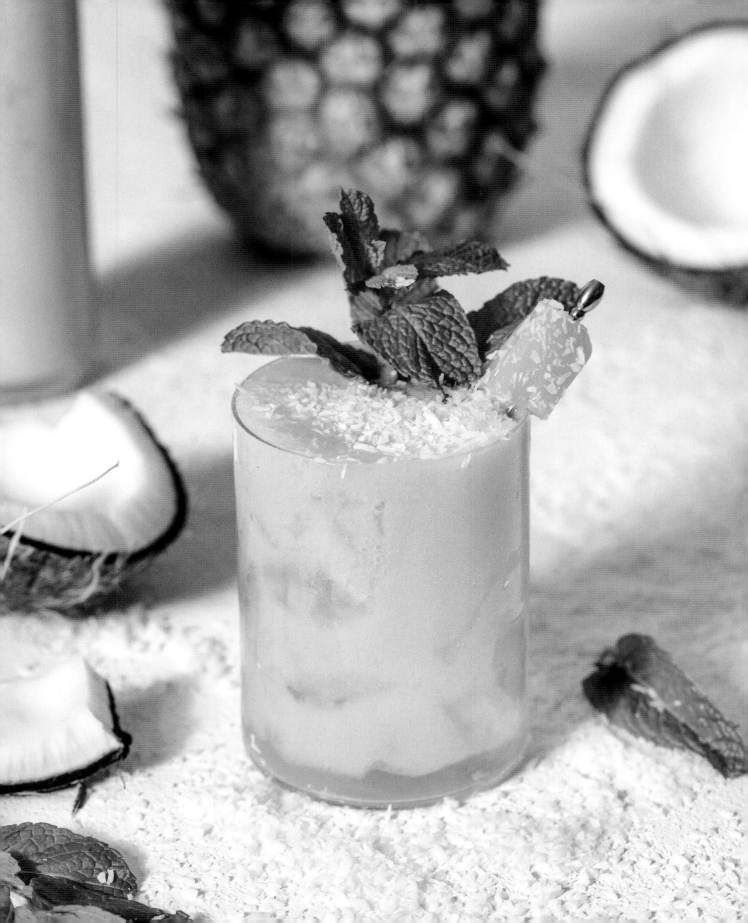

Vegan Maple
CHAI LATTE

MAKES
two 8-ounce
servings

PREP TIME
5 minutes,
plus 6 minutes
to steep

COOK TIME
5 minutes

Chai lattes are my go-to in the mornings. Usually, I purchase the biggest size I can get at my local coffee shop; however, on days when I don't feel like going out, this homemade version is my backup plan. This vegan and gluten-free latte is made with only a handful of ingredients and comes together in a few short minutes. It is bursting with bold chai spices and maple flavors, which work so well together; adding maple syrup to the mix has been my best decision yet!

LATTE:

2 cups unsweetened almond milk

3 black tea bags

3 tablespoons pure maple syrup

1 tablespoon chai spice mix, homemade (page 40) or store-bought

1 tablespoon vanilla extract

TOPPINGS:

Coconut whipped cream

Cinnamon sticks

Pinch of chai spice mix (page 40) (optional)

1. Bring the almond milk to a boil in a medium-size saucepan over high heat. Remove the pan from the heat and add the tea bags, lifting each bag up and down a few times before resting it in the milk to steep for 5 to 6 minutes.

2. Once fully steeped, remove the tea bags from the pan and whisk in the maple syrup, chai spice mix, and vanilla extract until everything is smooth and combined. You can reheat the mixture for another minute or so if you prefer to serve the lattes really hot.

3. To serve, pour the chai latte into two 8-ounce mugs and top each with coconut whipped cream, a cinnamon stick, and, if desired, a sprinkle of chai spice mix.

Tip: While I enjoy the slow and old-fashioned method of making this recipe on the stovetop, it can also be made in a high-powered blender with a heating mode, which will heat up the milk so that you can steep your tea right in the blender. After removing the tea bags, add the rest of the latte ingredients and pulse until combined.

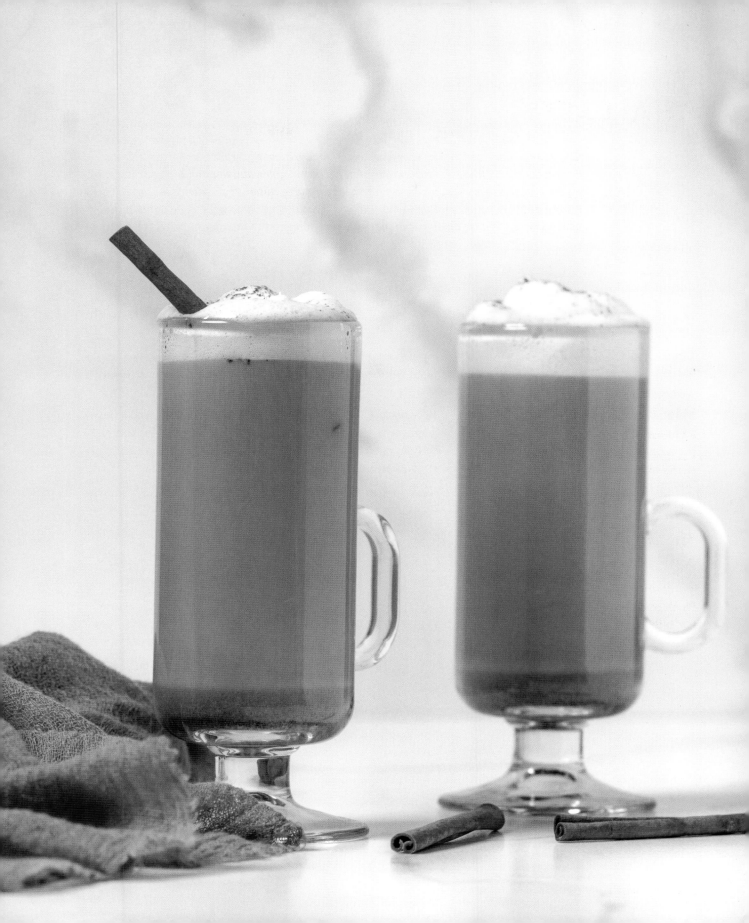

Apple Cinnamon Tea

MAKES
two 8-ounce servings

PREP TIME
5 minutes,
plus 10 minutes
to steep

COOK TIME
10 minutes

Have you ever tried apple cinnamon tea? If not, you're missing something good! I can't start my morning without something hot, and my beverage of choice is tea. I'm not sure if it has to do with my Jamaican background and the teaching of tea being the most important thing next to breakfast, but I enjoy tea on a daily basis. This recipe is a healthy combination of sweet, tart, and warm spice flavors and is perfect for any season. The naturally sweetened tea has so many great qualities: it serves up a powerful dose of antioxidants, boosts digestion, and has anti-inflammatory properties, thanks to the apples and cinnamon combo.

3 cups water

3 Gala apples, sliced, plus more for garnish if desired

2 cinnamon sticks

2 tablespoons agave syrup, plus more if desired

Whole cloves, for garnish (optional)

1. Bring the water, apple slices, and cinnamon sticks to a boil in a medium-size saucepan over high heat. Continue boiling for 3 to 4 minutes. Remove the pan from the heat and let steep, covered, for 8 to 10 minutes.

2. Once fully steeped, remove the apples and cinnamon sticks from the pan and whisk in the agave until fully dissolved and the tea is sweetened to your liking. You can reheat the tea for another minute or so if you prefer to serve it really hot.

3. To serve, pour the tea into two 8-ounce mugs and garnish with apple slices and cloves, if desired.

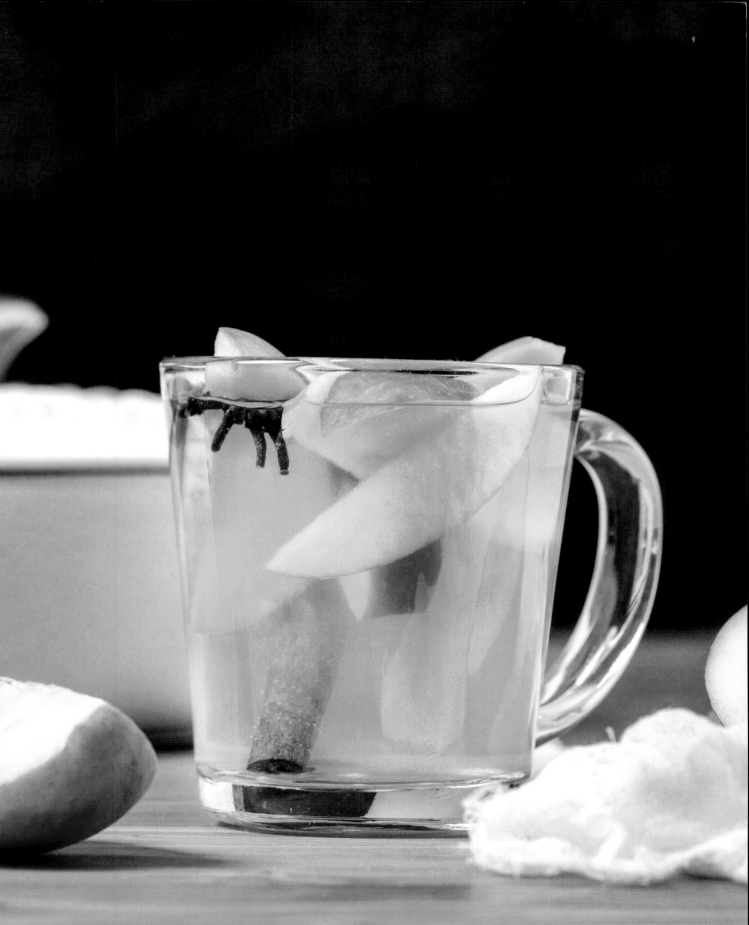

Cranberry Lemon Tea

MAKES
two 8-ounce
servings

PREP TIME
5 minutes,
plus 10 minutes
to steep

COOK TIME
10 minutes

Around the holiday season, I find myself enjoying cranberry scones, pancakes, waffles, cheesecake, cake, pie—you name it. However, I had never thought about enjoying cranberries in a tea. In case you didn't know, cranberries have amazing healing properties; therefore, enjoying this tea has added benefits besides tasting great. Grab your favorite mug and let's begin!

3 cups water

2 cups fresh or frozen cranberries, plus more for topping if desired

2 lemons, sliced, plus more for topping if desired

¼ cup agave syrup, plus more if desired

Pinch of ground cinnamon

1. Bring the water, cranberries, and lemon slices to a boil in a medium-size saucepan over high heat. Continue boiling for 3 to 4 minutes. Remove the pan from the heat and let steep, covered, for 8 to 10 minutes.

2. Once fully steeped, remove the cranberries and lemon slices from the pan and whisk in the agave and cinnamon until fully dissolved and the tea is sweetened to your liking. You can reheat the tea for another minute or so if you prefer to serve it really hot.

3. To serve, pour the tea into two 8-ounce mugs and top with cranberries and lemon slices, if desired.

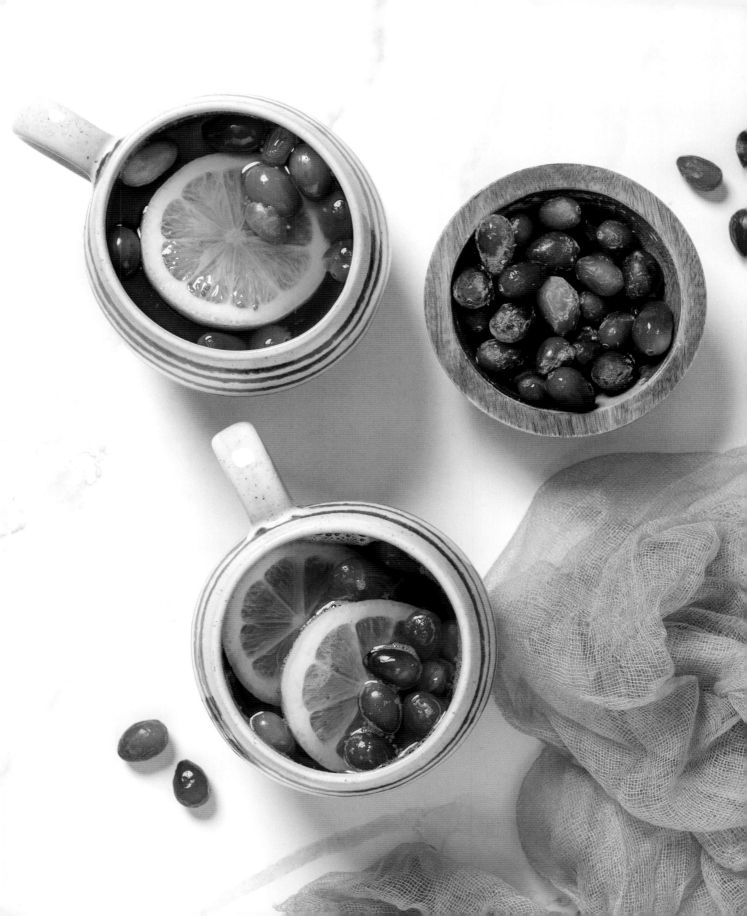

Southern Peach
SWEET TEA

MAKES
sixteen 8-ounce
servings

PREP TIME
5 minutes, plus
about 1 hour to
steep and chill

COOK TIME
20 minutes

This sweet tea recipe is special to me. For one, my blog, Orchids + Sweet Tea, *is named after this drink because it is tied so heavily to my Southern roots. Secondly, sweet tea has been a favorite of mine for as long as I can remember; therefore, every sip of this drink brings back amazing memories. This refreshing home-brewed tea boasts notes of peach and lemon and a whole lot of sweetness—just as they like it down South! A true Southern staple, where conversations cannot happen without a glass of sweet tea. Cheers!*

1 gallon water

8 to 10 black tea bags

2 lemons, sliced

2 peaches, sliced, plus more for topping if desired

2 cups lightly packed brown sugar, plus more if desired

¼ teaspoon baking soda (see Tip)

Ice cubes, for serving

Fresh mint leaves, for topping (optional)

1. Bring the water, tea bags, lemon slices, and peaches to a boil in a large pot over high heat. Remove the pot from the heat and let steep, covered, for 15 to 30 minutes.

2. Once fully steeped, remove the tea bags, lemon slices, and peaches from the pan and whisk in the brown sugar and baking soda until fully dissolved and the tea is sweetened to your liking.

3. Pour the sweet tea into a gallon-size pitcher and refrigerate for 30 minutes to 1 hour, until it's well chilled.

4. To serve, pour the tea into ice-filled glasses. Garnish with sliced peaches and mint leaves, if desired.

Tip: Adding baking soda to sweet tea prevents the tea from getting cloudy and bitter. If you've ever left your leftover sweet tea in the refrigerator only to find that after a day or so, it's become bitter and less enjoyable, know that adding a small amount of baking soda will do the trick.

The longer the tea bags are steeped, the stronger the tea flavor. You can let them steep for up to 30 minutes; longer than that, the tea will start to become bitter.

Leftover tea can be stored in a sealed jar in the refrigerator for up to 3 days.

I like to use brown sugar in my sweet tea as opposed to the traditional choice of white because of its taste and greater health value. You can always substitute organic cane sugar or stevia or allulose for an even healthier option.

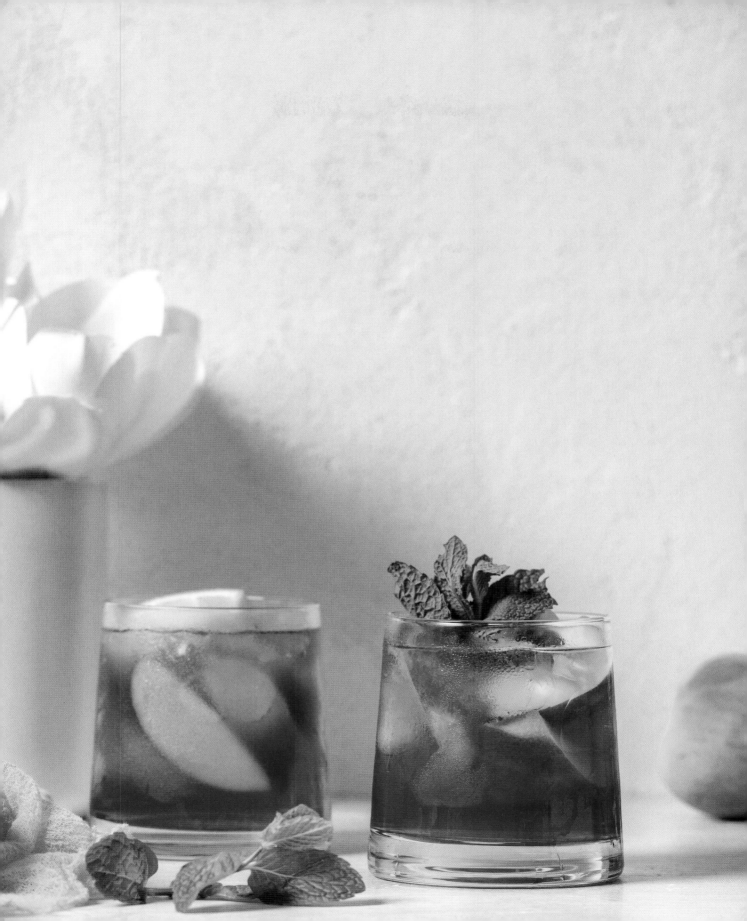

Vegan Jamaican
SEA MOSS DRINK

MAKES
two 4-ounce
servings

PREP TIME
12 minutes, plus
24 hours to soak
sea moss and 10
minutes to soak
dates

This recipe is a vegan take on Irish moss, a Jamaican staple enjoyed by many on a daily basis. In Jamaican culture, Irish moss is known for "putting things back in order"—meaning, restoring your immune system after fighting an illness or preventing future illness. Like the original, this sweet drink is deliciously creamy and thick and flavored with aromatic spices. Unlike the original, I chose to keep things healthier by using dates as the sweetener, which are soaked to hydrate and soften them so that they blend more easily. Don't worry—preparing the sea moss gel is really simple, and it can be stored for up to a month.

IRISH (SEA) MOSS GEL:

(Makes 1½ cups)

1 ounce dried Irish (sea) moss

1 cup water, plus more for rinsing and soaking

4 to 5 Medjool dates, pitted

Boiling water, for soaking the dates

1 cup unsweetened almond milk

1 teaspoon vanilla extract

½ teaspoon ground cinnamon, plus more for topping if desired

¼ teaspoon ground nutmeg

⅛ teaspoon ground allspice

1. Make the Irish (sea) moss gel: Rinse the dried sea moss thoroughly and place it in a medium-size bowl. Cover with water and soak for 24 hours, changing the water every 4 to 6 hours. Make sure the sea moss is fully covered with water while it soaks. Drain the sea moss and rinse thoroughly again, then place it in a blender along with 1 cup of fresh water. Blend on high speed until the mixture becomes gelatinous. Store leftovers in an airtight sterile container or jar in the refrigerator for up to 1 month or freeze for up to 3 months.

2. Soak the dates: Put the dates in a small heatproof bowl and pour boiling water over them until completely covered. Let soak for 10 minutes or so, then drain and rinse.

3. In a high-powered blender, blend the almond milk, 2 tablespoons of the sea moss gel, the soaked dates, vanilla extract, cinnamon, nutmeg, and allspice on high speed until smooth and thick, 2 to 3 minutes.

4. To serve, pour the drink into two 4-ounce glasses and sprinkle the tops with cinnamon, if desired.

5. If you'd like to make a larger amount to sip on throughout the week, you can store sea moss drink in a pitcher covered with plastic wrap or a sealed jar in the refrigerator for up to 1 week. To freeze the drink, place in tightly sealed freezer-safe jars or containers and freeze for up to 3 months. When you are ready to use it, remove the stored portions from the freezer and thaw them in the refrigerator overnight.

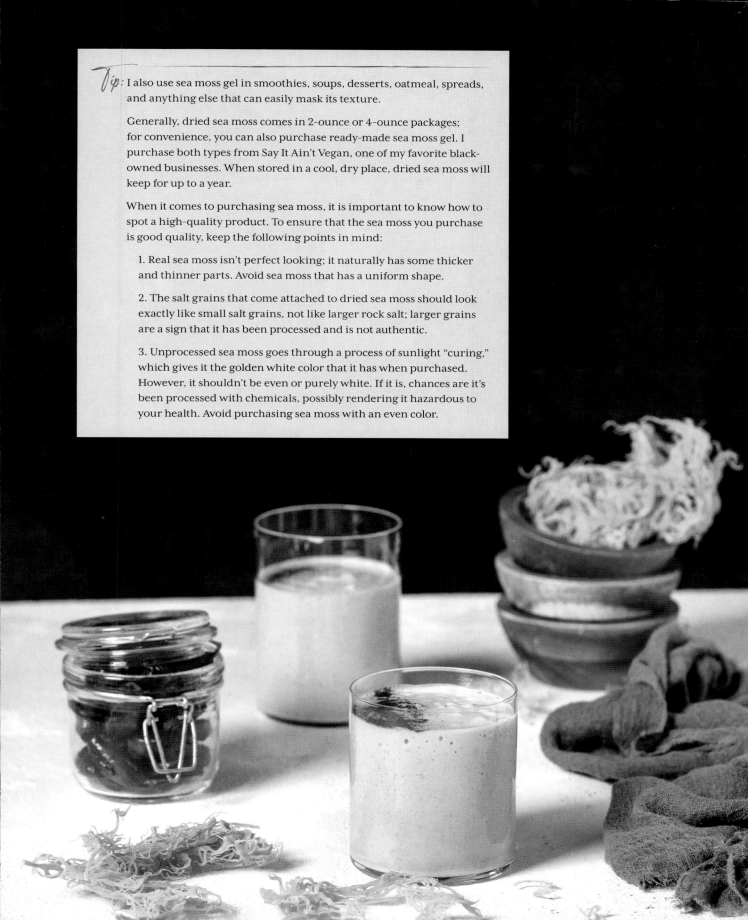

Tip: I also use sea moss gel in smoothies, soups, desserts, oatmeal, spreads, and anything else that can easily mask its texture.

Generally, dried sea moss comes in 2-ounce or 4-ounce packages; for convenience, you can also purchase ready-made sea moss gel. I purchase both types from Say It Ain't Vegan, one of my favorite black-owned businesses. When stored in a cool, dry place, dried sea moss will keep for up to a year.

When it comes to purchasing sea moss, it is important to know how to spot a high-quality product. To ensure that the sea moss you purchase is good quality, keep the following points in mind:

1. Real sea moss isn't perfect looking; it naturally has some thicker and thinner parts. Avoid sea moss that has a uniform shape.

2. The salt grains that come attached to dried sea moss should look exactly like small salt grains, not like larger rock salt; larger grains are a sign that it has been processed and is not authentic.

3. Unprocessed sea moss goes through a process of sunlight "curing," which gives it the golden white color that it has when purchased. However, it shouldn't be even or purely white. If it is, chances are it's been processed with chemicals, possibly rendering it hazardous to your health. Avoid purchasing sea moss with an even color.

FOOD LOVE AFFAIRS

With so many delicious options to choose from, I created this section of the book to show you a few of my favorite food and drink combos. Some of these pairings are obvious when it comes to foods that have a history of going great together, while others might be a surprise, but they are all sure to blow your mind once you give them a try! Let the love affairs begin....

AFFAIR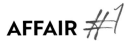

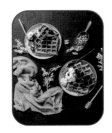

+

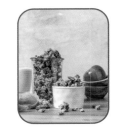

**Brown Butter
Blueberry Waffles
(page 112)**

**Apple Cinnamon
Granola (page 74)**

AFFAIR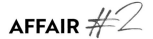

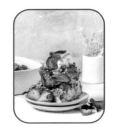

+

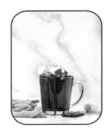

**Dairy-Free Strawberry
Pecan Maple French Toast
Casserole (page 124)**

**Vegan Spiced
Hot Chocolate
(page 278)**

AFFAIR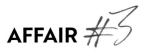

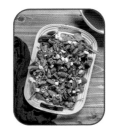

+

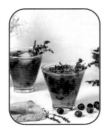

**Roasted Jerk Butternut
Squash, Tomato &
Veggie Salad (page 192)**

**Blueberry Thyme
Mocktail (page 290)**

AFFAIR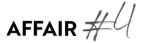

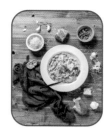

+

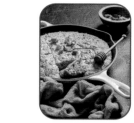

Creamy Tortellini Soup
with Kale & Roasted
Garlic (page 186)

Hot Honey Skillet
Cornbread (page 174)

AFFAIR #5

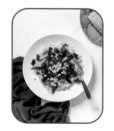

+

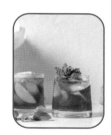

Creamy Southern Grits
with Sautéed Collards,
Candied Bacon &
Roasted Corn (page 234)

Southern Peach
Sweet Tea (page 310)

AFFAIR #6

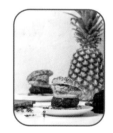

+

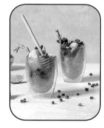

Jerk BBQ Pineapple
Black Bean Burgers
(page 220)

Slim's Grapefruit
Rosemary Mocktail
(page 294)

AFFAIR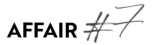

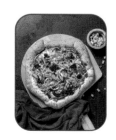

+

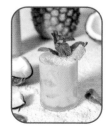

Jerk BBQ Chicken &
Veggie Pizza (page 208)

Piña Colada Mocktail
(page 300)

AFFAIR 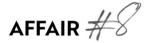 #8

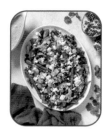

Roasted Vegetable
Green Goddess Salad
(page 194)

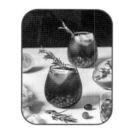

Healthy Cranberry
Pomegranate Juice
(page 282)

AFFAIR #9

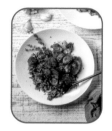

Maple Brown Butter Chicken
& Wild Rice Skillet with
Brussels Sprouts (page 224)

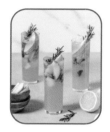

Apple Ginger Peach
Mocktail (page 298)

AFFAIR #10

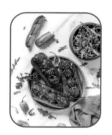

Plant-Based Jerk BBQ
Meatball Po' Boys (page 230)

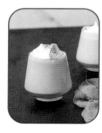

Vegan Jamaican Peanut
Punch (page 270)

AFFAIR #11

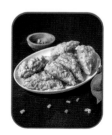

Jerk Chicken
White Cheddar Scallion
Scones (page 144)

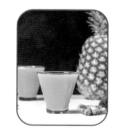

Carrot, Sweet Potato,
Pineapple & Ginger
Juice (page 286)

AFFAIR 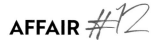#12

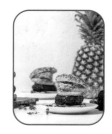

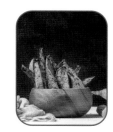

Jerk BBQ Pineapple Black
Bean Burgers (page 220)

Jerk Sweet Potato
Wedges (page 160)

AFFAIR #13

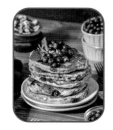

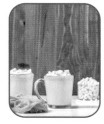

Vegan Blueberry
Whole-Wheat Pancakes
(page 104)

White Hot Chocolate
(page 276)

AFFAIR #14

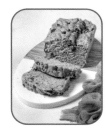

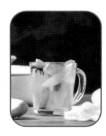

Rum Raisin Bread
(page 152)

Apple Cinnamon Tea
(page 304)

AFFAIR #15

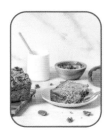

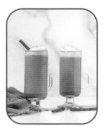

Vegan Pecan Chia
Banana Bread (page 134)

Vegan Maple Chai
Latte (page 302)

ACKNOWLEDGMENTS

In writing this book, I learned a lot about myself, my purpose, and the hard work that it takes to produce anything with greatness. In this process, I've never felt more rewarded than I feel now, and without the people who both played a hand (physically) or as inspiration, I wouldn't have this amazing project completed. Therefore, I want to thank:

God—Who in all His greatness chose me, trusted me, and gave me such an opportunity to share my personal story and path in both food and life, which isn't as conventional and "straight-pathed" as others. Thank you, Jesus.

My husband, Darnell—who has been my photographer, cheerleader, second opinion in both life and many projects related to *Orchids + Sweet Tea,* including this one. I honestly don't know what I would be or do without your partnership, love, and reassurance that I can do anything even when I didn't believe in myself.

My grandfather, Slim—who is no longer living on this Earth but continues to watch over me in every season. Thank you for being my biggest inspiration in life, in love, and in the way that I find resilience despite life's unfavorable circumstances.

My step-grandmother, Christine—while we no longer are connected with time, you've played a major role in the way that I enjoy food (especially within my Southern roots), understand true love/sacrifice, the importance of being my best self & respectable, and dedication to making an impact even in the smallest of ways.

My son, Kameron—who has been one of my biggest present inspirations and motivations for doing things to the best of my ability, so that I can show you that it's possible. I hope to be the best model that you appreciate once you're older. This one's for you!

My parents.

My brothers and sisters.

My friends.

My aunties.

My uncles.

My publishing family at Victory Belt—for believing in me, taking a chance on me, and allowing me to be as authentic and transparent with my journey with food and life in this book. I truly appreciate you all!

The entire editorial team, especially Holly and Pam—for the countless late nights, edit sessions, back and forths, and understanding throughout this entire process. You've made this all worth it!

To Susan and the marketing/communications team—who have always been just an email or phone call away, a second opinion on ideas, and so much more. You guys rock, truly!

The entire design team for your amazing work and dedication.

Matt Ellis—my Street photographer, who is so dope and talented and captured the most amazing parts of Brooklyn, which tells a story of old/new stomping grounds and brings this all together.

Every blogging friend who said "yes" to supporting this, sharing this, advice with this, and using this. THANK YOU! xx

And last but not least, to ALL OF MY AMAZING READERS/FOLLOWERS—thank you for rocking with me, supporting me, choosing to make my recipes, telling your friends/family about my content, coming to my defense at any given time, and so much more! *Orchids + Sweet Tea* would be nothing without you all.

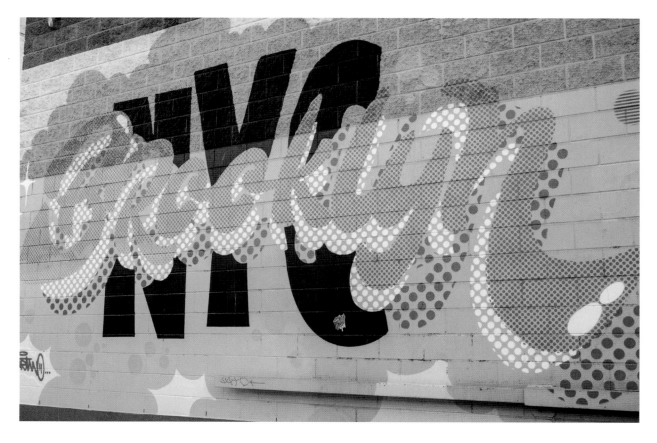

RECISE INDEX

Chapter 3: ESSENTIAL RECIPES

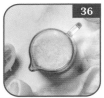
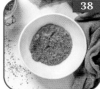
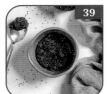

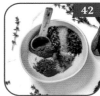
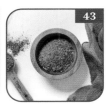
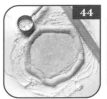

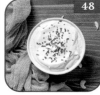
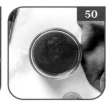
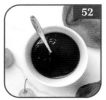

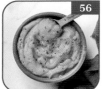

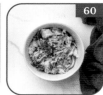
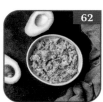
Chapter 4: MORNING EATS

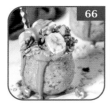
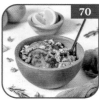
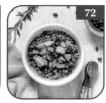
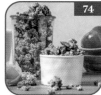
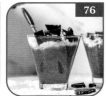
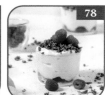

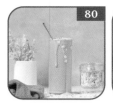
80
Peanut Butter
Banana Oat Smoothie

82
Sweet Potato Oat
Smoothie

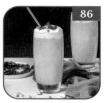
84
Sunrise Smoothie
(Carrot, Strawberry &
Orange)

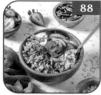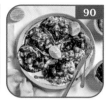
86
Cashew Date
Morning Shake

88
Dairy-Free
Strawberry-Peach
Crisp Yogurt Bowl

90
Meatless
Breakfast Tacos

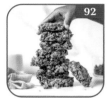
92
Kam's Superfood
Breakfast Cookies

94
Creamy Cornmeal
Porridge

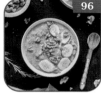
96
Jamaican-Inspired
Banana Oatmeal
Porridge

Chapter 5: **BRUNCH GOODNESS**

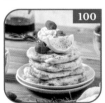
100
Lemon Raspberry
Poppy Seed Pancakes

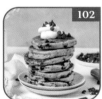
102
Vegan Peanut Butter
Chocolate Chip
Pancakes

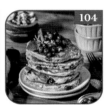
104
Vegan Blueberry
Whole-Wheat
Pancakes

106
Easy Dairy-Free
Pecan Pancakes

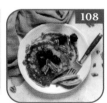
108
Vegan Sweet Potato
Pancakes

110
Banana Oat Flourless
Blender Waffles

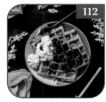
112
Brown Butter
Blueberry Waffles

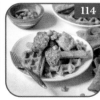
114
Flourless Sweet Potato
Waffles & Hot Maple
Cauliflower Bites

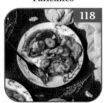
118
Dairy-Free Spiced
Banana French Toast

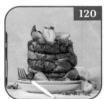
120
Strawberry Balsamic
Brioche French Toast

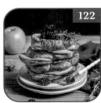
122
Apple Blackberry
Brioche French Toast

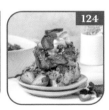
124
Dairy-Free Strawberry
Pecan French Toast
Casserole

Chapter 6: BREADS, MUFFINS & SCONES

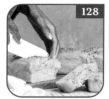
128
Easy Vegan Brioche Bread

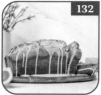
132
Citrus Whole-Wheat Breakfast Loaf

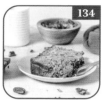
134
Vegan Pecan Chia Banana Bread

136
Garlic Cheese Herb Zucchini Bread

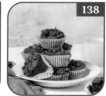
138
Gluten-Free Double Chocolate Muffins

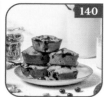
140
Jumbo Blueberry Walnut Muffins

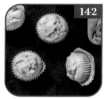
142
Sweet Cornmeal Rum Muffins

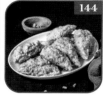
144
Jerk Chicken White Cheddar Scallion Scones

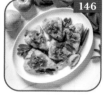
146
Brown Butter Apple Pie Scones with Caramelized Apples

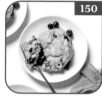
150
Maple Blueberry Scones

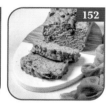
152
Rum Raisin Bread

Chapter 7: BITS & PIECES

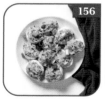
156
Spicy Avocado Deviled Eggs

158
Dairy-Free Crispy Buffalo Cauliflower Bites

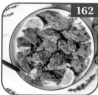
160
Jerk Sweet Potato Wedges

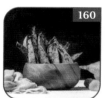
162
Crispy Lemon Pepper Smashed Potatoes with Pesto

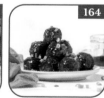
164
Spicy Vegan Jerk BBQ Meatballs

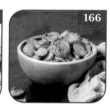
166
Baked Cajun Carrot Chips

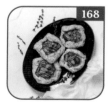
168
Mini Garlic Herb Tomato Galettes

170
Jamaican Rice & Peas

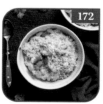
172
Creamy Cajun Pumpkin Mac & "Cheese"

174
Hot Honey Skillet Cornbread

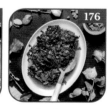
176
Southern Collard Greens

Chapter 8: SOUPS & SALADS

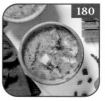 180
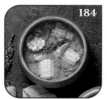 182
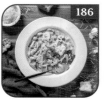 184
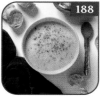 186
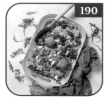 188
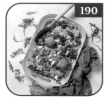 190

Plant-Based Jamaican "Pepperpot" Soup

Hearty Quinoa Veggie Soup

Jamaican Spiced Corn Soup

Creamy Tortellini Soup with Kale & Roasted Garlic

Cheesy Cauliflower & White Bean Soup

Creamy Cajun Roasted Corn, Tomato & Arugula Pasta Salad

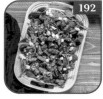 192
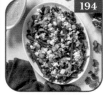 194
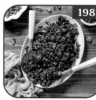 196
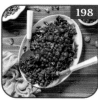 198

Roasted Jerk Butternut Squash & Veggie Salad

Roasted Vegetable Green Goddess Salad

Jerk Shrimp Asparagus Salad

Buffalo Chickpea Kale Salad

Chapter 9: DELICIOUS DINNERS

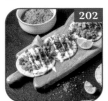 202
 204
 206
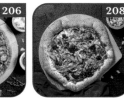 208
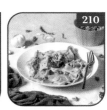 210
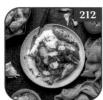 212

Roasted Bean, Quinoa & Sweet Potato Tacos

Buffalo Cauliflower Tacos

BBQ Loaded Veggie Pizza

Jerk BBQ Chicken & Veggie Pizza

Dairy-Free Garlic Alfredo Spinach Pasta

Fire-Roasted Tomato Deconstructed Stuffed Shells

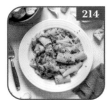 214
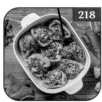 216
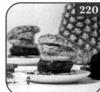 218
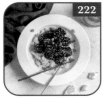 220
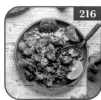 222
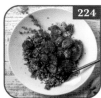 224

Cajun Sweet Potato Rigatoni with Kale

Creamy Lemon-Kale Orzo with Roasted Tomatoes & Vegetables

Cajun Quinoa & Brown Rice Stuffed Peppers

Jerk BBQ Pineapple Black Bean Burgers

Spicy Sesame Plant-Based Meatballs with Cauliflower Rice

Maple Brown Butter Chicken & Wild Rice Skillet with Brussels Sprouts

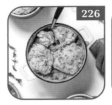
226

230

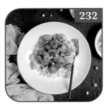
232

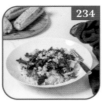
234

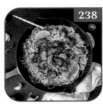
238

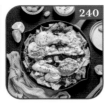
240

Savory Vegetarian
Jerk Pot Pies

Plant-Based Jerk BBQ
Meatball Po' Boys

Curry Shrimp with
Cauliflower Rice

Creamy Southern Grits
with Sautéed Collards,
Candied Bacon &
Roasted Corn

Cajun Shrimp
with Garlic Butter
Zucchini Noodles &
Tomatoes

Vegan Loaded
Quinoa Nachos

Chapter 10: SWEETS & DECADENT DRINKS

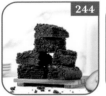
244

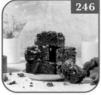
246

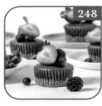
248

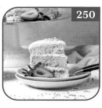
250

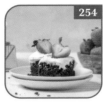
254

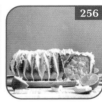
256

Easy Fudgy Vegan
Avocado Brownies

Vegan Sweet Potato
Pecan Brownies

Chocolate
Cheesecake Bites
with Mixed Berries

Vegan Strawberry
Funfetti
Birthday Cake

Vegan Red Velvet
Sheet Cake with
Bourbon Buttercream

Coconut Lime
Pound Cake

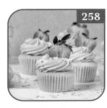
258

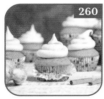
260

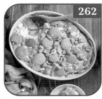
262

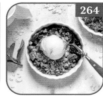
264

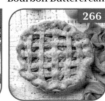
266

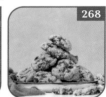
268

Vegan Oat Cupcakes
with Strawberry
Buttercream

Ginger Cupcakes
with Chai Cream
Cheese Frosting

Southern Banana
Pudding

Vegan Maple
Blackberry Crisps

Cheddar
Triple Apple Pie

Brown Butter Pecan
Chocolate Chip
Cookies

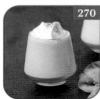
270

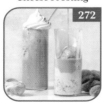
272

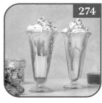
274

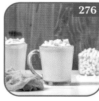
276

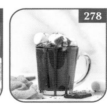
278

Vegan Jamaican
Peanut Punch

Vegan Chai Latte &
Salted Caramel Cashew
Ice Cream Float

Salted Caramel
Funfetti Milkshake

White Hot Chocolate

Vegan Spiced Hot
Chocolate

Chapter 11: HEALTHY JUICES, MOCKTAILS & TEAS

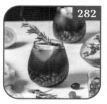
282
Healthy Cranberry Pomegranate Juice

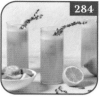
284
Cucumber Ginger Lemon Detox Juice

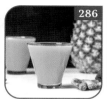
286
Carrot, Sweet Potato, Pineapple & Ginger Juice

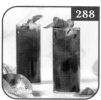
288
Jamaican Hibiscus Drink

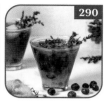
290
Blueberry Thyme Mocktail

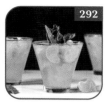
292
Citrus Cucumber Mocktail

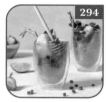
294
Slim's Grapefruit Rosemary Mocktail

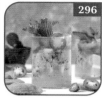
296
Spicy Kiwi Lime Mocktail

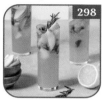
298
Apple Ginger Peach Mocktail

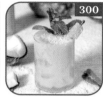
300
Piña Colada Mocktail

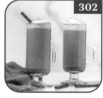
302
Vegan Maple Chai Latte

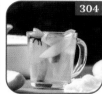
304
Apple Cinnamon Tea

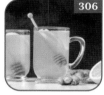
306
Honey Lemon Ginger Tea

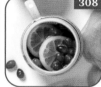
308
Cranberry Lemon Tea

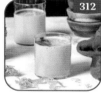
310
Southern Peach Sweet Tea

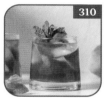
312
Vegan Jamaican Sea Moss Drink

GENERAL INDEX

I

ice cream
  Salted Caramel Funfetti
    Milkshake, 274–275
  substitutes for, 23
  Vegan Chai Latte & Salted
    Caramel Cashew Ice Cream
    Float, 272–273
  Vegan Maple Blackberry Crisps,
    264–265
ingredients, favorite
  Jamaican, 28–29
  miscellaneous, 33–34
  plant-forward, 30–32
  Southern, 26–27
Irish moss. *See* sea moss

J

jalapeño peppers
  Green Goddess Dressing, 194–195
  Meatless Breakfast Tacos, 90–91
  Spicy Kiwi Lime Mocktail,
    296–297
  Vegan Loaded Quinoa Nachos,
    240–241
Jamaican Hibiscus Drink, 288–289
Jamaican ingredients, 28–29
Jamaican Rice & Peas, 170–171
Jamaican Spiced Corn Soup,
  184–185
Jamaican-Inspired Banana
  Oatmeal Porridge, 96–97
Japanese sweet potato, 184
Jerk BBQ Chicken & Veggie Pizza,
  208–209
Jerk BBQ Pineapple Black Bean
  Burgers, 220–221
Jerk BBQ Sauce, 52–53
Jerk Chicken White Cheddar
  Scallion Scones, 144–145
Jerk Seasoning, 29, 42
Jerk Shrimp Asparagus Salad,
  196–197
Jerk Sweet Potato Wedges, 160–161
juices
  Carrot, Sweet Potato, Pineapple
    & Ginger Juice, 286–287
  Cucumber Ginger Lemon Detox
    Juice, 284–285
  Healthy Cranberry
    Pomegranate Juice, 282–283
Jumbo Blueberry Walnut Muffins,
  140–141
jumbo pasta shells
  Fire-Roasted Tomato
    Deconstructed Stuffed Shells,
    212–213

K

kale
  BBQ Loaded Veggie Pizza,
    206–207
  Buffalo Chicken Kale Salad,
    198–199
  Cajun Sweet Potato Rigatoni
    with Kale, 214–215
  Creamy Lemon-Kale Orzo
    with Roasted Tomatoes &
    Vegetables, 216–217
  Creamy Tortellini Soup with
    Kale & Roasted Garlic, 186–187
  Crispy Lemon Pepper Smashed
    Potatoes with Pesto, 162–163
  Hearty Quinoa Veggie Soup,
    182–183
  Plant-Based Jamaican
    "Pepperpot" Soup, 180–181
  Roasted Vegetable Green
    Goddess Salad, 194–195
Kam's Superfood Breakfast
  Cookies, 92–93
ketchup
  Smoky BBQ Sauce, 50–51
kidney beans
  Jamaican Rice & Peas, 170–171
kiwis
  Spicy Kiwi Lime Mocktail,
    296–297

L

leaveners, 32
legumes, 31
Lemon Raspberry Poppy Seed
  Pancakes, 100–101
lemons, 36
  Apple Ginger Peach Mocktail,
    298–299
  Cajun Shrimp with Garlic
    Butter Zucchini Noodles &
    Tomatoes, 238–239
  Carrot, Sweet Potato, Pineapple
    & Ginger Juice, 286–287
  Citrus Whole-Wheat Breakfast
    Loaf, 132–133
  Coconut Yogurt Parfaits with
    Raspberries & Granola, 78–79
  Cranberry Lemon Tea, 308–309
  Creamy Cajun Pumpkin Mac &
    "Cheese," 172–173
  Creamy Lemon-Kale Orzo
    with Roasted Tomatoes &
    Vegetables, 216–217
  Crispy Lemon Pepper Smashed
    Potatoes with Pesto, 162–163

Cucumber Ginger Lemon Detox
  Juice, 284–285
Dairy-Free Crispy Buffalo
  Cauliflower Bites, 158–159
Dairy-Free Garlic Alfredo
  Spinach Pasta, 210–211
Dairy-Free Strawberry-Peach
  Crisp Yogurt Bowl, 88–89
Fire-Roasted Tomato
  Deconstructed Stuffed Shells,
  212–213
Guacamole, 62–63
Healthy Cranberry
  Pomegranate Juice, 282–283
Hearty Quinoa Veggie Soup,
  182–183
Honey Lemon Ginger Tea,
  306–307
Lemon Raspberry Poppy Seed
  Pancakes, 100–101
Southern Peach Sweet Tea,
  310–311
Spicy Avocado Deviled Eggs,
  156–157
Spicy Sesame Plant-Based
  Meatballs with Cauliflower
  Rice, 222–223
Vegan Cream Cheese Sauce,
  48–49
Vegan Loaded Quinoa Nachos,
  240–241
Vegan Maple Blackberry Crisps,
  264–265
lentils, as meat substitutes, 20
lima beans
  Hearty Quinoa Veggie Soup,
    182–183
limes
  Blueberry Thyme Mocktail,
    290–291
  Coconut Lime Pound Cake,
    256–257
  Green Goddess Dressing, 194–195
  Meatless Breakfast Tacos, 90–91
  Roasted Bean, Quinoa & Sweet
    Potato Tacos, 202–203
  Slim's Grapefruit Rosemary
    Mocktail, 294–295
  Spicy Kiwi Lime Mocktail,
    296–297
  Vegan Loaded Quinoa Nachos,
    240–241

M

Maple Blueberry Scones, 150–151
Maple Brown Butter Chicken &
  Wild Rice Skillet with Brussels
  Sprouts, 224–225